ADHERENCE TO LONG-TERM THERAPIES
Evidence for action

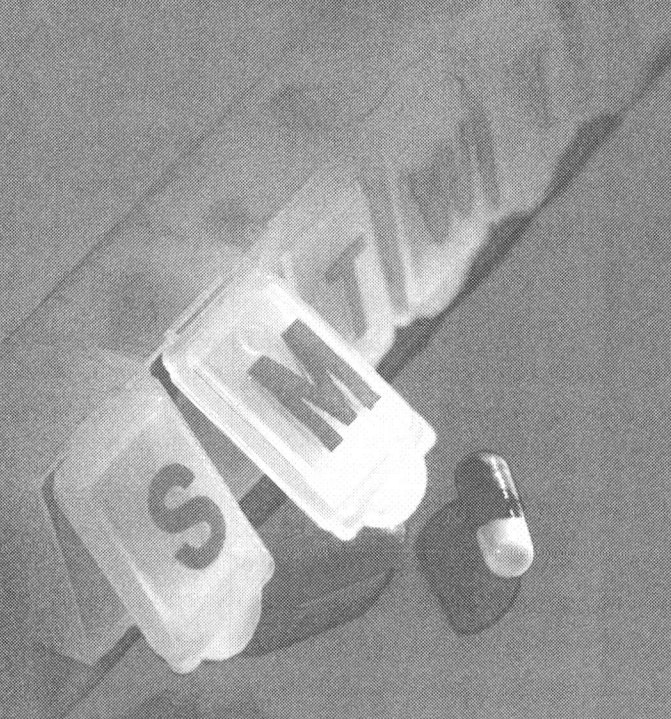

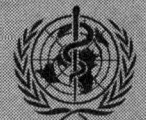

World Health Organization 2003

WHO Library Cataloguing-in-Publication Data

Adherence to long-term therapies : evidence for action.

1.Patient compliance 2.Long-term care 3.Drug therapy - utilization 4.Chronic disease - therapy 5.Health behavior 6.Evidence-based medicine I.WHO Adherence to Long Term Therapies Project II.Global Adherence Interdisciplinary Network.

ISBN 92 4 154599 2 (NLM classification: W 85)

© World Health Organization 2003

All rights reserved.
Publications of the World Health Organization can be obtained from Marketing and Dissemination, World Health Organization, 20 Avenue Appia, 1211 Geneva 27, Switzerland (tel: +41 22 791 2476; fax: +41 22 791 4857; email: bookorders@who.int). Requests for permission to reproduce or translate WHO publications – whether for sale or for noncommercial distribution – should be addressed to Publications, at the above address (fax: +41 22 791 4806; email: permissions@who.int).

The designations employed and the presentation of the material in this publication do not imply the expression of any opinion whatsoever on the part of the World Health Organization concerning the legal status of any country, territory, city or area or of its authorities, or concerning the delimitation of its frontiers or boundaries. Dotted lines on maps represent approximate border lines for which there may not yet be full agreement.

The mention of specific companies or of certain manufacturers' products does not imply that they are endorsed or recommended by the World Health Organization in preference to others of a similar nature that are not mentioned. Errors and omissions excepted, the names of proprietary products are distinguished by initial capital letters.

The World Health Organization does not warrant that the information contained in this publication is complete and correct and shall not be liable for any damages incurred as a result of its use.

Printed in Switzerland.

All correspondence should be sent to the author. Eduardo Sabaté, World Health Organization, 20 Avenue Appia, CH-1211 Geneva 27, Switzerland (sabatee@who.int). Requests for free electronic copies (pdf format only) should be sent to: adherence@who.int

CONTENTS

Preface	V
Ackowledgement	VII
Scientific writers	VIII
Introduction	XI
Take-home messages	XIII

Section I – Setting the scene — 1
Chapter I – Defining adherence — 3
Chapter II – The magnitude of the problem of poor adherence — 7
Chapter III – How does poor adherence affect policy makers and health managers? — 11

Section II – Improving adherence rates: guidance for countries — 17
Chapter IV – Lessons learned — 19
Chapter V – Towards the solution — 27
Chapter VI – How can improved adherence be translated into health and economics benefits? — 39

Section III – Disease-specific reviews — 45
Chapter VII – Asthma — 47
Chapter VIII – Cancer (palliative care) — 59
Chapter IX – Depression — 65
Chapter X – Diabetes — 71
Chapter XI – Epilepsy — 87
Chapter XII – HIV/AIDS — 95
Chapter XIII – Hypertension — 107
Chapter XIV – Tobacco smoking cessation — 115
Chapter XV – Tuberculosis — 123

Annexes — 133
Annex I – Behavioural mechanisms explaining adherence — 135
Annex II – Statements by stakeholders — 151
Annex III – Table of reported factors by condition and dimension — 162
Annex IV – Table of reported interventions by condition and dimension — 166
Annex V – Global adherence interdisciplinary network (GAIN) — 171

Where to find a copy of this book — 177
Official designated depositories libraries for WHO publications — 179
Reference libraries for WHO publications — 183
WHO official sales agents world wide — 195
Selected WHO publications of related interest — 197
A ready-to-use pamphlet for partners willing to promote this book — 199

Preface

Over the past few decades we have witnessed several phases in the development of approaches aimed at ensuring that patients continue therapy for chronic conditions for long periods of time. Initially the patient was thought to be the source of the "problem of compliance". Later, the role of the providers was also addressed. Now we acknowledge that a systems approach is required. The idea of compliance is associated too closely with blame, be it of providers or patients and the concept of adherence is a better way of capturing the dynamic and complex changes required of many players over long periods to maintain optimal health in people with chronic diseases.

This report provides a critical review of what is known about adherence to long-term therapies. This is achieved by looking beyond individual diseases. By including communicable diseases such as tuberculosis and human immunodeficiency virus/acquired immunodeficiency syndrome; mental and neurological conditions such as depression and epilepsy; substance dependence (exemplified by smoking cessation); as well as hypertension, asthma and palliative care for cancer, a broad range of policy options emerges. Furthermore, this broader focus highlights certain common issues that need to be addressed with respect to all chronic conditions regardless of their cause. These are primarily related to the way in which health systems are structured, financed and operated.

We hope that readers of this report will recognize that simplistic approaches to improving the quality of life of people with chronic conditions are not possible. What is required instead, is a deliberative approach that starts with reviewing the way health professionals are trained and rewarded, and includes systematically tackling the many barriers patients and their families encounter as they strive daily to maintain optimal health.

This report is intended to make a modest contribution to a much-needed debate about adherence. It provides analysis and solutions, it recommends that more research be conducted, but critically acknowledges the abundance of what we already know but do not apply. The potential rewards for patients and societies of addressing adherence to long-term therapies are large. WHO urges the readers of this report to work with us as we make the rewards real.

Derek Yach
January 2003

Acknowledgements

This report was edited by Eduardo Sabaté, WHO Medical Officer responsible for coordinating the WHO Adherence to Long-term Therapies Project, Management of Noncommunicable Diseases Department.

Deep appreciation is due to Rafael Bengoa, who envisioned the project and shaped the most crucial elements of the report, Derek Yach, who provided consistent support, intellectual stimulation and leadership to the project and Silvana De Castro, who provided valuable assistance with the many bibliographical reviews and with the writing of specific sections of this report.

Special appreciation goes to the scientific writers who provided their ideas and the material for the report. Their dedication and voluntary contributions have been central to this work. Thanks are also due to all the participants from WHO and the Global Adherence Interdisciplinary Network (GAIN) who by their continuous involvement and input during the planning, resource collection and writing phases of this project have given breadth and depth to the report.

Special thanks go to Steve Hotz for his intellectual support and hard work in helping to integrate the information on behavioural knowledge and its practical implications. Several international professional associations, in particular the International Society of Behavioural Medicine, the International Council of Nurses, the International Union of Psychological Sciences, the International Pharmaceutical Federation, and the World Organization of Family Doctors have played an important role in providing moral support and valuable input to the report.

Thanks are also due to Susan Kaplan, who edited the final text, and Tushita Bosonet, who was responsible for the artistic design.

The production of this report was made possible through the generous financial support of the governements of United Kingdom, Finland and Netherlands.

Scientific writers

The scientific writers who were invited to contribute to the report are recognized scientists in adherence-related issues. Their contributions were made voluntarily and have been incorporated following the directions of the editor of the report. All of them signed a Declaration of Interest. They are listed below in alphabetical order by topic. (Team leaders are indicated with an asterisk.)

Asthma

Bender, Bruce • Head • Pediatric Behavioral Health, National Jewish Medical and Research Center • USA

Boulet, Louis-Philippe • Professor • Laval University, Laval Hospital • Canada

Chaustre, Ismenia • Attending Physician and Professor • "JM de los Ríos" Children's Hospital • Venezuela

Rand, Cynthia* • Associate Professor • Johns Hopkins University • USA

Weinstein, Andrew • Researcher and Clinical Practitioner • Christiana Medical Center • USA

With the active support of the WHO-NMH/MNC/Chronic Respiratory Diseases unit

Behavioural mechanisms

Hotz Stephen* • University Research Fellow • University of Ottawa • Canada

Kaptein, Ad A. • Head • Psychology unit, Leiden University Medical Centre • The Netherlands

Pruitt, Sheri • Director of Behavioral Medicine • Permanente Medical Group • USA

Sanchez Sosa, Juan • Professor • National University of Mexico • Mexico

Willey, Cynthia • Professor of Pharmacoepidemiology • University of Rhode Island • USA

Cancer

De Castro, Silvana* • Technical Officer • Adherence Project, Department of Managment of Communicable Diseases, WHO • Switzerland

Sabaté, Eduardo • Medical Officer • Adherence Project, Department of Managment of Communicable Diseases, WHO • Switzerland

With the active support of the WHO-NMH/MNC/Program on Cancer Control unit

Depression

Peveler, Robert* • Head • Mental Health Group, Community Clinical Sciences Division, School of Medicine, University of Southampton • England

Tejada, Maria Luisa • Clinical practitioner • Hospital of Nyon • Switzerland

With the active support of the WHO-NMH/MSD/Mental and behavioural disorders unit

Diabetes

Karkashian, Christine* • Dean • School of Psychology, Latina University • Costa Rica

Schlundt, David • Associate Professor of Psychology • Vanderbilt University • USA

With the active support of the WHO-NMH/MNC/Diabetes unit

Epilepsy

Avanzini, Giuliano • President • International League against Epilepsy • Italy

de Boer, Hanneke M. • Global Campaign Co-Chair • The International Bureau for Epilepsy/Stichting Epilepsie Instellingen Nederland • the Netherlands

De Castro, Silvana* • Technical Officer • Adherence Project, Department of Managment of Communicable Diseases, WHO • Switzerland

Engel, Jerome Jr • Global Campaign Co-Chair • International League against Epilepsy and Director of the Seizure Disorder Center, University of California at Los Angeles School of Medicine • USA

Lee, Philip • President • International Bureau for Epilepsy • Ireland

Sabaté, Eduardo • Medical Officer • Adherence Project, Department of Managment of Communicable Diseases, WHO • Switzerland

With the active support of the WHO-NMH/MSD/Epilepsy unit, the International League Against Epilepsy and the International Bureau for Epilepsy

Human immunodeficiency virus (HIV)/acquired immunodeficiency syndrome (AIDS)

Chesney, Margaret A.* • Professor of Medicine • University of California at San Francisco, Prevention Sciences Group • USA

Farmer, Paul • Director • Partners in health • Harvard University • USA

Leandre, Fernet • Director • Zanmi Lazante Health Care • Haiti

Malow, Robert • Professor and Director • AIDS Prevention Program, Florida International University • USA

Starace, Fabrizio • Director • Consultation Psychiatry and Behavioural Epidemiology Service, Cotugno Hospital • Italy

With the active support of the WHO-HIV/AIDS care unit

Hypertension

Mendis, Shanti* • Coordinator • Cardiovascular diseases • WHO-HQ

Salas, Maribel • Senior Researcher • Caro Research Institute • USA

Smoking cessation

De Castro, Silvana • Technical Officer • Adherence Project, Department of Managment of Communicable Diseases, WHO • Switzerland

Lam, Tai Hing • Professor • Head Department of Community Medicine and Behavioural Sciences, University of Hong Kong • China

Sabaté, Eduardo* • Medical Officer • Adherence Project, Department of Managment of Communicable Diseases, WHO • Switzerland

Smirnoff, Margaret • Nurse Practitioner • Mount Sinai Center • USA

With the active support of the WHO-NMH/Tobacco Free Initiative department

Tuberculosis

Dick, Judy* • Senior Researcher • Medical Research Center of South Africa • South Africa

Jaramillo, Ernesto • Medical Officer • Stop TB, WHO • Switzerland

Maher, Dermot • Medical Officer • Stop TB, WHO • Switzerland

Volmink, Jimmy • Director of Research and Analysis • Global Health Council • USA

Special topics

Children and adolescents

Burkhart, Patricia • Assistant Professor and Nurse Researcher • University of Kentucky • USA

With the active support of the WHO-FCH/Child and adolescent health unit

Elderly patients

Di Pollina, Laura • Chief • Clinical Geriatrics, Geneva University Hospital • Switzerland

Health Economics

Kisa, Adnan • Associate Professor • Baskent University • Turkey

Nuño, Roberto • Health Economist • Spain

Sabaté, Eduardo* • Medical Officer • Adherence Project, Department of Managment of Communicable Diseases, WHO • Switzerland

Patients' perception of illness

Horne, Rob • Director and Professor of Psychology in Health Care • Centre for Health Care Research, University of Brighton • England

Introduction

Objectives and target audience

This report is part of the work of the Adherence to Long-term Therapies Project, a global initiative launched in 2001 by the Noncommunicable Diseases and Mental Health Cluster of the World Health Organization.

The main target audience for this report are policy-makers and health managers who can have an impact on national and local policies in ways that will benefit patients, health systems and societies with better health outcomes and economic efficiency. This report will also be a useful reference for scientists and clinicians in their daily work.

The main objective of the project is to improve worldwide rates of adherence to therapies commonly used in treating chronic conditions.

The four objectives of this report are to:

- summarize the existing knowledge on adherence, which will then serve as the basis for further policy development;

- increase awareness among policy-makers and health managers about the problem of poor rates of adherence that exists worldwide, and its health and economic consequences;

- promote discussion of issues related to adherence; and

- provide the basis for policy guidance on adherence for use by individual

- articulating consistent, ethical and evidence-based policy and advocacypositions; and

- managing information by assessing trends and comparing performance, setting the agenda for, and stimulating, research and involvement.

How to read this report

As this report intends to reach a wide group of professionals, with varied disciplines and roles, the inclusion of various topics at different levels of complexity was unavoidable. Also, during the compilation of the report, contributions were received from eminent scientists in different fields, who used their own technical languages, classifications and *definitions* when discussing adherence.

For the sake of simplicity, a table has been included for each disease reviewed in section III, showing the factors and interventions cited in the text, classified according to the five dimensions proposed by the project group and explained later in this report:

– social- and economic-related factors/interventions;

– health system/health care team-related factors/interventions;

– therapy-related factors/interventions;

– condition-related factors/interventions; and

– patient-related factors/interventions.

The section entitled "Take-home messages" summarizes the main findings of this report and indicates how readers could make use of them.

Section I:
Setting the scene, discusses the main concepts leading to the definition of adherence and its relevance to epidemiology and economics.

Section II:
Improving adherence rates: guidance for countries, summarizes the lessons learned from the reviews studied for this report and puts into context the real impact of adherence on health and economics for those who can make a change.

Section III:
Disease-specific reviews, discusses nine chronic conditions that were reviewed in depth. Readers with clinical practice or disease-oriented programmes will find it useful to read the review related to their current work. Policy-makers and health managers may prefer to move on to the Annexes.

Annex I:
Behavioural mechanisms explaining adherence, provides an interesting summary of the existing models for explaining people's behaviour (adherence or nonadherence), and explores the behavioural interventions that have been tested for improving adherence rates.

Annex II:
Statements by stakeholders, looks at the role of the stakeholder in improving adherence as evaluated by the stakeholders themselves.

Annexes III and IV:
Table of reported factors by condition and dimension and Table of reported interventions by condition and dimension, provide a summary of all the factors and interventions discussed in this report. These tables may be used to look for commonalities among different conditions.

Annex V:
Global Adherence Interdisciplinary network (GAIN), lists the members of this network.

Take-home messages

Poor adherence to treatment of chronic diseases is a worldwide problem of striking magnitude
Adherence to long-term therapy for chronic illnesses in developed countries averages 50%. In developing countries, the rates are even lower. It is undeniable that many patients experience difficulty in following treatment recommendations.

The impact of poor adherence grows as the burden of chronic disease grows worldwide
Noncommunicable diseases and mental disorders, human immunodeficiency virus/acquired immunodeficiency syndrome and tuberculosis, together represented 54% of the burden of all diseases worldwide in 2001 and will exceed 65% worldwide in 2020. The poor are disproportionately affected.

The consequences of poor adherence to long-term therapies are poor health outcomes and increased health care costs
Poor adherence to long-term therapies severely compromises the effectiveness of treatment making this a critical issue in population health both from the perspective of quality of life and of health economics. Interventions aimed at improving adherence would provide a significant positive return on investment through primary prevention (of risk factors) and secondary prevention of adverse health outcomes.

Improving adherence also enhances patients' safety
Because most of the care needed for chronic conditions is based on patient self-management (usually requiring complex multi-therapies), use of medical technology for monitoring, and changes in the patient's lifestyle, patients face several potentially life-threatening risks if not appropriately supported by the health system.

Adherence is an important modifier of health system effectiveness
Health outcomes cannot be accurately assessed if they are measured predominantly by resource utilization indicators and efficacy of interventions. The population health outcomes predicted by treatment efficacy data cannot be achieved unless adherence rates are used to inform planning and project evaluation.

"Increasing the effectiveness of adherence interventions may have a far greater impact on the health of the population than any improvement in specific medical treatments"[1]
Studies consistently find significant cost-savings and increases in the effectiveness of health interventions that are attributable to low-cost interventions for improving adherence. Without a system that addresses the determinants of adherence, advances in biomedical technology will fail to realize their potential to reduce the burden of chronic illness. Access to medications is necessary but insufficient in itself for the successful treatment of disease.

Health systems must evolve to meet new challenges
In developed countries, the epidemiological shift in disease burden from acute to chronic diseases over the past 50 years has rendered acute care models of health service delivery inadequate to address the health needs of the population. In developing countries, this shift is occurring at a much faster rate.

---

1 Haynes RB. Interventions for helping patients to follow prescriptions for medications. *Cochrane Database of Systematic Reviews*, 2001, Issue 1.

Patients need to be supported, not blamed
Despite evidence to the contrary, there continues to be a tendency to focus on patient-related factors as the causes of problems with adherence, to the relative neglect of provider and health system-related determinants. These latter factors, which make up the health care environment in which patients receive care, have a major effect on adherence.

Adherence is simultaneously influenced by several factors
The ability of patients to follow treatment plans in an optimal manner is frequently compromised by more than one barrier, usually related to different aspects of the problem. These include: the social and economic factors, the health care team/system, the characteristics of the disease, disease therapies and patient-related factors. Solving the problems related to each of these factors is necessary if patients' adherence to therapies is to be improved.

Patient-tailored interventions are required
There is no single intervention strategy, or package of strategies that has been shown to be effective across all patients, conditions and settings. Consequently, interventions that target adherence must be tailored to the particular illness-related demands experienced by the patient. To accomplish this, health systems and providers need to develop means of accurately assessing not only adherence, but also those factors that influence it.

Adherence is a dynamic process that needs to be followed up
Improving adherence requires a continuous and dynamic process. Recent research in the behavioural sciences has revealed that the patient population can be segmented according to level-of-readiness to follow health recommendations. The lack of a match between patient readiness and the practitioner's attempts at intervention means that treatments are frequently prescribed to patients who are not ready to follow them. Health care providers should be able to assess the patient's readiness to adhere, provide advice on how to do it, and follow up the patient's progress at every contact.

Health professionals need to be trained in adherence
Health providers can have a significant impact by assessing risk of nonadherence and delivering interventions to optimize adherence. To make this practice a reality, practitioners must have access to specific training in adherence management, and the systems in which they work must design and support delivery systems that respect this objective. For empowering health professionals an "adherence counselling toolkit" adaptable to different socioeconomic settings is urgently needed. Such training needs to simultaneously address three topics: knowledge (information on adherence), thinking (the clinical decision-making process) and action (behavioural tools for health professionals).

Family, community and patients' organizations: a key factor for success in improving adherence
For the effective provision of care for chronic conditions, it is necessary that the patient, the family and the community who support him or her all play an active role. Social support, i.e. informal or formal support received by patients from other members of their community, has been consistently reported as an important factor affecting health outcomes and behaviours. There is substantial evidence that peer support among patients can improve adherence to therapy while reducing the amount of time devoted by the health professionals to the care of chronic conditions.

A multidisciplinary approach towards adherence is needed
A stronger commitment to a multidisciplinary approach is needed to make progress in this area. This will require coordinated action from health professionals, researchers, health planners and policy-makers.

Section I

Setting the scene

CHAPTER I

Defining adherence

1. What is adherence? 3

2. The state-of-the-art measurement 4

3. References 5

1. What is adherence?

Although most research has focused on adherence to medication, adherence also encompasses numerous health-related behaviours that extend beyond taking prescribed pharmaceuticals. The participants at the WHO Adherence meeting in June 2001 *(1)* concluded that defining adherence as "the extent to which the patient follows medical instructions" was a helpful starting point. However, the term "medical" was felt to be insufficient in describing the range of interventions used to treat chronic diseases. Furthermore, the term "instructions" implies that the patient is a passive, acquiescent recipient of expert advice as opposed to an active collaborator in the treatment process.

In particular, it was recognized during the meeting that adherence to any regimen reflects behaviour of one type or another. Seeking medical attention, filling prescriptions, taking medication appropriately, obtaining immunizations, attending follow-up appointments, and executing behavioural modifications that address personal hygiene, self-management of asthma or diabetes, smoking, contraception, risky sexual behaviours, unhealthy diet and insufficient levels of physical activity are all examples of therapeutic behaviours.

The participants at the meeting also noted that the relationship between the patient and the health care provider (be it physician, nurse or other health practitioner) must be a partnership that draws on the abilities of each. The literature has identified the quality of the treatment relationship as being an important determinant of adherence. Effective treatment relationships are characterized by an atmosphere in which alternative therapeutic means are explored, the regimen is negotiated, adherence is discussed, and follow-up is planned.

The adherence project has adopted the following definition of adherence to long-term therapy, a merged version of the definitions of Haynes *(2)* and Rand *(3)*:

> *the extent to which a person's behaviour — taking medication, following a diet, and/or executing lifestyle changes, corresponds with agreed recommendations from a health care provider.*

Strong emphasis was placed on the need to differentiate adherence from compliance. The main difference is that adherence requires the patient's agreement to the recommendations. We believe that patients should be active partners with health professionals in their own care and that good communication between patient and health professional is a must for an effective clinical practice.

In most of the studies reviewed here, it was not clear whether or not the "patient's previous agreement to recommendations" was taken into consideration. Therefore, the terms used by the original authors for describing compliance or adherence behaviours have been reported here.

A clear distinction between the concepts of acute as opposed to *chronic*, and *communicable* (infectious) as opposed to *noncommunicable*, diseases must also be established in order to understand the type of care needed. Chronic conditions, such as human immunodeficiency virus (HIV), acquired immunodeficiency syndrome (AIDS) and tuberculosis, may be infectious in origin and will need the same kind of care as many other chronic noncommunicable diseases such as hypertension, diabetes and depression.

The adherence project has adopted the following definition of chronic diseases:

> *"Diseases which have one or more of the following characteristics: they are permanent, leave residual disability, are caused by nonreversible pathological alteration, require special training of the patient for rehabilitation, or may be expected to require a long period of supervision, observation or care" (4).*

2. The state-of-the-art measurement

Accurate assessment of adherence behaviour is necessary for effective and efficient treatment planning, and for ensuring that changes in health outcomes can be attributed to the recommended regimen. In addition, decisions to change recommendations, medications, and/or communication style in order to promote patient participation depend on valid and reliable measurement of the adherence construct. Indisputably, there is no "gold standard" for measuring adherence behaviour *(5,6)* and the use of a variety of strategies has been reported in the literature.

One measurement approach is to ask providers and patients for their subjective ratings of adherence behaviour. However, when providers rate the degree to which patients follow their recommendations they overestimate adherence *(7,8)*. The analysis of patients' subjective reports has been problematic as well. Patients who reveal they have not followed treatment advice tend to describe their behaviour accurately *(9)*, whereas patients who deny their failure to follow recommendations report their behaviour inaccurately *(10)*. Other subjective means for measuring adherence include standardized, patient-administered questionnaires *(11)*. Typical strategies have assessed global patient characteristics or "personality" traits, but these have proven to be poor predictors of adherence behaviour *(6)*. There are no stable (i.e. trait) factors that reliably predict adherence. However, questionnaires that assess specific behaviours that relate to specific medical recommendations (e.g. food frequency questionnaires *(12)* for measuring eating behaviour and improving the management of obesity) may be better predictors of adherence behaviour *(13)*.

Although objective strategies may initially appear to be an improvement over subjective approaches, each has drawbacks in the assessment of adherence behaviours. Remaining dosage units (e.g. tablets) can be counted at clinic visits; however, counting inaccuracies are common and typically result in overestimation of adherence behaviour *(14)*, and important information (e.g. timing of dosage and patterns of missed dosages) is not captured using this strategy. A recent innovation is the electronic monitoring device (medication event monitoring system (MEMS)) which records the time and date when a medication container was opened, thus better describing the way patients take their medications *(9)*.

Unfortunately, the expense of these devices precludes their widespread use. Pharmacy databases can be used to check when prescriptions are initially filled, refilled over time, and prematurely discontinued. One problem with this approach is that obtaining the medicine does not ensure its use. Also, such information can be incomplete because patients may use more than one pharmacy or data may not be routinely captured.

Independently of the measurement technique used, thresholds defining "good" and "bad" adherence are widely used despite the lack of evidence to support them. In practice, "good" and "bad" adherence might not really exist because the dose–response phenomenon is a continuum function.

Although dose–response curves are difficult to construct for real-life situations, where dosage, timing and others variables might be different from those tested in clinical trials, they are needed if sound policy decisions are to be made when defining operational adherence thresholds for different therapies.

Biochemical measurement is a third approach for assessing adherence behaviours. Non-toxic biological markers can be added to medications and their presence in blood or urine can provide evidence that a patient recently received a dose of the medication under examination. This assessment strategy is not without drawbacks as findings can be misleading and are influenced by a variety of individual factors including diet, absorption and rate of excretion *(15)*.

In summary, measurement of adherence provides useful information that outcome-monitoring alone cannot provide, but it remains only an estimate of a patient's actual behaviour. Several of the measurement strategies are costly (e.g. MEMS) or depend on information technology (e.g. pharmacy databases) that is unavailable in many countries. Choosing the "best" measurement strategy to obtain an approximation of adherence behaviour must take all these considerations into account. Most importantly, the strategies employed must meet basic psychometric standards of acceptable reliability and validity *(16)*. The goals of the provider or researcher, the accuracy requirements associated with the regimen, the available resources, the response burden on the patient and how the results will be used should also be taken into account. Finally, no single measurement strategy has been deemed optimal. A multi-method approach that combines feasible self-reporting and reasonable objective measures is the current state-of-the-art in measurement of adherence behaviour.

3. References

1. Sabate E. *WHO Adherence Meeting Report*. Geneva, World Health Organization, 2001.
2. Haynes RB. *Determinants of compliance: The disease and the mechanics of treatment*. Baltimore MD, Johns Hopkins University Press, 1979.
3. Rand CS. Measuring adherence with therapy for chronic diseases: implications for the treatment of heterozygous familial hypercholesterolemia. *American Journal of Cardiology*, 1993, 72:68D-74D.
4. *Dictionary of health services management*, 2nd ed. Owing Mills, MD, National Health Publishing, 1982.
5. Timmreck TC, Randolph JF. Smoking cessation: clinical steps to improve compliance. *Geriatrics*, 1993, 48:63-66.
6. Farmer KC. Methods for measuring and monitoring medication regimen adherence in clinical trials and clinical practice. *Clinical Therapeutics*, 1999, 21:1074-1090.
7. DiMatteo MR, DiNicola DD. *Achieving patient compliance*. New York, Pergamon, 1982.
8. Norell SE. Accuracy of patient interviews and estimates by clinical staff in determining medication compliance. *Social Science & Medicine - Part E, Medical Psychology*, 1981, 15:57-61.
9. Cramer JA, Mattson RH. Monitoring compliance with antiepileptic drug therapy. In: Cramer JA, Spilker B, eds. *Patient compliance in medical practice and clinical trials*. New York, Raven Press, 1991:123-137.
10. Spector SL et al. Compliance of patients with asthma with an experimental aerosolized medication: implications for controlled clinical trials. *Journal of Allergy & Clinical Immunology*, 1986, 77:65-70.
11. Morisky DE, Green LW, Levine DM. Concurrent and predictive validity of a self-reported measure of medication adherence. *Medical Care*, 1986, 24:67-74.
12. Freudenheim JL. A review of study designs and methods of dietary assessment in nutritional epidemiology of chronic disease. *Journal of Nutrition*, 1993, 123:401-405.
13. Sumartojo E. When tuberculosis treatment fails. A social behavioral account of patient adherence. *American Review of Respiratory Disease*, 1993, 147:1311-1320.
14. Matsui D et al. Critical comparison of novel and existing methods of compliance assessment during a clinical trial of an oral iron chelator. *Journal of Clinical Pharmacology*, 1994, 34:944-949.
15. Vitolins MZ et al. Measuring adherence to behavioral and medical interventions. *Controlled Clinical Trials*, 2000, 21:188S-194S.
16. Nunnally JC, Bernstein IH. *Psychometric theory*, 3rd ed. New York, McGraw-Hill, 1994.

CHAPTER II

The magnitude of the problem of poor adherence

1. A worldwide problem of striking magnitude   7

2. The impact of poor adherence grows as the burden of chronic diseases grows worldwide   8

3. The poor are disproportionately affected   8

4. References   9

1. A worldwide problem of striking magnitude

A number of rigorous reviews have found that, in developed countries, adherence among patients suffering chronic diseases averages only 50% *(1, 2)*. The magnitude and impact of poor adherence in developing countries is assumed to be even higher given the paucity of health resources and inequities in access to health care.

For example, in China, the Gambia and the Seychelles, only 43%, 27% and 26%, respectively, of patients with hypertension adhere to their antihypertensive medication regimen *(3–6)*. In developed countries, such as the United States, only 51% of the patients treated for hypertension adhere to the prescribed treatment *(7)*. Data on patients with depression reveal that between 40% and 70% adhere to antidepressant therapies *(8)*. In Australia, only 43% of the patients with asthma take their medication as prescribed all the time and only 28% use prescribed preventive medication *(9)*. In the treatment of HIV and AIDS, adherence to antiretroviral agents varies between 37% and 83% depending on the drug under study *(10, 11)* and the demographic characteristics of patient populations *(12)*. This represents a tremendous challenge to population health efforts where success is determined primarily by adherence to long-term therapies.

Although extremely worrying, these indicators provide an incomplete picture. To ascertain the true extent of adherence, data on developing countries and important subgroups, such as adolescents, children and marginal populations are urgently required. A full picture of the magnitude of the problem is critical to developing effective policy support for efforts aimed at improving adherence.

> *In developed countries, adherence to long-term therapies in the general population is around 50% and is much lower in developing countries.*

2. The impact of poor adherence grows as the burden of chronic diseases grows worldwide

Noncommunicable diseases, mental health disorders, HIV/AIDS and tuberculosis, *combined* represented 54% of the burden of all illness worldwide in 2001 *(13)* and will exceed 65% of the global burden of disease in 2020 (Fig. 1) *(14)*. Contrary to popular belief, noncommunicable diseases and mental health problems are also prevalent in developing countries, representing as much as 46% of the total burden of disease for the year 2001 *(13)*, and predicted to rise to 56% by 2020 (Fig. 2) *(1F4)*.

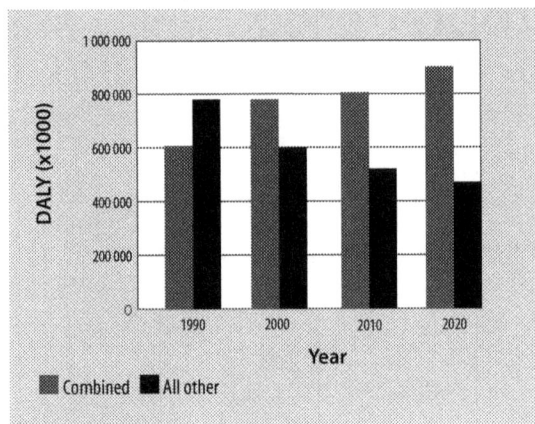

Figure 1   Burden of chronic conditions – world (Murray and Lopez, 1996)

Source: reference *(30)*
DALY, disability-adjusted life year;
Combined, noncommunicable diseases + mental disorders +AIDS + TB.

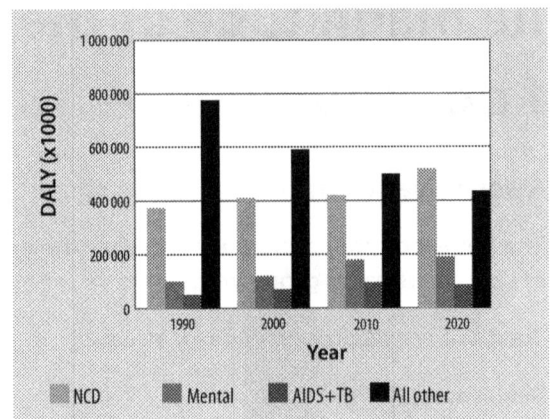

Figure 2   Burden of chronic conditions – developing countries (Murray and Lopez, 1996)

Source: reference *(30)*
DALY, disability-adjusted life year;
Mental, mental disorders;
NCD, noncommunicable diseases.

3. The poor are disproportionately affected

> *When we are sick, working is hard and learning is harder still. Illness blunts our creativity, cuts out opportunities. Unless the consequences of illness are prevented, or at least minimized, illness undermines people, and leads them into suffering, despair and poverty.*
>
> *Kofi Annan, Secretary-General of the United Nations on the occasion of the release of the Report of the Commission on Macroeconomics and Health, in London, 20 December 2001.*

There is a two-way interdependent relationship between economic poverty and chronic disease. Many of the world's poor, despite regional differences in geography, culture and commerce, experience the same discouraging cycle: being healthy requires money for food, sanitation and medical care, but to earn money, one must be healthy. The lack of adequate care for chronic conditions forces poor families to face a particularly heavy burden of caring for their loved ones that undermines the development of their most basic roles. Women are particularly "taxed" by the lack of a health care system that deals effectively with chronic diseases *(15-17)*. Competing needs in populations suffering from chronic poverty undermine efforts to address the needs of patients requring long-term care, including the problem of adherence to medications and therapies.

Poor adherence compounds the challenges of improving health in poor populations, and results in waste and underutilization of already limited treatment resources.

4. References

1. Haynes RB. Interventions for helping patients to follow prescriptions for medications. *Cochrane Database of Systematic Reviews*, 2001 Issue1.
2. Sackett D et al. Patient compliance with antihypertensive regimens. *Patient Counselling & Health Education*, 1978, 11:18-21.
3. Bovet P et al. Monitoring one-year compliance to antihypertension medication in the Seychelles. *Bulletin of the World Health Organization*, 2002, 80:33-39.
4. Graves JW. Management of difficult-to-control hypertension *Mayo Clinic Proceedings*, 2000, 75:278-284 [erratum published in *Mayo Clinical Proceedings*, 2000, 75:542].
5. van der Sande MA et al. Blood pressure patterns and cardiovascular risk factors in rural and urban Gambian communities. *Journal of Human Hypertension*, 2000, 14:489-496.
6. Guo H, He H, Jiang J. [Study on the compliance of antihypertensive drugs in patients with hypertension.] [Chinese] *Chung-Hua Liu Hsing Ping Hsueh Tsa Chih [Chinese Journal of Epidemiology]*, 2001, 22:418-420.
7. Anonymous. Critical overview of antihypertensive therapies: what is preventing us from getting there? Based on a presentation by Mark A. Munger, PharmD. *American Journal of Managed Care*, 2000, 6 (4 Suppl):S211-S221.
8. Demyttenaere K. Noncompliance with antidepressants: who's to blame? *International Clinical Psychopharmacology*, 1998, 13 (Suppl 2):S19-S25.
9. Reid D et al. Management and treatment perceptions among young adults with asthma in Melbourne: the Australian experience from the European Community Respiratory Health Survey. *Respirology*, 2000, 5:281-287.
10. Markowitz AJ, Winawer SJ. Screening and surveillance for colorectal cancer. *Seminars in Oncology*, 1999, 26:485-498.
11. Stein MD et al. Adherence to antiretroviral therapy among HIV-infected methadone patients: effect of ongoing illicit drug use. *American Journal of Drug & Alcohol Abuse*, 2000, 26:195-205.
12. Laine C et al. Adherence to antiretroviral therapy by pregnant women infected with human immunodeficiency virus: a pharmacy claims-based analysis. *Obstetrics & Gynecology*, 2000, 95:167-173.
13. *The World Health Report 2002: Reducing Risks, Promoting Healthy Life.* Geneva, World Health Organization, 2002.
14. Murray CJL, Lopez A. *The global burden of disease.* Geneva, World Health Organization, 1996.
15. Timmreck TC, Randolph JF. Smoking cessation: clinical steps to improve compliance. *Geriatrics*, 1993, 48:63–66.
16. Farmer KC. Methods for measuring and monitoring medication regimen adherence in clinical trials and clinical practice. *Clinical Therapeutics*, 1999, 21:1074–1090.
17. Robinson KM. Family caregiving: who provides the care, and at what cost? *Nurse Economics*, 1997, 15:243-247.

CHAPTER III

How does poor adherence affect policy-makers and health managers?

1. Diabetes   11

2. Hypertension   12

3. Asthma   13

4. References   14

There is strong evidence that many patients with chronic illnesses including asthma, hypertension, diabetes and HIV/AIDS, have difficulty adhering to their recommended regimens. This results in less than optimal management and control of the illness. Poor adherence is the primary reason for suboptimal clinical benefit (1,2). It causes medical and psychosocial complications of disease, reduces patients' quality of life, and wastes health care resources. Taken together, these direct consequences impair the ability of health care systems around the world to achieve population health goals.

The conclusions of research in this area are unequivocal – adherence problems are observed in all situations where the self-administration of treatment is required, regardless of type of disease, disease severity and accessibility to health resources. While it may seem to be a simple issue, many factors contribute to adherence problems. Although some of these factors are patient-related, the characteristics of the disease and its treatment, and attributes of the health care system and service delivery also have great influence. Adherence problems have generally been overlooked by health stakeholders, and as a result have received little direct, systematic, intervention. Three prevalent chronic diseases, diabetes, hypertension and asthma provide compelling illustrations of different facets of these issues.

1. Diabetes

Poor adherence to the treatment for diabetes results in avoidable suffering for the patients and excess costs to the health system. The CODE-2 study (Cost of Diabetes in Europe – type 2) found that, in Europe, only 28% of patients treated for diabetes achieved good glycaemic control (3,4). The control of diabetes requires more than just taking medicine. Other aspects of self-management such as self-monitoring of blood glucose, dietary restrictions, regular foot care and ophthalmic examinations have all been shown to markedly reduce the incidence and progression of complications of diabetes. In the United States, less than 2% of adults with diabetes perform the full level of care that has been recommended by the American Diabetes Association (5). Poor adherence to recognized standards of care is the principal cause of development of complications of diabetes and their associated individual, societal and economic costs.

The CODE-2 study was done in countries with nearly full access to medicines. The picture in developing countries, where many fewer patients have their diabetes well-controlled, is cause for even greater concern.

Patients with diabetes usually have co-morbidities that make their treatment regimens even more complex. In particular, other commonly associated diseases such as hypertension, obesity and depression are themselves known to be characterized by poor rates of adherence, and serve to further increase the likelihood of poor treatment outcomes (6,7).

The combined health and economic burden of diabetes is huge and increasing. The CODE-2 study showed that the total cost of treating more than 10 million patients with type 2 diabetes in the countries studied was approximately US 29 billion, which represents an average of 5% of the total health care expenditure in each country. The overall cost to the health care system of treating patients with type 2 diabetes is on average over 1.5 times higher than per capita health care expenditure, an excess cost-burden of 66% over the general population. Furthermore, that cost increases 2- to 3.5-fold once patients develop preventable microvascular and macrovascular complications. Hospitalization costs, which include the treatment of long-term complications such as heart disease, account for 30–65% of the overall costs of the disease – the largest proportion of costs.

The direct costs of complications attributable to poor control of diabetes are 3–4 times higher than those of good control. The indirect costs (production losses due to sick leave, early retirement and premature death) are of approximately the same magnitude as these direct costs. Similar findings have been reported in other studies (8-10). Clearly, if health systems could be more effective in promoting adherence to self-management of diabetes, the human, social and economic benefits would be substantial.

2. Hypertension

It is well known that high blood pressure increases the risk of ischaemic heart disease 3- to 4-fold (27) and of overall cardiovascular risk by 2- to 3-fold (11). The incidence of stroke increases approximately 3-fold in patients with borderline hypertension and approximately 8-fold in those with definite hypertension (12). It has been estimated that 40% of cases of acute myocardial infarction or stroke are attributable to hypertension (13-15).

Despite the availability of effective treatments, studies have shown that in many countries less than 25% of patients treated for hypertension achieve optimum blood pressure (16). For example, in the United Kingdom and the United States, only 7% and 30% of patients, respectively, had good control of blood pressure (17) and in Venezuela only 4.5% of the treated patients had good blood pressure control (18). Poor adherence has been identified as the main cause of failure to control hypertension (19–25). In one study, patients who did not adhere to beta-blocker therapy were 4.5 times more likely to have complications from coronary heart disease than those who did (26). The best available estimate is that poor adherence to therapy contributes to lack of good blood pressure control in more than two-thirds of people living with hypertension (20).

Considering that in many countries poorly controlled blood pressure represents an important economic burden (e.g. in the United States the cost of health care related to hypertension and its complications was 12.6% of total expenditure on health care in 1998) (28), improving adherence could represent for them an important potential source of health and economic improvement, from the societal (29), institutional (30) and employers' point of view (31,32).

3. Asthma

Research worldwide has documented poor adherence to treatments for asthma although there are large variations between countries *(33)*. Rates of nonadherence among patients with asthma range from 30% to 70%, whether adherence is measured as percentage of prescribed medication taken, serum theophylline levels, days of medication adherence, or percentage of patients who failed to reach a clinically estimated adherence minimum *(34)*. Evidence shows that adherence rates for the regular taking of preventive therapies are as low as 28% in developed countries *(35,36)*.

Adherence is also a serious problem in particular populations such as children and adolescents. In adolescents, adherence to prescribed pulmonary medication may be as low as 30% in general practice *(37)*. The complexity of optimum routine management of the disease – almost one hundred per cent self-managed – results in reduced adherence *(38)*.

Failure to adhere to a regular self-management plan for asthma (including the regular taking of preventive therapies) results in poor asthma control which has clinical consequences, such as exacerbation of asthma, and decreased quality of life for the patients, as well as economic consequences, such as increased hospitalization and emergency department visits, resulting in unnecessarily high costs of health care.

There is a large variation between countries in the costs associated with asthma, but there are several outstanding commonalities: the total cost of asthma as a single condition currently comprises up to 1 to 2% of health care expenditures; hospitalization and emergency care are consistently, disproportionately high, and there is a nearly 1:1 relationship between direct and indirect costs. The available data suggest that this distribution of excess costs is attributable to nonscheduled acute or emergency care, indicating poor asthma management and control *(39)*. Such data highlight the significant cost of hospital care for asthma, compared to the costs of the more frequently used and less costly outpatient and pharmaceutical services.

Economic studies consistently show that the costs incurred by an adult with poorly controlled asthma are higher than those for a well-controlled patient with the same severity of disease. For severe asthma, it has been estimated that the savings produced by optimal control would be around 45% of the total medical costs *(39)*. Poorer adherence to medication among elderly patients with moderate-to-severe asthma was associated with a 5% increase in annual physician visits, whereas better adherence was associated with a 20% decrease in annual hospitalization *(40)*. This represents a significant potential cost saving to society in addition to the improvement in the quality of life and productive output of the affected individuals.

To the individual with asthma, or his or her family, the costs of asthma can be immense. For example, studies have demonstrated that the average amount spent by a family on medical treatments for children with asthma in the United States ranged between 5.5 and 14.5% of family income *(41)*. In India, a study in the state of Andhra Pradesh estimated that the average expenditure for asthma treatment was about 9% of per capita income *(42)*.

The above discussion shows that when asthma is not well controlled, it is likely to affect the social functioning of a country, impairing not only child development and education but also causing disruption in job training or ongoing employment for millions of adults worldwide.

4. References

1. Rybacki JJ. Improving cardiovascular health in postmenopausal women by addressing medication adherence issues. *Journal of the American Pharmaceutical Association*, 2002, 42:63-71.

2. Dunbar-Jacob J et al. Adherence in chronic disease. *Annual Review of Nursing Research*, 2000, 18:48-90.

3. Liebl A et al. [Costs of type 2 diabetes in Germany. Results of the CODE-2 study.] [German] *Deutsche Medizinische Wochenschrift*, 2001, 126:585-589.

4. Liebl A et al. Complications, co-morbidity, and blood glucose control in type 2 diabetes mellitus patients in Germany - results from the CODE-2 study. *Experimental & Clinical Endocrinology & Diabetes*, 2002, 110:10-16.

5. Beckles GL et al. Population-based assessment of the level of care among adults with diabetes in the U.S. *Diabetes Care*, 1998, 21:1432-1438.

6. Lustman PJ, Griffith LS, Clouse RE. Depression in adults with diabetes. *Seminars in Clinical Neuropsychiatry*, 1997, 2:15-23.

7. Ciechanowski PS, Katon WJ, Russo JE. Depression and diabetes: impact of depressive symptoms on adherence, function, and costs. *Archives of Internal Medicine*, 2000, 27:3278-3285.

8. Kangas T et al. Direct costs of health care of drug-treated diabetic patients in Finland in 1989. In: Kangas T. *The Finndiab Report*. Stakes, Research Reports 58, 1995.

9. Henriksson F et al. Direct medical costs for patients with type 2 diabetes in Sweden. *Journal of Internal Medicine*, 2000, 248:387-396.

10. Herman WH, Eastman RC. The effects of treatment on the direct costs of diabetes. *Diabetes Care*, 1998, 21 (Suppl 3):C19-C24.

11. Berenson GS et al. Association between multiple cardiovascular risk factors and atherosclerosis in children and young adults. The Bogalusa Heart Study. *New England Journal of Medicine*, 1998, 338:1650-1656.

12. Thompson DW, Furlan AJ. Clinical epidemiology of stroke. *Neurologic Clinics*, 1996, 14:309-315.

13. al Roomi KA, Heller RF, Wlodarczyk J. Hypertension control and the risk of myocardial infarction and stroke: a population-based study. *Medical Journal of Australia*, 1990, 153:595-599.

14. Borghi C et al. Effects of the administration of an angiotensin-converting enzyme inhibitor during the acute phase of myocardial infarction in patients with arterial hypertension. SMILE Study Investigators. Survival of Myocardial Infarction Long-term Evaluation. *American Journal of Hypertension*, 1999, 12:665-672.

15. Marmot MG, Poulter NR. Primary prevention of stroke. *Lancet*, 1992, 339:344-347.

16. Burt VL et al. Prevalence of hypertension in the US adult population. Results from the Third National Health and Nutrition Examination Survey, 1988-1991. *Hypertension*, 1995, 25:305-313.

17. Heller RF et al. Blood pressure measurement in the United Kingdom Heart Disease Prevention Project. *Journal of Epidemiology & Community Health*, 1978, 32:235-238.

18. Sulbaran T et al. Epidemiologic aspects of arterial hypertension in Maracaibo, Venezuela. *Journal of Human Hypertension*, 2000, 14 (Suppl 1):S6-S9.

19. Waeber B, Burnier M, Brunner HR. How to improve adherence with prescribed treatment in hypertensive patients? *Journal of Cardiovascular Pharmacology*, 2000, 35 (Suppl 3):S23-S26.

20. *The sixth report of the joint national committee on prevention, detection, evaluation, and treatment of high blood pressure*. Bethesda, MD, National High Blood Pressure Education Program, National Heart, Lung, and Blood Institute, National Institutes of Health. 1997.

21. Burt VL et al. Prevalence of hypertension in the US adult population: results from the Third National Health and Nutrition Examination Survey 1988-1991. *Hypertension*, 1995, 25:305-313.

22. Hershey JC et al. Patient compliance with antihypertensive medication. *American Journal of Public Health*, 1980, 70:1081-1089.

23. Luscher TF et al. Compliance in hypertension: facts and concepts. *Journal of Hypertension*, 1985, 3:3-9.

24. Hughes DA et al. The impact of non-compliance on the cost-effectiveness of pharmaceuticals: a review of the literature. *Health Economics*, 2001, 10:601-615.

25. Morisky DE et al. Five-year blood pressure control and mortality following health education for hypertensive patients. *American Journal of Public Health*, 1983, 73:153-162.

26. Psaty BM et al. The relative risk of incident coronary heart disease associated with recently stopping the use of beta-blockers. *Journal of the American Medical Association*, 1990, 263:1653-1657.

27. Spector SL et al. Compliance of patients with asthma with an experimental aerosolized medication: implications for controlled clinical trials. *Journal of Allergy and Clinical Immunology*. 1986;77:6-70.

28. Hodgson TA, Cai L. Medical care expenditures for hypertension, its complications, and its comorbidities. *Medical Care*, 2001, 39:599-615.

29. Piatrauskene I. [Hypertension: economic aspects.] [Russian] *Sovetskoe Zdravookhranenie*, 1991, 4:22-25.

30. McCombs JS et al. The costs of interrupting antihypertensive drug therapy in a Medicaid population. *Medical Care*, 1994, 32:214-226.

31. Tulenbaev MZ et al. [Economic efficacy of implementing a program to control arterial hypertension among industrial workers.] [Russian] *Terapevticheskii Arkhiv*, 1987, 59:50-52.

32. Rizzo JA, Abbott TA, III, Pashko S. Labour productivity effects of prescribed medicines for chronically ill workers. *Health Economics*, 1996, 5:249-265.

33. Cerveri I et al. International variations in asthma treatment compliance: the results of the European Community Respiratory Health Survey (ECRHS). *European Respiratory Journal*, 1999, 14:288-294.

34. Bender B, Milgrom H, Rand C. Nonadherence in asthmatic patients: is there a solution to the problem? *Annals of Allergy, Asthma, & Immunology*, 1997, 79:177-185.

35. Reid D et al. Management and treatment perceptions among young adults with asthma in Melbourne: the Australian experience from the European Community Respiratory Health Survey. *Respirology*, 2000, 5:281–287.

36. Pearson MH, Bucknall CE. *Measuring clinical outcomes in asthma*. London, Royal College of Physicians, 1999.

37. Dekker FW et al. Compliance with pulmonary medication in general practice. *European Respiratory Journal*, 1993, 6:886-890.

38. Slack MK, Brooks AJ. Medication management issues for adolescents with asthma. *American Journal of Health-System Pharmacy*, 1995, 52:1417-1421.

39. *GINA Project (Global Initiative for Asthma)*. 2002, http://www.ginasthma.com.

40. Balkrishnan R, Christensen DB. Inhaled corticosteroid use and associated outcomes in elderly patients with moderate to severe chronic pulmonary disease. *Clinical Therapeutics*, 2000, 22:452-469.

41. Marion RJ, Creer TL, Reynolds RV. Direct and indirect costs associated with the management of childhood asthma. *Annals of Allergy*, 1985, 54:31-34.

42. Mahapatra P. *Social, economic and cultural aspects of asthma: an exploratory study in Andhra Pradesh, India*. Hyderabad, India, Institute of Health Systems, 1993.

Section II

Improving adherence rates: guidance for countries

CHAPTER IV

Lessons learned

1. Patients need to be supported, not blamed   19
2. The consequences of poor adherence to long-term therapies are poor health outcomes and increased health care costs   20
3. Improving adherence also enhances patient safety   21
4. Adherence is an important modifier of health system effectiveness   22
5. Improving adherence might be the best investment for tackling chronic conditions effectively   22
6. Health systems must evolve to meet new challenges   23
7. A multidisciplinary approach towards adherence is needed   24
8. References   24

Over the past 40 years, health, behavioural and social scientists have been accumulating knowledge concerning the prevalence of poor adherence, its determinants and interventions. This report is an attempt to integrate diverse findings across a number of diseases in order to stimulate intersectoral awareness of the magnitude and impact of poor adherence to therapies for chronic conditions, to catalyse discussion, and to identify specific targets for further research and intervention.

Several key lessons have emerged or have been reinforced by evidence from the reviews discussed in this report. These are described below.

1. Patients need to be supported, not blamed

Despite evidence to the contrary, there continues to be a tendency to focus on patient-related factors as the causes of problems with adherence, to the relative neglect of provider and health system-related determinants. These latter factors make up the health care environment in which patients receive care and have a considerable effect on adherence. Interventions that target the relevant factors in the health care environment are urgently required.

Patients may also become frustrated if their preferences in treatment-related decisions are not elicited and taken into account. For example, patients who felt less empowered in relation to treatment decisions had more negative attitudes towards prescribed antiretroviral therapy and reported lower rates of adherence (1).

Adherence is related to the way in which individuals judge personal need for a medication relative to their concerns about its potential adverse effects (2). Horne et al. proposed a simple necessity-concerns framework to help clinicians elicit and address some of the key beliefs that influence patients' adherence to medication. Necessity beliefs and concerns are evaluative summations of the personal salience of the potential costs and benefits or pros and cons of the treatment (3).

2. The consequences of poor adherence to long-term therapies are poor health outcomes and increased health care costs

Adherence is a primary determinant of the effectiveness of treatment (4,5) because poor adherence attenuates optimum clinical benefit (6,7). Good adherence improves the effectiveness of interventions aimed at promoting healthy lifestyles, such as diet modification, increased physical activity, non-smoking and safe sexual behaviour (8-10), and of the pharmacological-based risk-reduction interventions (4,11-13). It also affects secondary prevention and disease treatment interventions.

For example, low adherence has been identified as the primary cause of unsatisfactory control of blood pressure (14). Good adherence has been shown to improve blood pressure control (15) and reduce the complications of hypertension (16-18). In Sudan, only 18% of nonadherent patients achieved good control of blood pressure compared to 96% of those who adhered to their prescribed treatment (19,20).

In studies on the prevention of diabetes type 2, adherence to a reduced-fat diet (21) and to regular physical exercise (22) has been effective in reducing the onset of the disease. For those already suffering the disease, good adherence to treatment, including suggested dietary modifications, physical activity, foot care and ophthalmological check-ups, has been shown to be effective in reducing complications and disability, while improving patients' quality of life and life expectancy (23).

Level of adherence has been positively correlated with treatment outcomes in depressed patients, independently of the anti-depressive drugs used (24). In communicable chronic conditions such as infection with HIV, good adherence to therapies has been correlated with slower clinical progression of the disease as well as lower virological markers (25-32).

In addition to their positive impact on the health status of patients with chronic illnesses, higher rates of adherence confer economic benefits. Examples of these mechanisms include direct savings generated by reduced use of the sophisticated and expensive health services needed in cases of disease exacerbation, crisis or relapse. Indirect savings may be attributable to enhancement of, or preservation of, quality of life and the social and vocational roles of the patients.

There is strong evidence to suggest that self-management programmes offered to patients with chronic diseases improve health status and reduce utilization and costs. When self-management and adherence programmes are combined with regular treatment and disease-specific education, significant improvements in health-promoting behaviours, cognitive symptom management, communication and disability management have been observed. In addition, such programmes appear to result in a reduction in the numbers of patients being hospitalized, days in hospital and outpatient visits. The data suggest a cost to savings ratio of approximately 1:10 in some cases, and these results persisted over 3 years (33). Other studies have found similarly positive results when evaluating the same or alternative interventions (28,34-47).

It has been suggested that good adherence to treatment with antiretroviral agents might have an important impact on public health by breaking the transmission of the virus because of the lower viral load found in highly adherent patients (12).

The development of resistance to therapies is another serious public health issue related to poor adherence, among other factors. In addition to years of life lost due to premature mortality and health care costs attributable to preventable morbidity, the economic consequences of poor adherence include stimulating the need for ongoing investment in research and development of new compounds to fight new resistant variants of the causative organisms.

In patients with HIV/AIDS, the resistance of the virus to antiretroviral agents has been linked to lower levels of adherence (29) by some researchers, while others have suggested that resistant virus is more likely to emerge at higher levels of adherence (48,49). Although they appear to be contradictory, both describe the same phenomenon from a different starting point. At the lower end of the spectrum of adherence, there is insufficient antiretroviral agent to produce selective pressure, so the more adherence rates increase the higher the likelihood that resistance will appear. At the higher levels of adherence, there is not enough virus to become resistant, thus the less adherent the patient, the greater the viral load and the likelihood of resistance. Some of the published research has suggested that when adherence rates are between 50% and 85%, drug resistance is more likely to develop (50,51). Unfortunately, a significant proportion of treated patients fall within this range (52). The "chronic" investment in research and development could be avoided if adherence rates were higher, and the resources could be better used in the development of more effective and safer drugs, or by being directed to the treatment of neglected conditions.

There is growing evidence to suggest that because of the alarmingly low rates of adherence, increasing the effectiveness of adherence interventions may have a far greater impact on the health of the population than any improvement in specific medical treatments (53).

We strongly support the recommendations of the Commission on Macroeconomics and Health on investing in operational research "at least 5% of each country proposal for evaluating health interventions in practice, including adherence as an important factor influencing the effectiveness of interventions" (12).

3. Improving adherence also enhances patient safety

Because most of the care needed for chronic conditions is based on patient self-management (usually requiring complex multi-therapies (54), the use of medical technology for monitoring and changes in the patient's lifestyle (55), patients face several potentially life-threatening risks if health recommendations are not followed as they were prescribed. Some of the risks faced by patients who adhere poorly to their therapies are listed below.

More intense relapses. Relapses related to poor adherence to prescribed medication can be more severe than relapses that occur while the patient is taking the medication as recommended, so persistent poor adherence can worsen the overall course of the illness and may eventually make the patients less likely to respond to treatment (56).

Increased risk of dependence. Many medications can produce severe dependence if taken inappropriately by patients. Good examples are diazepam (57) and opioid-related medications.

Increased risk of abstinence and rebound effect. Adverse effects and potential harm may occur when a medication is abruptly discontinued or interrupted. Good adherence plays an important role in avoiding problems of withdrawal (e.g. as seen in thyroid hormone replacement therapy) and rebound effect (e.g. in patients being treated for hypertension and depression), and consequently decreases the likelihood that a patient will experience adverse effects of discontinuation (58,59).

Increased risk of developing resistance to therapies. In patients with HIV/AIDS, the resistance to antiretroviral agents has been linked to lower levels of adherence *(48,60)*. Partial or poor adherence at levels less than 95% can lead to the resumption of rapid viral replication, reduced survival rates, and the mutation to treatment-resistant strains of HIV *(61)*. The same happens in the treatment of tuberculosis where poor adherence is recognized as a major cause of treatment failure, relapse and drug resistance *(62,63)*.

Increased risk of toxicity. In the case of over-use of medicines (a type of nonadherence), patients are at an increased risk of toxicity, especially from drugs with accumulative pharmacodynamics and/or a low toxicity threshold (e.g. lithium). This is particularly true for elderly patients (altered pharmacodynamics) and patients with mental disorders (e.g. schizophrenia).

Increased likelihood of accidents. Many medications need to be taken in conjunction with lifestyle changes that are a precautionary measure against the increased risk of accidents known to be a side-effect of certain medications. Good examples are medications requiring abstinence from alcohol (metronidazole) or special precautions while driving (sedatives and hypnotics).

4. Adherence is an important modifier of health system effectiveness

Health outcomes cannot be accurately assessed if they are measured predominantly by resource utilization indicators and efficacy of interventions.

The economic evaluation of nonadherence requires the identification of the associated costs and outcomes. It is logical that nonadherence entails a cost due to the occurrence of the undesired effects that the recommended regimen tries to minimize. In terms of outcomes, nonadherence results in increased clinical risk and therefore in increased morbidity and mortality.

For health professionals, policy-makers and donors, measuring the performance of their health programmes and systems using resource utilization end-points and the efficacy of interventions is easier than measuring the desired health outcomes. While such indicators are important, over-reliance on them can bias evaluation towards the process of *health care provision*, missing indicators of *health care uptake* which would make accurate estimates of *health outcomes* possible *(64)*.

The population-health outcomes predicted by treatment efficacy data will not be achieved unless adherence rates are used to inform planning and project evaluation.

5. Improving adherence might be the best investment for tackling chronic conditions effectively

Studies consistently find significant cost-savings and increases in the effectiveness of health interventions that are attributable to low-cost interventions for improving adherence. In many cases investments in improving adherence are fully repaid with savings in health care utilization *(33)* and, in other instances, the improvement in health outcomes fully justifies the investment. The time is ripe for large-scale, multidisciplinary field studies aimed at testing behaviourally sound, multi-focal interventions, across diseases and in different service-delivery environments.

Interventions for removing barriers to adherence must become a central component of efforts to improve population health worldwide. Decision-makers need not be concerned that an undesired increase in health budget will occur due to increasing consumption of medications, because adherence to those medicines already prescribed will result in a significant decrease in the overall health budget due to the reduction in the need for other more costly interventions. Rational use of medicines means good prescribing and full adherence to the prescriptions.

Interventions that promote adherence can help close the gap between the clinical efficacy of interventions and their effectiveness when used in the field, and thus increase the overall effectiveness and efficiency of the health system.

For outcomes to be improved, changes to health policy and health systems are essential. Effective treatment for chronic conditions requires a transfer of health care away from a system that is focused on episodic care in response to acute illness towards a system that is proactive and emphasizes health throughout a lifetime.

Without a system that addresses the determinants of adherence, advances in biomedical technology will fail to realize their potential to reduce the burden of chronic illness. Access to medications is necessary, but insufficient in itself to solve the problem *(12)*.

> *Increasing the effectiveness of adherence interventions might have a far greater impact on the health of the population than any improvement in specific medical treatments (65).*

6. Health systems must evolve to meet new challenges

In developed countries, the epidemiological shift in disease burden from acute to chronic diseases over the past 50 years has rendered acute care models of health service delivery inadequate to address the health needs of the population. In developing countries this shift is occurring at a much faster rate.

The health care delivery system has the potential to affect patients' adherence behaviour. Health care systems control access to care. For example, health systems control providers' schedules, length of appointments, allocation of resources, fee structures, communication and information systems, and organizational priorities. The following are examples of the ways in which systems influence patients' behaviour:

- Systems direct appointment length, and providers report that their schedules do not allow time to adequately address adherence behaviour *(66)*.

- Systems determine fee structures, and in many systems (e.g. fee-for-service) the lack of financial reimbursement for patient counselling and education seriously threatens adherence-focused interventions.

- Systems allocate resources in a way that may result in high stress and increased demands upon providers which, in turn, have been associated with decreased adherence in their patients *(67)*.

- Systems determine continuity of care. Patients demonstrate better adherence behaviour when they receive care from the same provider over time *(68)*.

- Systems direct information sharing. The ability of clinics and pharmacies to share information on patients' behaviour regarding prescription refills has the potential to improve adherence.

- Systems determine the level of communication with patients. Ongoing communication efforts (e.g. telephone contacts) that keep the patient engaged in health care may be the simplest and most cost-effective strategy for improving adherence *(69)*.

Few studies have evaluated programmes that have used such interventions, and this is a serious gap in the applied knowledge base. For an intervention to be truly multi-level, systemic barriers must be included. Unless variables such as these are addressed, it would be expected that the impact of the efforts of providers and patients would be limited by the external constraints.

The changing nature of disease prevalence also influences activities at the system level. Continued reliance on acute models has delayed the reforms necessary to address longer-term interventions for chronic conditions. In developing countries this shift is occurring at a much faster rate at a time when the battle against communicable diseases is still being fought.

In some countries, the attention of the policy-makers may remain focused on communicable diseases, for example HIV/AIDS and tuberculosis. However, these diseases are not effectively addressed by the acute care model. Even if it were to provide full and unrestricted access to appropriate drugs, the acute care model would lack impact because it does not address the broad determinants of adherence.

7. A multidisciplinary approach towards adherence is needed

The problem of nonadherence has been much discussed, but has been relatively neglected in the mainstream delivery of primary care health services. Despite an extensive knowledge base, efforts to address the problem have been fragmented, and with few exceptions have failed to harness the potential contributions of the diverse health disciplines. A stronger commitment to a multidisciplinary approach is needed in order to make progress in this area. This will require coordinated action from health professionals, researchers, health planners and policy-makers.

8. References

1. Webb DG, Horne R, Pinching AJ. Treatment-related empowerment: preliminary evaluation of a new measure in patients with advanced HIV disease. *International Journal of STD & AIDS*, 2001, 12:103-107.

2. Horne R, Weinman J. Patients' beliefs about prescribed medicines and their role in adherence to treatment in chronic physical illness. *Journal of Psychosomatic Research*, 1999, 47:555-567.

3. Horne R. Patients' beliefs about treatment: the hidden determinant of treatment outcome? *Journal of Psychosomatic Research*, 1999, 47:491-495.

4. *The World Health Report 2002: Reducing Risks, Promoting Healthy Life.* Geneva, World Health Organization, 2002.

5. Cramer JA. Consequences of intermittent treatment for hypertension: the case for medication compliance and persistence. *American Journal of Managed Care*, 1998, 4:1563-1568.

6. Dunbar-Jacob J et al. Adherence in chronic disease. *Annual Review of Nursing Research*, 2000, 18:48-90.

7. Sarquis LM et al. [Compliance in antihypertensive therapy: analyses in scientific articles.] [Portuguese] *Revista Da Escola de Enfermagem Da USP,* 1998, 32:335-353.

8. Clark DO. Issues of adherence, penetration, and measurement in physical activity effectiveness studies. *Medical Care*, 2001, 39:409-412.

9. Green CA. What can patient health education coordinators learn from ten years of compliance research? *Patient Education & Counseling*, 1987, 10:167-174.

10. Rayman RB. Health promotion: a perspective. *Aviation Space & Environmental Medicine*, 1988, 59:379-381.

11. Scheen AJ. [Therapeutic non-compliance: a major problem in the prevention of cardiovascular diseases.] [French] *Revue Medicale de Liege*, 1999, 54:914-920.

12. *Macroeconomics and Health: Investing in Health for Economic Development – Report of the Commission on Macroeconomics and Health.* Geneva, World Health Organization, 2001.

13. Burke LE, Dunbar-Jacob JM, Hill MN. Compliance with cardiovascular disease prevention strategies: a review of the research. *Annals of Behavioral Medicine*, 1997, 19:239-263.

14. Waeber B, Burnier M, Brunner HR. How to improve adherence with prescribed treatment in hypertensive patients? *Journal of Cardiovascular Pharmacology*, 2000, 35 (Suppl 3):S23-S26.

15. Luscher TF et al. Compliance in hypertension: facts and concepts. *Journal of Hypertension* (Suppl), 1985, 3:S3-S9.

16. Psaty BM et al. The relative risk of incident coronary heart disease associated with recently stopping the use of beta-blockers. *Journal of the American Medical Association*, 1990, 263:1653-1657.

17. Rogers PG, Bullman W. Prescription medicine compliance: review of the baseline of knowledge – report of the National Council on Patient Information and Education. *Journal of Pharmacoepidemiology*, 1995, 3:3-36.

18. Beckles GL et al. Population-based assessment of the level of care among adults with diabetes in the U.S. *Diabetes Care*, 1998, 21:1432-1438.

19. Khalil SA, Elzubier AG. Drug compliance among hypertensive patients in Tabuk, Saudi Arabia. *Journal of Hypertension*, 1997, 15:561-565.

20. Elzubier AG et al. Drug compliance among hypertensive patients in Kassala, eastern Sudan. *Eastern Mediterranean Health Journal*, 2000, 6:100-105.

21. Swinburn BA, Metcalf PA, Ley SJ. Long-term (5-year) effects of a reduced-fat diet intervention in individuals with glucose intolerance. *Diabetes Care*, 2001, 24:619-624.

22. Foreyt JP, Poston WS. The challenge of diet, exercise and lifestyle modification in the management of the obese diabetic patient. *International Journal of Obesity*, 1999, 23 (Suppl 7):S5-S11.

23. Anderson BJ, Vangsness L, Connell A. Family conflict, adherence, and glycaemic control in youth with short duration Type 1 diabetes. *Diabetic Medicine*, 2002, 19:635-642.

24. Thompson C et al. Compliance with antidepressant medication in the treatment of major depressive disorder in primary care: a randomized comparison of fluoxetine and a tricyclic antidepressant. *American Journal of Psychiatry*, 2000, 157:338-343.

25. Stein MD et al. Adherence to antiretroviral therapy among HIV-infected methadone patients: effect of ongoing illicit drug use. *American Journal of Drug & Alcohol Abuse*, 2000, 26:195-205.

26. Gifford AL et al. Predictors of self-reported adherence and plasma HIV concentrations in patients on multidrug antiretroviral regimens. *Journal of Acquired Immune Deficiency Syndromes*, 2000, 23:386-395.

27. Paterson DL et al. Adherence to protease inhibitor therapy and outcomes in patients with HIV infection. *Annals of Internal Medicine*, 2000, 133:21-30.

28. Tuldra A et al. Prospective randomized two-arm controlled study to determine the efficacy of a specific intervention to improve long-term adherence to highly active antiretroviral therapy. *Journal of Acquired Immune Deficiency Syndromes*, 2000, 25:221-228.

29. Bangsberg DR et al. Adherence to protease inhibitors, HIV-1 viral load, and development of drug resistance in an indigent population. *AIDS*, 2000, 14:357-366.

30. Chesney MA. Factors affecting adherence to antiretroviral therapy. *Clinical Infectious Disease*, 2000, 30 (Suppl 2):S171-S176.

31. Murri R et al. Patient-reported nonadherence to HAART is related to protease inhibitor levels. *Journal of Acquired Immune Deficiency Syndromes*, 2000, 24:123-128.

32. Chesney MA, Morin M, Sherr L. Adherence to HIV combination therapy. *Social Science and Medicine*, 2000, 50:1599-1605.

33. Holman HR et al. Evidence that an education program for self-management of chronic disease can improve health status while reducing health care costs: a randomized trial. *Abstract Book/Association for Health Services Research*, 1997, 14:19-20.

34. Gibson PG et al. Self-management education and regular practitioner review for adults with asthma. *Cochrane Database of Systematic Reviews*, 2001.

35. Sloss EM et al. Selecting target conditions for quality of care improvement in vulnerable older adults. *Journal of the American Geriatrics Society*, 2000, 48:363-369.

36. Mar J, Rodriguez-Artalejo F. Which is more important for the efficiency of hypertension treatment: hypertension stage, type of drug or therapeutic compliance? *Journal of Hypertension* (Suppl), 2001, 19:149-155.

37. Massanari MJ. Asthma management: curtailing cost and improving patient outcomes. *Journal of Asthma*, 2000, 37:641-651.

38. Balkrishnan R, Christensen DB. Inhaled corticosteroid use and associated outcomes in elderly patients with moderate to severe chronic pulmonary disease. *Clinical Therapeutics*, 2000, 22:452-469.

39. Kokubu F et al. [Hospitalization reduction by an asthma tele-medicine system.] [Japanese] *Arerugi – Japanese Journal of Allergology*, 2000, 49:19-31.

40. On-demand use of 2 agonists led to better asthma control than did regular use in moderate-to-severe asthma. *ACP Journal Club*, 2001, 134:17.

41. Valenti WM. Treatment adherence improves outcomes and manages costs. *AIDS Reader*, 2001, 11:77-80

42. McPherson-Baker S et al. Enhancing adherence to combination antiretroviral therapy in nonadherent HIV-positive men. *AIDS Care*, 2000, 12:399-404.

43. Ostrop NJ, Hallett KA, Gill MJ. Long-term patient adherence to antiretroviral therapy. *Annals of Pharmacotherapy*, 2000, 34:703-709.

44. Desvarieux M et al. A novel approach to directly observed therapy for tuberculosis in an HIV-endemic area. *American Journal of Public Health*, 2001, 91:138-141.

45. Put C et al. A study of the relationship among self-reported noncompliance, symptomatology, and psychological variables in patients with asthma. *Journal of Asthma*, 2000, 37:503-510.

46. Ciechanowski PS, Katon WJ, Russo JE. Depression and diabetes: impact of depressive symptoms on adherence, function, and costs. *Archives of Internal Medicine*, 2000, 27:3278-3285.

47. Rohland BM, Rohrer JE, Richards CC. The long-term effect of outpatient commitment on service use. *Administration & Policy in Mental Health*, 2000, 27:383-394.

48. Bangsberg DR et al. Adherence to protease inhibitors, HIV-1 viral load, and development of drug resistance in an indigent population. *AIDS*, 2000, 14:357-366.

49. Gallego O et al. Drug resistance in patients experiencing early virological failure under a triple combination including indinavir. *AIDS*, 2001, 15:1701-1706.

50. Chesney MA. Factors affecting adherence to antiretroviral therapy. *Clinics in Infectious Disease*, 2000, 30:S171-S176.

51. Wahl LM, Nowak MA. Adherence and drug resistance: predictions for therapy outcome. *Proceedings of the Royal Society of London – Series B: Biological Sciences*, 2000, 267:835-843.

52. Markowitz M. Resistance, fitness, adherence, and potency: mapping the paths to virologic failure. *Journal of the American Medical Association*, 2000, 283:250-251.

53. Haynes RB. Interventions for helping patients to follow prescriptions for medications. *Cochrane Database of Systematic Reviews*, 2001.

54. Chesney MA, Morin M, Sherr L. Adherence to HIV combination therapy. *Social Science & Medicine*, 2000, 50:1599-1605.

55. Johnson KH, Bazargan M, Bings EG. Alcohol consumption and compliance among inner-city minority patients with type 2 diabetes mellitus. *Archives of Family Medicine*, 2000, 9:964-970.

56. Weiden P. Adherence to antipsychotic medication: key facts. *Schizophrenia Home Page*, 2002 (www.schizophrenia.com/ami/coping/noncompli2.htm).

57. Bush PJ, Spector KK, Rabin DL. Use of sedatives and hypnotics prescribed in a family practice. *Southern Medical Journal*, 1984, 77:677-681.

58. Demyttenaere K, Haddad P. Compliance with antidepressant therapy and antidepressant discontinuation symptoms. *Acta Psychiatrica Scandinavica*, 2000, 403:50-56.

59. Kaplan EM. Antidepressant noncompliance as a factor in the discontinuation syndrome. *Journal of Clinical Psychiatry*, 1997, 58:31-35.

60. Wahl LM, Nowak MA. Adherence and drug resistance: predictions for therapy outcome. *Proceedings of the Royal Society of London – Series B: Biological Sciences*, 2000, 267:835-843.

61. Paterson DL et al. Adherence to protease inhibitor therapy and outcomes in patients with HIV infection. *Annals of Internal Medicine*, 2000, 133:21-30.

62. Yach D. Tuberculosis in the Western Cape health region of South Africa. *Social Science & Medicine*, 1988, 27:683-689.

63. Bell J, Yach D. Tuberculosis patient compliance in the western Cape, 1984. *South African Medical Journal*, 1988, 73:31-33.

64. Ehiri BI. Improving compliance among hypertensive patients: a reflection on the role of patient education. *International Journal of Health Promotion & Education*, 2000, 38:104-108.

65. Haynes RB et al. Interventions for helping patients follow prescriptions for medications. *Cochrane Database of Systematic Reviews*, 2001.

66. Ammerman AS et al. Physician-based diet counseling for cholesterol reduction: current practices, determinants, and strategies for improvement. *Preventive Medicine*, 1993, 22:96-109.

67. DiMatteo MR, DiNicola DD. *Achieving patient compliance.* New York, Pergamon, 1982.

68. Meichenbaum D, Turk DC. *Facilitating treatment adherence: A practitioner's guidebook.* New York, Plenum Press, 1987.

69. Haynes RB, McKibbon KA, Kanani R. Systematic review of randomised trials of interventions to assist patients to follow prescriptions for medications. *Lancet*, 1996, 348:383-386 [erratum published in *Lancet*, 1997, 3499059:1180].

CHAPTER V

Towards the solution

1. Five interacting dimensions affect adherence   27

2. Intervening in the five dimensions   31

3. Reference   36

1. Five interacting dimensions affect adherence

Adherence is a multidimensional phenomenon determined by the interplay of five sets of factors, here termed "dimensions", of which patient-related factors are just one determinant (Figure 3). The common belief that patients are solely responsible for taking their treatment is misleading and most often reflects a misunderstanding of how other factors affect people's behaviour and capacity to adhere to their treatment.

The five dimensions are briefly discussed below. The length of the discussion on each dimension reflects the quantity of evidence available, which is biased by the traditional misconception that adherence is a patient-driven problem. Therefore, the size of the section does not reflect its importance.

Figure 3   The five dimensions of adherence

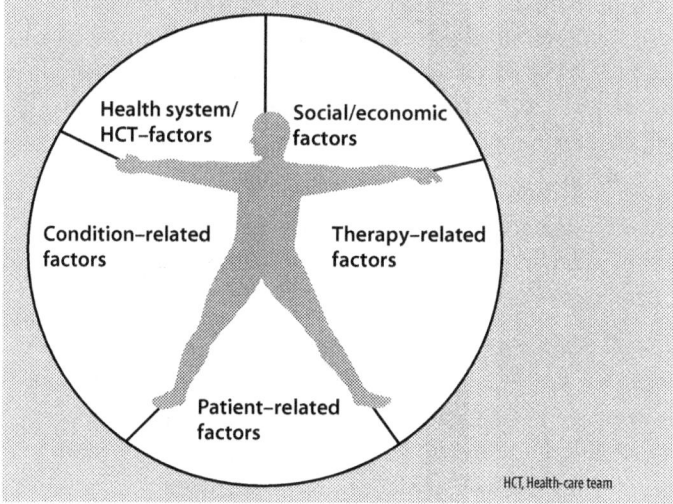

HCT, Health-care team

A. Social and economic factors

Although socioeconomic status has not consistently been found to be an independent predictor of adherence, in developing countries low socioeconomic status may put patients in the position of having to choose between competing priorities. Such priorities frequently include demands to direct the limited resources available to meet the needs of other family members, such as children or parents for whom they care.

Some factors reported to have a significant effect on adherence are: poor socioeconomic status, poverty, illiteracy, low level of education, unemployment, lack of effective social support networks, unstable living conditions, long distance from treatment centre, high cost of transport, high cost of medication, changing environmental situations, culture and lay beliefs about illness and treatment, and family dysfunction. Various sociodemographic and economic variables are discussed in the course of this report (see also Annex 3).

Some studies have reported that organizational factors are more related to adherence than sociodemographic ones, but this might differ from one setting to another. An interesting study by Albaz in Saudi Arabia concluded that organizational variables (time spent with the doctor, continuity of care by the doctor, communication style of the doctor and interpersonal style of the doctor) are far more important than sociodemographic variables (gender, marital status, age, educational level and health status) in affecting patients' adherence *(1)*.

Race has frequently been reported to be a predictor of adherence, regardless of whether the members of a particular race are living in their country of origin or elsewhere as immigrants. Often, cultural beliefs are the reason behind these racial differences *(2)*, but, no less often, social inequalities confound these findings *(3)*. For example, in the United Kingdom, HIV-positive black Africans have been found to have a different experience of treatment because of their fear of being experimented on, distrust of the medical profession and fears of discrimination *(4)*. In the United States, African Americans have been reported to express significantly more doubt regarding their ability to use protease inhibitors and adhere to the treatment, and about the competence of their physicians than do the white population *(5)*.

War has also been reported to have an influence on adherence to therapies, even after the war is over. This is mainly the result of war experiences such as economic hardship, lack of medical control, fatalism and anarchy *(6)*.

Age is a factor reported as affecting adherence, but inconsistently. It should be evaluated separately for each condition, and, if possible, by the characteristics of the patient and by developmental age group (i.e. children dependent on parent, adolescents, adults and elderly patients).

Adherence to treatment by *children and adolescents* ranges from 43% to 100%, with an average of 58% in developed countries *(7)*. Several studies have suggested that adolescents are less adherent than younger children *(8)*. The adherence of infants and toddlers to recommended treatment regimens is largely determined by the ability of the parent or guardian to understand and follow through with the recommended management. As age increases, children have the cognitive ability to carry out treatment tasks, but continue to need parental supervision.

School-aged children engage in the developmental task of industry, learning to regulate their own behaviour and control the world around them. As children enter school, they spend less time at home with their parents and are increasingly influenced by their peers and the social environment.

At the same time, increasing numbers of single and working parents have shifted more of the responsibility for disease management to the child. Assigning too much responsibility to a child for management of his or her treatment can lead to poor adherence. For example, studies indicate that, like adults, children exaggerate their adherence behaviours in their self-reports *(9)*. Parents need to understand that inaccurate diary reporting may hinder appropriate disease management by clinicians. These findings underscore the value of parental supervision and guidance of children in their health behaviours. Shared family responsibility for treatment tasks and continuous reinforcement appear to be important factors in the enhancement of adherence to prescribed treatment for the paediatric population. In addition to parental supervision, behavioural techniques designed to help children, such as goal-setting, cueing, and rewards or tokens, have been found to improve adherence in the school-aged population (10).

Adolescents, though capable of greater autonomy in following treatment recommendations, struggle with self-esteem, body image, social role definition and peer-related issues. Poor adherence in adolescents may reflect rebellion against the regimen's control over their lives. Most studies indicate that children and adolescents who assume early sole responsibility for their treatment regimen are less adherent and in poorer control of their disease management. Both sustaining parental involvement and minimizing conflict between adolescents and their parents are valuable in encouraging adherence to treatment regimens. Providing families with information on forming a partnership between the parent(s) and the adolescent is of considerable importance in promoting adherence to treatment for this age group. Educational efforts focusing on adolescents' attitudes towards their disease and its management, instead of predominantly on knowledge acquisition, may be beneficial.

Elderly people represent 6.4 % of the world's population and their numbers are increasing by 800 000 every month. They have become the fastest-growing segment of the population in many developing countries (11,12).

This demographic transition has led to an increased prevalence of chronic illnesses that are particularly common in the elderly. These include Alzheimer disease, Parkinson disease, depression, diabetes, congestive heart failure, coronary artery disease, glaucoma, osteoarthritis, osteoporosis and others.

Many elderly patients present with multiple chronic diseases, which require complex long-term treatment to prevent frailty and disability. Furthermore, the elderly are the greatest consumers of prescription drugs. In developed countries, people over 60 years old consume approximately 50% of all prescription medicines (as much as three times more per capita than the general population) and are responsible for 60% of medication-related costs even though they represent only 12% to 18% of the population in these countries (13).

Adherence to treatments is essential to the well-being of elderly patients, and is thus a critically important component of care. In the elderly, failure to adhere to medical recommendations and treatment has been found to increase the likelihood of therapeutic failure (14), and to be responsible for unnecessary complications, leading to increased spending on health care, as well as to disability and early death (15).

Poor adherence to prescribed regimens affects all age groups. However, the prevalence of cognitive and functional impairments in elderly patients (16) increases their risk of poor adherence. Multiple co-morbidities and complex medical regimens further compromise adherence. Age-related alterations in pharmacokinetics and pharmacodynamics make this population even more vulnerable to problems resulting from nonadherence.

B. Health care team and system-related factors

Relatively little research has been conducted on the effects of health care team and system-related factors on adherence. Whereas a good patient-provider relationship may improve adherence (17), there are many factors that have a negative effect. These include, poorly developed health services with inadequate or non-existent reimbursement by health insurance plans, poor medication distribution systems, lack of knowledge and training for health care providers on managing chronic diseases, overworked health care providers, lack of incentives and feedback on performance, short consultations, weak capacity of the system to educate patients and provide follow-up, inability to establish community support and self-management capacity, lack of knowledge on adherence and of effective interventions for improving it.

C. Condition-related factors

Condition-related factors represent particular illness-related demands faced by the patient. Some strong determinants of adherence are those related to the severity of symptoms, level of disability (physical, psychological, social and vocational), rate of progression and severity of the disease, and the availability of effective treatments. Their impact depends on how they influence patients' risk perception, the importance of following treatment, and the priority placed on adherence. Co-morbidities, such as depression *(18)* (in diabetes or HIV/AIDS), and drug and alcohol abuse, are important modifiers of adherence behaviour.

D. Therapy-related factors

There are many therapy-related factors that affect adherence. Most notable are those related to the complexity of the medical regimen, duration of treatment, previous treatment failures, frequent changes in treatment, the immediacy of beneficial effects, side-effects, and the availability of medical support to deal with them.

Unique characteristics of diseases and/or therapies do not outweigh the common factors affecting adherence, but rather modify their influence. Adherence interventions should be tailored to the needs of the patient in order to achieve maximum impact.

E. Patient-related factors

Patient-related factors represent the resources, knowledge, attitudes, beliefs, perceptions and expectations of the patient.

Patients' knowledge and beliefs about their illness, motivation to manage it, confidence (self-efficacy) in their ability to engage in illness-management behaviours, and expectations regarding the outcome of treatment and the consequences of poor adherence, interact in ways not yet fully understood to influence adherence behaviour.

Some of the patient-related factors reported to affect adherence are: forgetfulness; psychosocial stress; anxieties about possible adverse effects; low motivation; inadequate knowledge and skill in managing the disease symptoms and treatment; lack of self-perceived need for treatment; lack of perceived effect of treatment; negative beliefs regarding the efficacy of the treatment; misunderstanding and non-acceptance of the disease; disbelief in the diagnosis; lack of perception of the health risk related to the disease; misunderstanding of treatment instructions; lack of acceptance of monitoring; low treatment expectations; low attendance at follow-up, or at counselling, motivational, behavioural, or psychotherapy classes; hopelessness and negative feelings; frustration with health care providers; fear of dependence; anxiety over the complexity of the drug regimen, and feeling stigmatized by the disease.

Perceptions of personal need for medication are influenced by symptoms, expectations and experiences and by illness cognitions *(19)*. Concerns about medication typically arise from beliefs about side-effects and disruption of lifestyle, and from more abstract worries about the long-term effects and dependence. They are related to negative views about medicines as a whole and suspicions that doctors over-prescribe medicines *(20,21)* as well as to a broader "world view" characterized by suspicions of chemicals in food and the environment *(22)* and of science, medicine and technology *(23)*.

A patient's motivation to adhere to prescribed treatment is influenced by the value that he or she places on following the regimen (cost-benefit ratio) and the degree of confidence in being able to follow it *(24)*. Building on a patient's intrinsic motivation by increasing the perceived importance of adherence, and strengthening confidence by building self-management skills, are behavioural treatment targets that must be addressed concurrently with biomedical ones if overall adherence is to be improved.

2. Intervening in the five dimensions

The ability of patients to follow treatments in an optimal manner is frequently compromised by more than one barrier. Interventions to promote adherence require several components to target these barriers, and health professionals must follow a systematic process to assess all the potential barriers.

Given that interventions are available, why has the adherence problem persisted? One answer concerns their implementation. There has been a tendency to focus on unidimensional factors (primarily patient-related factors). All five dimensions (social and economic factors, health care team and systems-related factors, therapy-related factors, condition-related factors and patient-related factors), should be considered in a systematic exploration of the factors affecting adherence and the interventions aimed at improving it.

While many interventions (e.g. education in self-management *(25-34)*; pharmacy management programmes *(35,36)*; nurse, pharmacist and other non-medical health professional intervention protocols *(37-43)*; counselling *(44,45)*; behavioural interventions *(46,47)*; follow-up *(48,49)* and reminders, among others), have been shown to be effective in significantly improving adherence rates *(50-54)*, they have tended to be used alone. A single-factor approach might be expected to have limited effectiveness, if the factors determining adherence interact and potentiate each other's influence as they are likely to do.

The most effective approaches have been shown to be multi-level – targeting more than one factor with more than one intervention. Several programmes have demonstrated good results using multi-level team approaches *(55-57)*. Examples include the Multiple Risk Factor Intervention Trial Research Group, 1982 *(58)* and the Hypertension Detection and Follow-up Program Cooperative Group, 1979 *(59)*. In fact, adequate evidence exists to support the use of innovative, modified health care system teams rather than traditional, independent physician practice and minimally structured systems *(60,61)*.

Various interventions are already being implemented by many different health care actors. Although not all of these actors are directly responsible for providing health care, they nevertheless have an important role in improving adherence because they can influence one or more of the factors that determine adherence.

The work that is being done to improve adherence and the persons performing the work are described below.

A. Social and economic interventions

Policy-makers who have the major responsibility for designing and managing the health care environment need to understand the ways in which social and economic factors influence adherence.

The main economic and social concerns that should be addressed in relation to adherence are poverty *(62)*, access to health care and medicines, illiteracy *(62)*, provision of effective social support networks and mechanisms for the delivery of health services that are sensitive to cultural beliefs about illness and treatment. (For more information see Annex 4.)

The high cost of medicines and care is consistently reported as an important cause of nonadherence in developing countries. Universal and sustainable financing, affordable prices and reliable supply systems are required if good rates of adherence to therapies are to be achieved. Considerable efforts are being made by WHO's partners to improve access to medicines and care worldwide.

Community-based organizations, education of illiterate patients, assessment of social needs *(63)* and family preparedness have been reported to be effective social interventions for improving adherence *(64)*.

Social support (i.e. informal or formal support received by patients from other members of their community), has been consistently reported as an important factor affecting health outcomes and behaviours *(65,66)*. It has also been reported to improve adherence to prescribed recommendations for treating chronic conditions *(67)*, such as diabetes *(68-78)*, hypertension *(79,80)*, epilepsy *(81-86)*, asthma *(87)* and HIV/AIDS *(88-92)*, and to some preventive interventions such as breast cancer screening guidelines *(93)* and follow-up for abnormal Pap smears *(94,95)*. So far, social support has not been shown to affect adherence to smoking cessation therapies *(96-98)*.

Good examples of successfully implemented community-based programmes are the medication groups *(99)* and the peer/community support groups. The objectives of these programmes are:

– to promote the exchange of experiences of dealing with a disease and its treatment;

– to provide comprehensive medical information; and

– to promote patients' responsibility for their own care.

There is substantial evidence that peer support among patients can improve adherence to therapy *(88,100-107)* while reducing the amount of time devoted by health professionals to the care of patients with chronic conditions *(107-109)*. Many other community interventions have also been shown to result in economic and health benefits by improving patients' self-management capacities *(110-117)* and/or by the integration of the provision of care *(57,118-121)*.

The participation of patients' organizations, with the support of community health professionals *(122)*, has been shown to be effective in promoting the maintenance and motivation required for the self-management of chronic diseases, as well as keeping the patient active in the knowledge of his or her disease and in the acquisition of new habits *(110,111,113-115,123,124)*.

There are three different types of patients' organization (PO):

– Patient's organizations directly owned and managed by the health care provider (e.g. health maintenance organizations (HMOs) in the United States);

– Patient's organizations directly owned by patients, but promoted, organized and supported by public health care providers (as in Mexico); and

– independent Patient's organizations with no ties with health care providers.

Unfortunately, the Patient's organizations that have no ties with health care providers usually lack the health care programmes required for supporting patients' self-management. Their effectiveness has not been evaluated and such organizations usually focus mainly on patient advocacy.

Although well-established group interventions do exist, few patients are informed by health professionals of the benefits of joining support groups for improving self-management of chronic conditions. Further evaluation is needed to assess the effectiveness and cost-effectiveness of these organizations in enhancing adherence.

WHO, ministries of health and development agencies have a major role in promoting and coordinating community-based efforts to tackle social and economic factors affecting adherence to therapies.

B. Health care team and health system interventions

The issue of nonadherence has caught the attention of front-line health service providers and health researchers for a long time. However, opinion leaders among policy-makers have yet to adopt the issue as a policy target. This report can be used to focus attention on the consequences of poor adherence not only for population health, but for the efficiency of the health care system and to demonstrate the key role that policy-makers have to play.

> *Adherence is a multidimensional issue where different health care actors' efforts meet.*

Health leaders at many different levels contribute to shaping a health system to meet the needs of its constituents. The way that health systems operate, the types of services and resources that are available and accessible to the population, and the ways in which health providers deliver treatments are of primary concern here.

This review found five major barriers inextricably linked to health system and team factors:

– lack of awareness and knowledge about adherence;

– lack of clinical tools to assist health professionals in evaluating and intervening in adherence problems;

– lack of behavioural tools to help patients develop adaptive health behaviours or to change maladaptive ones;

– gaps in the provision of care for chronic conditions; and

– suboptimal communication between patients and health professionals.

No single intervention or package of interventions has been shown to be effective across all patients, conditions and settings. Consequently, interventions that target adherence must be tailored to the particular illness-related demands experienced by the patient. To accomplish this, health systems and providers need to develop means of accurately assessing not only adherence, but also those factors that contribute to it.

Because health care providers could be expected to play a significant role in promoting adherence, designing and implementing interventions to influence what they do would seem a reasonable strategy. Although there have been efforts in this area, it is possible that they have had less-than-optimal power because they have not conveyed a sufficiently powerful skill set and/or the skills have not been widely adopted in practice.

To make this way of practice a reality, practitioners must have access to specific training in adherence management, and the systems in which they work must design and support delivery systems that respect this objective. For empowering health professionals an "adherence counselling toolkit" adaptable to different socioeconomic settings is urgently needed that will systematically assess, suggest interventions and follow up patients' adherence.

Such training needs to address three main topics simultaneously.

The information on adherence. A summary of the factors that have been reported to affect adherence, the effective interventions available, the epidemiology and economics of adherence and behavioural mechanisms driving patient-related adherence.

A clinically useful way of using this information and thinking about adherence. This should encompass assessment tools and strategies to promote change. Any educational intervention should provide answers to the following questions: How should patients be interviewed to assess adherence? How can one learn from local factors and interventions? How should priorities be ranked and the best available interventions chosen? How should the patients' progress be followed up and assessed?

Behavioural tools for creating or maintaining habits. This component should be taught using "role-play" and other educational strategies to ensure that health professionals incorporate behavioural tools for enhancing adherence into their daily practice.

Some information is available on training health professionals to perform patient-tailored interventions effectively. Ockene et al. *(125)* reported the effectiveness of short patient-centred interventions in three different randomized clinical trials: the WATCH study (diet) *(126,127)*, the Project Health (alcohol) *(128)*, the Nurse-Delivery Diabetic Smoking Intervention Project *(129)* and the Physician-Delivered Smoking Intervention Project (smoking cessation) *(130)*. The latter found a statistically significant improvement in smoking quitting rates associated with 5-9 minutes of intervention.

It is clear from these studies that good adherence requires a continuous and dynamic process. Practitioners (and other health enablers) often assume that the patient is, or should be, motivated to follow a best-practice protocol. However, recent research in the behavioural sciences reveals this to be an erroneous assumption. The patient population can be segmented according to level-of-readiness to follow health recommendations *(131-133)*. The lack of a match between the patient's readiness and the practitioner's attempts at intervention means that treatments are frequently prescribed to patients who are not ready to follow them.

Although adherence interventions directed towards patients have typically focused on providing education to increase knowledge, the available evidence shows that knowledge alone is not enough. Roter et al. published a meta-analysis of adherence-enhancing interventions which concluded that "no single strategy or programmatic focus showed any clear advantage compared with another and that comprehensive interventions combining cognitive, behavioural, and affective [motivational] components were more effective than single-focus interventions" *(134)*. Information alone is not enough for creating or maintaining good adherence habits. First-line interventions to optimize adherence must go beyond the provision of advice and prescriptions. If either the perceived value of adhering, or confidence, is low, the likelihood of adherence will also be low.

Health care providers can learn to assess the potential for nonadherence, and to detect nonadherence itself. They can then use this information to implement brief interventions to encourage and support progress towards adherence. A conceptual framework that explains how patients progress to adherence will help practitioners to tailor their interventions to the needs of the patient.

More research is required in this area. New, sustainable initiatives targeting providers could aim to impart knowledge about the broad determinants of the problem and of specific strategies for addressing them, in ways that can be systematically implemented in practice.

The evidence reviewed for this report suggests that it would be helpful to create a shift in provider perspective that supports tailoring of interventions to the needs of individual patients, and to teach specific strategies to address those needs. One of the problems in this area has been the relatively low levels of knowledge transfer. The results of effective studies have not been widely implemented in practice. This highlights the need for educational programmes that go beyond describing the problem, and that convey solutions to everyday problems in practice.

WHO and many ministries of health are working to improve the provision of health care, but a lot of work still needs to be done on the development of appropriate care for chronic conditions.

C. Therapy-related interventions

In studies of therapy-related interventions, the main barriers to adherence were found to be the dose frequency and the incidence of side-effects. Pharmaceutical companies in partnership with health professionals and researchers are addressing these problems. The health system has an important role in minimizing the impact of side-effects on patients.

D. Condition-related interventions

Disease-specific demands, symptoms and impairments are the targets of health professionals. These actors could provide optimal care by identifying and treating these problems, as well as identifying and treating co-morbidities that affect adherence. For example, because of the high prevalence of depression and its considerable effect on adherence, adherence counselling interventions should include systematic screening for depression.

E. Patient-related interventions

The major barriers to adherence described in the literature reviewed for this report were lack of information and skills as they pertain to self-management, difficulty with motivation and self-efficacy, and lack of support for behavioural changes.

These barriers were especially significant for those interventions intended to change habits and/or lifestyles, but also affected medication use. WHO acknowledges the necessity of supporting patients' efforts at self-management. Many researchers are working to develop or improve and disseminate self-management guidelines.

Global changes in the delivery of health services and shrinking health care budgets have also contributed to a need for patients to become more able to manage their own treatments. The development of self-management interventions aimed at improving motivation and adherence, based on the best available evidence, will help to fill this need. This work can support efforts by patients' organizations to engage and support their members.

Increasing the impact of interventions aimed at patient-related factors is essential. There is a wealth of data from the behavioural sciences demonstrating the efficacy of specific strategies. Although it is well known that education alone is a weak intervention, many interventions continue to rely on patient education to encourage patients to adhere to their treatment. Patients need to be informed, motivated and skilled in the use of cognitive and behavioural self-regulation strategies if they are to cope effectively with the treatment-related demands imposed by their illness. For the effective provision of care for chronic conditions it is necessary to activate the patient and the community who support him or her *(135)*.

A continuous effort is being made to improve the provision of information to patients, but motivation, which drives sustainable good adherence, is one of the most difficult elements for the health care system to provide in the long term. Although health professionals have an important role in promoting optimism, providing enthusiasm, and encouraging maintenance of health behaviours among their patients *(136)*, the health systems and health care teams experience difficulties in constantly motivating patients with chronic conditions. These difficulties have led to an increased interest during the past decade, in the role of community-based educational and/or self-management programmes aimed at the creation and maintenance of healthy habits, including adherence to health recommendations.

3. References

1. Albaz RS. Factors affecting patient compliance in Saudi Arabia. *Journal of Social Sciences*, 1997, 25:5-8.

2. Morgan M. Managing hypertension: belief and responses to medication among cultural groups. *Sociology of Health & Illness*, 1988, 10:561-578.

3. Belgrave LL. Race and compliance with hypertension treatment. Sociological Abstracts no. 45. *American Sociological Association*, 1997.

4. Erwin J. Treatment issues for HIV+ Africans in London. *Social Science & Medicine*, 1999, 49: 1519-1528.

5. Siegel K. Racial differences in attitudes toward protease inhibitors among older HIV-infected men. *AIDS Care*, 2000, 12,423-434.

6. Schwalm DU. Effects of war on compliance. *Curare*, 1997, 20:101-107.

7. Burkhart P, Dunbar-Jacob J. Adherence research in the pediatric and adolescent populations: A decade in review. In: Hayman L, Mahom M, Turner R, eds. *Chronic illness in children: An evidence-based approach*. New York, Springer, 2002:199-229.

8. Fotheringham MSM. Adherence to recommended medical regimens in childhood and adolescence. *Journal of Pediatrics and Child Health*, 1995, 31:72-78.

9. Burkhart PV, Dunbar-Jacob JM, Rohay JM. Accuracy of children's self-reported adherence to treatment. *Journal of Nursing Scholarship*, 2001, 33:27-32.

10. Rapoff M. *Adherence to pediatric medical regimens*. New York, Plenum, 1999.

11. Coutts JA, Gibson NA, Paton JY. Measuring compliance with inhaled medication in asthma. *Archives of Disease in Childhood*, 1992, 67:332-333.

12. Courteheuse C. [Reciprocal responsibility: the case with asthma.] [French] *Revue Medicale de la Suisse Romande*, 1992, 112:235-238.

13. Eney RD, Goldstein EO. Compliance of chronic asthmatics with oral administration of theophylline as measured by serum and salivary levels. *Pediatrics*, 1976, 57:513-517.

14. Jernigan JA. Update on drugs and the elderly. *American Family Physician*, 1984, 29:238-247.

15. Johnson MJ, Williams M, Marshall ES. Adherent and nonadherent medication-taking in elderly hypertensive patients. *Clinical Nursing Research*, 1999, 8:318-335.

16. Pinzone HA et al. Prediction of asthma episodes in children using peak expiratory flow rates, medication compliance, and exercise data. *Annals of Allergy*, 1991, 67:481-486.

17. Rose LE et al. The contexts of adherence for African Americans with high blood pressure. *Journal of Advanced Nursing*, 2000, 32:587-594.

18. Ciechanowski, PS, Katon, WJ, and Russo, JE Depression and diabetes: impact of depressives symptoms on adherence, function, and costs. Archives of Internal Medicine, 2000, 27:3278-3285.

19. Horne R. Patients' beliefs about treatment: the hidden determinant of treatment outcome? *Journal of Psychosomatic Research*, 1999, 47:491-495.

20. Horne R, Hankins M, Jenkins R. The satisfaction with information about medicines scale (SIMS): A new measurement tool for audit and research. *Quality in Health Care*, 2001, 10:135-140.

21. Horne R, Weinman J. Patients' beliefs about prescribed medicines and their role in adherence to treatment in chronic physical illness. *Journal of Psychosomatic Research*, 1999, 47:555-567.

22. Gupta K, Horne R. The influence of health beliefs on the presentation and consultation outcome in patients with chemical sensitivities. *Journal of Psychosomatic Research*, 2001, 50:131-137.

23. Petrie KJ, Wessely S. Modern worries, new technology, and medicine. *British Medical Journal*, 2002, 324:690-691.

24. Miller W, Rollnick S. *Motivational interviewing*. New York, Guilford Press, 1999.

25. Gut-Gobert C et al. [Current trends in asthma management.] [French] *Presse Medicale*, 2000, 29:761-765.

26. Weinstein AG. Asthma treatment and noncompliance. *Delaware Medical Journal*, 2000, 72:209-213.

27. Gibson PG. Self-management education and regular practitioner review for adults with asthma. *Cochrane Database of Systematic Reviews*, 2001, Issue 1.

28. Tuldra A et al. Prospective randomized two-arm controlled study to determine the efficacy of a specific intervention to improve long-term adherence to highly active antiretroviral therapy. *Journal of Acquired Immune Deficiency Syndromes*, 2000, 25:221-228.

29. Sebastian MS, Bothamley GH. Tuberculosis preventive therapy: perspective from a multi-ethnic community. *Respiratory Medicine*, 2000, 94:648-653.

30. Walsh S, Hagan T, Gamsu D. Rescuer and rescued: applying a cognitive analytic perspective to explore the 'mis-management' of asthma. *British Journal of Medical Psychology*, 2000, 73:151-168.

31. Renders C, Valk G, Griffin S. Interventions to improve the management of diabetes mellitus in primary care, outpatient and community settings. *Cochrane Database of Systematic Reviews*, 2001, Issue 1.

32. Haisch J, Remmele W. [Effectiveness and efficiency of ambulatory diabetes education programmes. A comparison of specialty practice and general practice.] [German] *Deutsche Medizinische Wochenschrift*, 2000, 125:171-176.

33. Shiffman S et al. The efficacy of computer-tailored smoking cessation material as a supplement to nicotine polacrilex gum therapy. *Archives of Internal Medicine*, 2000, 160:1675-1681.

34. Marquez CE et al. [Treatment compliance in arterial hypertension. A 2-year intervention trial through health education.] [Spanish] *Atencion Primaria*, 2000, 26:5-10.

35. Lowe CJ et al. Effects of a medicine review and education programme for older people in general practice. *British Journal of Clinical Pharmacology*, 2000, 50:172-175.

36. Sloss EM et al. Selecting target conditions for quality of care improvement in vulnerable older adults. *Journal of the American Geriatrics Society*, 2000, 48:363-369.

37. Richardson R et al. Learning curve. Hypertension: catch them when they're older. *Nursing Times*, 2000, 96:42-43.

38. Kokubu F et al. [Hospitalization reduction by an asthma tele-medicine system japanese]. *Arerugi – Japanese Journal of Allergology*, 2000, 49:19-31.

39. Serrier P et al. [Evaluation of an educational program on asthma for pharmacists.] [French] *Presse Medicale*, 2000, 29:1987-1991.

40. Strobach D et al. [Patient medication counselling – patient counselling about discharge medication]. [German] *Medizinische Klinik*, 2000, 95:548-551.

41. Piette JD et al. Do automated calls with nurse follow-up improve self-care and glycemic control among vulnerable patients with diabetes? *American Journal of Medicine*, 2000, 108:20-27.

42. Rice VH. Nursing interventions for smoking cessation. *Cochrane Database of Systematic Reviews*, 2001, Issue 1, 2001.

42. Banerjee A et al. Evaluation of a unified treatment regimen for all new cases of tuberculosis using guardian-based supervision. *International Journal of Tuberculosis & Lung Disease*, 2000, 4:333-339.

44. Rohland BM, Rohrer JE, Richards CC. The long-term effect of outpatient commitment on service use. *Administration & Policy in Mental Health*, 2000, 27:383-394.

45. Nisbeth O, Klausen K, Andersen LB. Effectiveness of counselling over 1 year on changes in lifestyle and coronary heart disease risk factors. *Patient Education & Counseling*, 2000, 40:121-31.

46. Nichols-English G, Poirier S. Optimizing adherence to pharmaceutical care plans. *Journal of the American Pharmaceutical Association*, 2000, 40:475-485.

47. Siegel K, Karus D, Schrimshaw EW. Racial differences in attitudes toward protease inhibitors among older HIV-infected men. *AIDS* Care, 2000, 12:423-434.

48. James M et al. Cost effectiveness analysis of screening for sight threatening diabetic eye disease. *British Medical Journal,* 2000, 320:1627-1631 [erratum published in *British Medical Journal,* 2000, 321:424].

49. McCulloch D. Managing diabetes for improved health and economic outcomes. *American Journal of Managed Care,* 2000, 6 (Suppl):S1089-S1095.

50. Ostrop NJ, Hallett KA, Gill MJ. Long-term patient adherence to antiretroviral therapy. *Annals of Pharmacotherapy,* 2000, 34:703-709.

51. Tutty S, Simon G, Ludman E. Telephone counseling as an adjunct to antidepressant treatment in the primary care system. A pilot study. *Effective Clinical Practice,* 2000, 3:170-178.

52. Solomon LJ et al. Free nicotine patches plus proactive telephone peer support to help low-income women stop smoking. *Preventive Medicine,* 2000, 31:68-74.

53. Norris SL et al. Effectiveness of physician-based assessment and counseling for exercise in a staff model HMO. *Preventive Medicine,* 2000, 30:513-523.

54. Salmon-Ceron D et al. [Adherence to antiretroviral treatments with a protease inhibitor in HIV-infected patients.] [French] *Annales de Medecine Interne,* 2000, 151:297-302.

55. Muller C, Hagele R, Heinl KW. [Differentiation and modification of compliance with reference to topical corticoid medication in patients with bronchial asthma.] [German] *Pneumologie,* 1996, 50:257-259.

56. Woller W et al. Cortisone image and emotional support by key figures in patients with bronchial asthma. An empirical study. *Psychotherapy & Psychosomatics,* 1993, 59:190-196.

57. Wagner EH et al. Chronic care clinics for diabetes in primary care: A system-wide randomized trial. *Diabetes Care,* 2001, 24:695-700.

58. Risk factor changes and mortality results. Multiple Risk Factor Intervention Trial Research Group. 1982. *Journal of the American Medical Association,* 1997, 277:582-594.

59. Five-year findings of the hypertension detection and follow-up program. I. Reduction in mortality of persons with high blood pressure, including mild hypertension. Hypertension Detection and Follow-up Program Cooperative Group. 1979. *Journal of the American Medical Association,* 1997, 277:157-166.

60. DeBusk RF et al. A case-management system for coronary risk factor modification after acute myocardial infarction. *Annals of Internal Medicine,* 1994, 120:721-729.

61. Peters AL, Davidson MB, Ossorio RC. Management of patients with diabetes by nurses with support of subspecialists. *HMO Practice,* 1995, 9:8-13.

62. Garnett WR. Antiepileptic drug treatment: outcomes and adherence. *Pharmacotherapy,* 2000, 20:191S-199S.

63. Ruggieron L et al. Impact of social support and stress on compliance in women with gestational diabetes. *Diabetes Care,* 1990, 13:441-443.

64. Glasgow RE, McCaul KD, Schafer LC. Self care behaviors and glycemic control in Type 1 diabetes. *Journal of Chronic Diseases,* 1987, 40:399-412.

65. MacLean D, Lo R. The non-insulin-dependent diabetic: success and failure in compliance. *Australian Journal of Advanced Nursing,* 1998, 15:33-42.

66. Kyngas H. Predictors of good compliance in adolescents with epilepsy. *Seizure,* 2001, 10:549-553.

67. Kyngas H, Rissanen M. Support as a crucial predictor of good compliance of adolescents with a chronic disease. *Journal of Clinical Nursing,* 2001, 10:767-774.

68. Pendley JS et al. Peer and family support in children and adolescents with type 1 diabetes. *Journal of Pediatric Psychology,* 2002, 27:429-438.

69. Burroughs TE et al. Research on social support in adolescents with IDDM: a critical review. *Diabetes Educator,* 1997, 23:438-448.

70. Fitzgerald JT et al. Differences in the impact of dietary restrictions on African Americans and Caucasians with NIDDM. *Diabetes Educator,* 1997, 23:41-47.

71. Wang CY, Fenske MM. Self-care of adults with non-insulin-dependent diabetes mellitus: influence of family and friends. *Diabetes Educator,* 1996, 22:465-470.

72. La Greca AM et al. I get by with a little help from my family and friends: adolescents' support for diabetes care. *Journal of Pediatric Psychology,* 1995, 20:449-476.

73. Garay-Sevilla ME et al. Adherence to treatment and social support in patients with non-insulin dependent diabetes mellitus. *Journal of Diabetes & its Complications,* 1995, 9:81-86.

74. Belgrave FZ, Lewis DM. The role of social support in compliance and other health behaviors for African Americans with chronic illnesses. *Journal of Health & Social Policy,* 1994, 5:55-68.

75. Ruggiero L et al. Self-reported compliance with diabetes self-management during pregnancy. *International Journal of Psychiatry in Medicine,* 1993, 23:195-207.

76. Sherbourne CD et al. Antecedents of adherence to medical recommendations: results from the Medical Outcomes Study. *Journal of Behavioral Medicine,* 1992, 15:447-468.

77. Nagasawa M et al. Meta-analysis of correlates of diabetes patients' compliance with prescribed medications. *Diabetes Educator,* 1990, 16:192-200.

78. Ruggiero L et al. Impact of social support and stress on compliance in women with gestational diabetes. *Diabetes Care,* 1990, 13:441-443.

79. Fishman T. The 90-Second Intervention: a patient compliance mediated technique to improve and control hypertension. *Public Health Reports,* 1995, 110:173-178.

80. Stanton AL. Determinants of adherence to medical regimens by hypertensive patients. *Journal of Behavioral Medicine,* 1987, 10:377-394.

81. Kyngas H. Compliance with health regimens of adolescents with epilepsy. *Seizure,* 2000, 9:598-604.

82. Kyngas HA, Kroll T, Duffy ME. Compliance in adolescents with chronic diseases: a review. *Journal of Adolescent Health,* 2000, 26:379-388.

83. Cameron C. Patient compliance: recognition of factors involved and suggestions for promoting compliance with therapeutic regimens. *Journal of Advanced Nursing,* 1996, 24:244-250.

84. Schlenk EA, Hart LK. Relationship between health locus of control, health value, and social support and compliance of persons with diabetes mellitus. *Diabetes Care,* 1984, 7:566-574.

85. Levy RL. Social support and compliance: a selective review and critique of treatment integrity and outcome measurement. *Social Science & Medicine,* 1983, 17:1329-1338.

86. Doherty WJ et al. Effect of spouse support and health beliefs on medication adherence. *Journal of Family Practice,* 1983, 17:837-841.

87. Kyngas HA. Compliance of adolescents with asthma. *Nursing & Health Sciences,* 1999, 1:195-202.

88. Weishut DJ. [Coping with AIDS in a support group – an encounter with the health system.] [Hebrew] *Harefuah,* 1996, 130:521-523.

89. Demas PA et al. Maternal adherence to the zidovudine regimen for HIV-exposed infants to prevent HIV infection: a preliminary study. *Pediatrics,* 2002, 110:e35.

90. Spire B et al. Adherence to highly active antiretroviral therapies (HAART) in HIV-infected patients: from a predictive to a dynamic approach. *Social Science & Medicine,* 2002, 54:1481-1496.

91. Roberts KJ. Barriers to and facilitators of HIV-positive patients' adherence to antiretroviral treatment regimens. *AIDS Patient Care & STDs,* 2000, 14:155-168.

92. Catz SL et al. Patterns, correlates, and barriers to medication adherence among persons prescribed new treatments for HIV disease. *Health Psychology,* 2000, 19:124-133.

93. Katapodi MC et al. The influence of social support on breast cancer screening in a multicultural community sample. *Oncology Nursing Forum*, 2002, 29:845-852.

94. Abercrombie PD. Improving adherence to abnormal Pap smear follow-up. *Journal of Obstetric, Gynecologic, & Neonatal Nursing*, 2001, 30:80-88.

95. Crane LA. Social support and adherence behavior among women with abnormal Pap smears. *Journal of Cancer Education*, 1996, 11:164-173.

96. Owen N, Brown SL. Smokers unlikely to quit. *Journal of Behavioral Medicine*, 1991, 14:627-636.

97. Dilorio C, Faherty B, Manteuffel B. Cognitive-perceptual factors associated with antiepileptic medication compliance. *Research in Nursing & Health*, 1991, 14:329-338.

98. Orleans CT et al. Self-help quit smoking interventions: effects of self-help materials, social support instructions, and telephone counseling. *Journal of Consulting & Clinical Psychology*, 1991, 59:439-448.

99. Guimon J. The use of group programs to improve medication compliance in patients with chronic diseases. *Patient Education & Counseling*, 1995, 26:189-193.

100. Broadhead RS et al. Increasing drug users' adherence to HIV treatment: results of a peer-driven intervention feasibility study. *Social Science & Medicine*, 2002, 55:235-246.

101. Magura S et al. Adherence to medication regimens and participation in dual-focus self-help groups. *Psychiatric Services*, 2002, 53:310-316.

102. Hoch C, Gobel U, Janssen G. [Psychosocial support of patients with homozygous beta-thalassaemia.] [German] *Klinische Padiatrie*, 2000, 212:216-219.

103. Richards W et al. A self-help program for childhood asthma in a residential treatment center. *Clinical Pediatrics*, 1981, 20:453-457.

104. Weishut DJ. [Coping with AIDS in a support group – an encounter with the health system.] [Hebrew] *Harefuah*, 1996, 130:521-523.

105. Getahun H, Maher D. Contribution of 'TB clubs' to tuberculosis control in a rural district in Ethiopia. *International Journal of Tuberculosis & Lung Disease*, 2000, 4:174-178.

106. Garay-Sevilla ME et al. Adherence to treatment and social support in patients with non-insulin dependent diabetes mellitus. *Journal of Diabetes & its Complications*, 1995, 9:81-86.

107. Kulcar Z. Self-help, mutual aid and chronic patients' clubs in Croatia, Yugoslavia: discussion paper. *Journal of the Royal Society of Medicine*, 1991, 84:288-291.

108. Boza RA et al. Patient noncompliance and overcompliance. Behavior patterns underlying a patient's failure to 'follow doctor's orders'. *Postgraduate Medicine*, 1987, 81:163-170.

109. Lilja P. Recognizing the effect of social support on compliance to medical regimen in the elderly chronically ill. *Home Healthcare Nurse*, 1984, 2:17-22.

110. Koch T, Selim P, Kralik D. Enhancing lives through the development of a community-based participatory action research programme. *Journal of Clinical Nursing*, 2002, 11:109-117.

111. Dias JC. [Community participation and control of endemic diseases in Brazil: problems and possibilities.] [Portuguese] *Cadernos de Saude Publica*, 1998, 14 (Suppl) 2:19-37.

112. Asthana S, Oostvogels R. Community participation in HIV prevention: problems and prospects for community-based strategies among female sex workers in Madras. *Social Science & Medicine*, 1996, 43:133-148.

113. Loue S, Lloyd LS, Phoombour E. Organizing Asian Pacific Islanders in an urban community to reduce HIV risk: a case study. *AIDS Education & Prevention*, 1996, 8:381-393.

114. Freudenberg N. A new role for community organizations in the prevention and control of tuberculosis. *Journal of Community Health*, 1995, 20:15-28.

115. Bermejo A, Bekui A. Community participation in disease control. *Social Science & Medicine*, 1993, 36:1145-1150.

116. Kuehnert PL. Community health nursing and the AIDS pandemic: case report of one community's response. *Journal of Community Health Nursing*, 1991, 8:137-146.

117. Delaney C. Reducing recidivism: medication versus psychosocial rehabilitation. *Journal of Psychosocial Nursing & Mental Health Services*, 1998, 36:28-34.

118. Davies M et al. Evaluation of a hospital diabetes specialist nursing service: a randomized controlled trial. *Diabetic Medicine*, 2001, 18:301-307.

119. Akbar DH, Al Gamdi AA. Common causes of admission in diabetics. *Saudi Medical Journal*, 2000, 21:539-542.

120. Gray A et al. Cost effectiveness of an intensive blood glucose control policy in patients with type 2 diabetes: economic analysis alongside randomised controlled trial (UKPDS 41). United Kingdom Prospective Diabetes Study Group. *British Medical Journal*, 2000, 320:1373-1378.

121. Steffens B. Cost-effective management of type 2 diabetes: providing quality care in a cost-constrained environment. *American Journal of Managed Care*, 2000, 6:S697-S703.

122. Feuerstein M et al. Compliance – a joint effort of the patient and his doctor. *Epilepsy Research*, 1988, (Suppl) 1:51-56.

123. Carter IR, Nash C, Ridgway A. On any Saturday – a practical model for diabetes education. *Journal of the National Medical Association*, 2002, 94:67-72.

124. O'Grady A et al. Effectiveness of changes in the delivery of diabetes care in a rural community. *Australian Journal of Rural Health*, 2001, 9:74-78.

125. Ockene J. Strategies to increase adherence to treatment. In: Burke LE, Ockene IS, eds. *Compliance in health care and research*. Armonk, New York, Futura, 2001:43-55.

126. Ockene IS et al. Effect of physician-delivered nutrition counseling training and an office-support program on saturated fat intake, weight, and serum lipid measurements in a hyperlipidemic population: Worcester Area Trial for Counseling in Hyperlipidemia (WATCH). *Archives of Internal Medicine*, 1999, 159:725-731.

127. Ockene IS et al. Effect of training and a structured office practice on physician-delivered nutrition counseling: the Worcester-Area Trial for Counseling in Hyperlipidemia (WATCH). *American Journal of Preventive Medicine*, 1996, 12:252-258.

128. Ockene JK et al. Provider training for patient-centered alcohol counseling in a primary care setting. *Archives of Internal Medicine*, 1997, 157:2334-2341.

129. Canga N et al. Intervention study for smoking cessation in diabetic patients: a randomized controlled trial in both clinical and primary care settings. *Diabetes Care*, 2000, 23:1455-1460.

130. Ockene JK et al. The Physician-Delivered Smoking Intervention Project: factors that determine how much the physician intervenes with smokers. *Journal of General Internal Medicine*, 1994, 9:379-384.

131. Prochaska JO, DiClemente CC. Stages of change in the modification of problem behaviors. *Progress In Behavior Modification*, 1992, 28:183-218.

132. Prochaska JO, DiClemente CC, Norcross JC. In search of how people change. Applications to addictive behaviors. *American Psychologist*, 1992, 47:1102-1114.

133. Prochaska JO, Redding C, Evers K. The Transtheoretical Model. In: Glanz K LF, Rimer BK, eds. *Health behavior and health education: theory, research, and practice*. San Francisco, Jossey-Bass, 1997.

134. Roter DL et al. Effectiveness of interventions to improve patient compliance: a meta-analysis. *Medical Care*, 1998, 36:1138-1161.

135. McCann K. AIDS in the nineties: from science to policy. Care in the community and by the community. *AIDS Care*, 1990, 2:421-424.

139. Lo R. Correlates of expected success at adherence to health regimen of people with IDDM. *Journal of Advanced Nursing*, 1999, 30:418-424.

CHAPTER VI

How can improved adherence be translated into health and economic benefits?

1. Diabetes   39

2. Hypertension   40

3. Asthma   41

4. References   43

Many studies have reported institutional changes in costs following changes in adherence rates. Some studies have shown that initial investments in interventions to enhance adherence are fully recovered within a few years and recurrent costs are fully covered by savings. These "cost-saving interventions" are firmly linked to the prevention of disease relapses, crises and/or complications.

From a societal point of view, most interventions aimed at enhancing adherence have been shown to result in cost-savings, due to the improvement in patients' quality of life, indirect costs avoided and increased productivity. Such savings are not reflected in economic studies with an institutional perspective.

1. Diabetes

Diabetes is a typical chronic disease that demonstrates the need for integrated and multifaceted approaches to achieve good control. Almost any intervention designed to improve metabolic control in diabetic patients, or to delay the onset of complications does so by supporting patients in developing appropriate self-management behaviours. Interventions to enhance adherence in patients with diabetes benefit from a comprehensive and multifactorial approach to providing better control of the disease.

For example, a systematic review by Renders and colleagues (1), of interventions to improve the management of diabetes mellitus in primary care, conducted in outpatient and community settings, analysed 41 heterogeneous studies of multifaceted intervention strategies. Some of these studies were targeted at health professionals, others at the organization of care, but most of them targeted both. In 15 studies, patient education was added to the professional and organizational interventions. The reviewers concluded that multifaceted professional interventions can enhance the performance of health professionals in managing diabetic patients. Organizational interventions that improve regular prompted recall and review of patients can also improve diabetes management. In addition, the inclusion of patient-oriented interventions can lead to improved health outcomes for the patients. Nurses can play an important role in patient-oriented interventions, through patient education and facilitating adherence to treatment.

A recent meta-analysis has shown that education about self-management improves glycaemic levels at immediate follow-up, and increased contact time increases this effect. However, the benefit declines 1-3 months after the intervention ceases, suggesting that learned behaviours change over time (2), and that some additional interventions are needed for maintaining them.

In a study in Switzerland, Gozzoli et al. estimated the impact of several alternative interventions for improving the control of complications of diabetes (3). They concluded that the implementation of multifactorial interventions, including improved control of cardiovascular risk factors, combined with early diagnosis and treatment of complications of diabetes, could save both costs and lives.

Nurse case-management (4-6), disease management (7,8) and population-based management (9) have all resulted in better adherence to recommended standards of care, sometimes with impressive clinical and economic outcomes. Moreover, the Chronic Care Model (CCM), a systematic approach to improving the quality of care for persons with chronic diseases, has shown promising results (10,11).

Positive results have also been reported from the United States by the Diabetes Roadmap of Group Health Cooperative of Puget Sound (GHC), an HMO serving about 400 000 people in western Washington state, which uses the strategy of population-based management of care to improve care and outcomes for its 13 000 diabetic patients (9). Population-based care uses guidelines, and epidemiological data and techniques to plan, organize, deliver and monitor care in specific clinical sub-populations such as patients with diabetes. This support programme is aimed at helping primary care teams to improve their ability to deliver population-based diabetes care. Based on an integrated CCM, the programme includes an on-line registry of diabetic patients, evidence-based guidelines for routine diabetes care, improved support for patient self-management and practice re-design including group visits. Also, members of a decentralized diabetes education team see patients jointly. Preliminary outcomes show that retinal screening rates have increased from 56% to 70%, renal screening rates from 18% to 68%, foot examination rates from 18% to 82% and patients being tested for glycosylated haemoglobin from 72% to 92%. The cost of care for the entire population of diabetic patients has decreased by 11%.

Most studies that reported cost-savings used a systematic approach to disease management (8,12). More research is needed to assess the cost-effectiveness of interventions aimed at improving adherence rates (13).

2. Hypertension

In patients with hypertension, adherence to treatment recommendations has a major impact on health outcomes and the costs of care. Some of the better recognized determinants of adherence to antihypertensive therapy are related to drug treatment such as drug tolerability and regimen complexity. Thus, reduced side-effects, fewer daily doses of antihypertensives, monotherapies and fewer changes in antihypertensive medications have all been associated with better adherence (14-16).

In a landmark study conducted by Morisky et al. (17), patients were assigned to three adherence-promoting interventions: physician counselling, family support for monitoring pill taking, group sessions with a social worker or to a control group. The 5-year analysis showed a continuing positive effect on appointment-keeping, weight control and blood-pressure control in the intervention groups. The all-cause life table mortality rate was 57.3% less for the intervention group than for the control group and the hypertension-related mortality rate was 53.2% less. The results from this longitudinal study provide evidence to support the use of adherence-enhancing interventions in patients with hypertension.

Another study used an educational programme to emphasize the importance of proper treatment. In the intervention groups, the systolic and diastolic blood pressure of both men and women decreased despite the 5-year increase in age; moreover, hypertension was better controlled after the programme (24.8% baseline; 39.7% at the end of the study), and substantial decreases in deaths due to cardiovascular disease were reported *(18)*.

Another intervention that has shown promising results is home recording of blood pressure. For example, one study showed that in patients who initially showed poor compliance, there was an increase in compliance from 0 to 70% after self-measuring of blood pressure was introduced. The authors concluded that self-recording of blood pressure may be of value in patients with unsatisfactory blood-pressure responses in whom poor compliance is suspected *(19)*.

Other studies have shown that care of patients by specially trained nurses resulted in increased adherence *(20-22)* and compelling evidence for the efficacy of brief, nurse-administered behavioural counselling comes from a study of 883 patients of physicians in Great Britain *(21)*. Another study also showed that adherence to hypertension therapy would benefit from intervention by nurses *(22)*.

Finally, Bogden et al. *(23)* tested the effect of physicians and pharmacists working together as a team on patients with uncontrolled hypertension. In a randomized, controlled trial, 95 adult patients with hypertension (more than twice as many patients in the intervention group as in the control group) attained blood pressure control.

3. Asthma

A systematic review by the Cochrane Airways Group has shown that training patients in asthma self-management which involves self-monitoring of either peak expiratory flow or symptoms, coupled with regular medical review and a written action plan appeared to improve health outcomes for adults with asthma. In addition, self-management education reduced hospitalizations, visits by the doctor, unscheduled visits to the doctor, days off work or school and nocturnal asthma. Finally, training programmes that enabled people to adjust their medication using a written action plan appeared to be more effective than other forms of asthma self-management and significant improvements in lung function were achieved *(24)*.

The Cochrane Airways Group has also shown that non-comprehensive approaches such as the use of limited education about asthma (information only) do not appear to improve health outcomes in adults with asthma although perceived symptoms may improve *(24)*.

Therefore, patient education and self-management should be integral components of any plan for long-term control of asthma. In particular, economic appraisals of asthma self-management programmes have shown them to be cost-effective both in terms of direct costs (mainly averted hospitalizations and reduced emergency department use) and in terms of indirect costs (e.g. productivity losses and missed school days). The cost-benefit ratios are between 1:2.5 and 1:7. Ratios are even better in programmes directed at high-risk groups and patients with severe asthma *(25-27)*. Some examples of studies that reported net cost-savings are described below.

The Open Airways programme of six 1-hour monthly sessions instructed low-income parents of 310 urban children with asthma in the management steps to be taken both by the children and their parents. The programme found that 44% of the parents lacked confidence in their ability to manage asthma attacks, believing they should take their children to the hospital emergency department for all episodes, whether mild or severe. Compared to a control group, participation in the Open Airways programme reduced emergency department visits and hospitalizations for asthma among those who had been hospitalized during the previous year by half, resulting in savings of US 11.22 for every dollar spent *(28)*.

An Italian study evaluated two structured educational programmes on asthma. The study found that the savings per patient in terms of reduced morbidity were US 1894.70 (for the intensive programme

(IP)) and US 1697.80 (for the brief programme (BP)). The net benefit was US 1181.50 for IP and US 1028.00 for BP and the cost-benefit ratio per dollar spent was 1:2.6 for IP and 1:2.5 for BP (29).

In a programme at Henry Ford Hospital in Detroit, Michigan, in 1986-1987 involving three, 1-hour, education sessions in small groups, a registered nurse taught patients about the importance of medication adherence, methods to control and prevent asthma attacks, relaxation exercises and smoking cessation. For just US 85 per person in annual programme costs, this intervention reduced the cost of emergency department visits by US 623 per person during the following year. The programme also reduced the number of days on which the activity of participants was limited because of asthma by 35% compared to a control group (30).

In Germany a structured intervention programme produced net benefits of DM 12 850 (in 1991 DM) per patient within 3 years. Within the health care sector, the net benefits were DM 5 900. Within 3 years, the paying bodies saved DM 2.70, and society as a whole saved DM 5.00 on each DM spent on the programme (cost-saving ratios 1:2.7 and 1:5). The authors concluded that the intervention produced net monetary benefits. This result was stable even when tested with different outcome measures. Such a programme is therefore worthwhile, not only for its demonstrated medical benefits, but also for its economic savings (31).

In a study in the United States, adult patients with asthma learned self-management skills in seven 90-minute, group sessions at Ohio University in Athens, Ohio. Participants were asked to keep a weekly record of peak flow rates and of any attacks they experienced. They also kept a workbook to record the information that was later used to calculate costs and benefits. At a programme cost of US 208 per patient, annual asthma-related costs for each patient were reduced by an average of nearly US 500 in the year following the programme, primarily from reductions in hospitalizations and work absences. The researchers have also adapted an individualized intervention for use in doctors' surgeries (32). The subsequent economic evaluation of this study showed that the programme was beneficial, reducing the cost of asthma to each patient by US 475.29. The benefit came primarily from reductions in hospital admissions (reduced from US 18 488 to US 1538) and income lost as a result of asthma (reduced from US 11 593 to US 4 589). The asthma self-management programme cost US 208.33 per patient. A comparison of the costs of the programme with the benefits produced a 1:2.28 cost-benefit ratio, demonstrating that the programme more than paid for itself (33).

The Harvard Community Health Plan, a large staff-model HMO, reduced the annual rate of paediatric emergency-department admissions related to asthma by 79% and hospital admissions by 86% using a single outreach nurse for 8 hours per week. In addition to instructing patients in asthma management, medications, triggers, and the use of inhalers and peak-flow meters, the nurse maintained regular telephone contact with the families to ensure compliance with individualized treatment plans. Patients participated for between 6 months and 2 years. At a cost of just US 11 115 per year, this intervention saved approximately US 87 000 in 1993 dollars (34).

In the Wee Wheezers programme, four small-group sessions of about 2 hours each were conducted to instruct parents of children under the age of 7 years how to help their children manage asthma attacks, communicate with health professionals, and promote the psychosocial well-being of the family unit. The last two sessions included 45 minutes of direct instruction for children aged 4-6 years. On average, the children reported 0.9 fewer sick days and 5.8 more symptom-free days, and their parents reported 4.4 more nights of uninterrupted sleep during the month preceding the follow-up questionnaire. The programme cost approximately US 26 per child (35).

To sum up, best practices in asthma control and in enhancement of adherence must include and reinforce the links between education and self-management. Not surprisingly, there is high quality evidence to support the efficacy and cost-effectiveness of guided self-management plans. Furthermore, most studies have reported net cost-savings.

4. References

1. Renders C, Valk G, Griffin S. Interventions to improve the management of diabetes mellitus in primary care, outpatient and community settings. *Cochrane Database of Systematic Reviews*, 2001.

2. Norris SLL et al. Self-management education for adults with type 2 diabetes: a meta-analysis of the effect on glycemic control. *Diabetes Care*, 2002, 25:1159-1171.

3. Gozzoli V et al. Economic and clinical impact of alternative disease management strategies for secondary prevention in type 2 diabetes in the Swiss setting. *Swiss Medical Weekly*, 2001, 131:303-310.

4. Aubert RE et al. Nurse case management to improve glycemic control in diabetic patients in a health maintenance organization. A randomized, controlled trial. *Annals of Internal Medicine*, 1998, 129:605-612.

5. Piette JD et al. Do automated calls with nurse follow-up improve self-care and glycemic control among vulnerable patients with diabetes? *American Journal of Medicine*, 2000, 108:20-27.

6. Weinberger M et al. A nurse-coordinated intervention for primary care patients with non-insulin-dependent diabetes mellitus: impact on glycemic control and health-related quality of life. *Journal of General Internal Medicine*, 1995, 10:59-66.

7. McCulloch DK et al. Improvement in diabetes care using an integrated population-based approach in a primary care setting. *Disease Management*, 2000, 3:75-82.

8. Sadur CN et al. Diabetes management in a health maintenance organization. Efficacy of care management using cluster visits. *Diabetes Care*, 1999, 22:2011-2017.

9. McCulloch DK et al. A population-based approach to diabetes management in a primary care setting: Early results and lessons learned. *Effective Clinical Practice*, 1998, 1:12-22.

10. Bodenheimer T, Wagner EH, Grumbach K. Improving primary care for patients with chronic illness: the chronic care model, Part 2. *Journal of the American Medical Association*, 2002, 288:1909-1914.

11. Bodenheimer T, Wagner EH, Grumbach K. Improving primary care for patients with chronic illness. *Journal of the American Medical Association*, 2002, 288:1775-1779.

12. Wagner EH et al. Effect of improved glycemic control on health care costs and utilization. *Journal of the American Medical Association*, 2001, 285:182-189.

13. Newell SA, Bowman JA, Cockburn JD. Can compliance with nonpharmacologic treatments for cardiovascular disease be improved?. *American Journal of Preventive Medicine*, 2000, 18:253-261.

14. Monane M et al. The effects of initial drug choice and comorbidity on antihypertensive therapy compliance. Results from a population-based study in the elderly. *American Journal of Hypertension*, 1997, 10:697-704.

15. Bloom BS. Continuation of initial antihypertensive medication after 1 year of therapy. *Clinical Therapeutics*, 1998, 20:671-681.

16. Hasford JM. A population-based European cohort study of persistence in newly diagnosed hypertensive patients. *Journal of Human Hypertension*, 2002, 16:569-575.

17. Morisky DE et al. Five-year blood pressure control and mortality following health education for hypertensive patients. *American Journal of Public Health*, 1983, 73:153-162

18. Kotchen JM et al. Impact of a rural high blood pressure control program on hypertension control and cardiovascular disease mortality. *Journal of the American Medical Association*, 1986, 255:2177-2182.

19. Edmonds D et al. Does self-measurement of blood pressure improve patient compliance in hypertension? *Journal of Hypertension*, 1985, (Suppl) 3:S31-S34.

20. Stason WB et al. Effectiveness and costs of veterans affairs hypertension clinics. *Medical Care*, 1994, 32:1197-1215.

21. Steptoe A et al. Behavioural counselling in general practice for the promotion of healthy behaviour among adults at increased risk of coronary heart disease: randomised trial. *British Medical Journal*, 1999, 319:943-947.

22. Richardson R et al. Learning curve. Hypertension: catch them when they're older. *Nursing Times*, 2000, 96:42-43.

23. Bogden PE et al. Comparing standard care with a physician and pharmacist team approach for uncontrolled hypertension. *Journal of General Internal Medicine*, 1998, 13:740-745.

24. Gibson PG et al. Limited (information only) patient education programs for adults with asthma. *Cochrane Database of Systematic Reviews*, 2002.

25. Taggart VS et al. You can control asthma: evaluation of an asthma education program for hospitalized inner-city children. *Patient Education & Counseling*, 1991, 17:35-47.

26. Sommaruga M et al. The effects of a cognitive behavioural intervention in asthmatic patients. *Monaldi Archives for Chest Disease*, 1995, 50:398-402.

27. Liljas B, Lahdensuo A. Is asthma self-management cost-effective? *Patient Education & Counseling*, 1997, 32:S97-S104.

28. Clark NM et al. The impact of health education on frequency and cost of health care use by low income children with asthma. *Journal of Allergy & Clinical Immunology*, 1986, 78:108-115.

29. Neri M et al. Economic analysis of two structured treatment and teaching programs on asthma. *Allergy*, 1996, 51:313-319.

30. Bolton MB et al. The cost and effectiveness of an education program for adults who have asthma. *Journal of General Internal Medicine*, 1991, 6:401-407.

31. Trautner C, Richter B, Berger M. Cost-effectiveness of a structured treatment and teaching programme on asthma. *European Respiratory Journal*, 1993, 6:1485-1491.

32. Kotses H et al. A self-management program for adult asthma. Part I: Development and evaluation. *Journal of Allergy & Clinical Immunology*, 1995, 95:529-540.

33. Taitel MS et al. A self-management program for adult asthma. Part II: Cost-benefit analysis. *Journal of Allergy & Clinical Immunology*, 1995, 95:672-676.

34. Greineder DK, Loane KC, Parks P. Reduction in resource utilization by an asthma outreach program. *Archives of Pediatrics & Adolescent Medicine*, 1995, 149:415-420.

35. Wilson SR et al. Education of parents of infants and very young children with asthma: a developmental evaluation of the Wee Wheezers program. *Journal of Asthma*, 1996, 33:239-254 [erratum published in *Journal of Asthma*, 1997, 34:261].

Section III

Disease-Specific Reviews

CHAPTER VII

Asthma

1. Defining nonadherence to asthma therapy 47
2. Rates of adherence to inhaled corticosteroids and other drugs for the prevention of asthma 48
3. Forms of nonadherence 50
4. Factors associated with adherence to asthma treatment 51
5. Adherence in special populations 52
6. Interventions to improve adherence to asthma therapy 53
7. Discussion 56
8. Conclusions 56
9. References 57

Asthma is a chronic, inflammatory disease of the airways that has dramatically increased in incidence over the past 15 years in both developed and developing countries. The global burden of asthma is considerable. Its effects include reduced quality of life, lost productivity, missed school days, increased health care costs, the risk of hospitalization and even death (1).

Although effective treatments that have been shown to dramatically reduce asthma morbidity are available, they are effective only when properly used by patients. Because human behaviour is the necessary interface between good therapies and therapeutic effectiveness, both clinical researchers and clinicians should understand the factors associated with patient adherence. This chapter discusses adherence issues in asthma, with a particular focus on adherence to preventive therapy, such as inhaled corticosteroids (ICSs). The prevalence of nonadherence to preventive therapy and patient factors associated with nonadherence are reviewed. Finally, we suggest some directions for future field research.

1. Defining nonadherence to asthma therapy

Assessing and understanding patient adherence in the management of asthma requires an appreciation of the diversity and complexity of adherence behaviour. Adherence to medication can be defined as the degree to which use of medication by the patient corresponds with the prescribed regimen.

Patients who regularly and consistently follow the prescribed regimen demonstrate adherent use. Adherence to medication is not a dichotomy, however, and patients can demonstrate a wide variety of patterns of medication use. The efficacy of asthma therapies can be modulated by these adherence patterns in several ways.

The most obvious form of nonadherence is chronic under-use, i.e. the patient consistently uses less medication than is prescribed. Chronic under-treatment of asthma may lead to poor control of symptoms and greater reliance on *pro re nata* (PRN) treatments for the relief of acute asthma symptoms.

Patients may also have an erratic pattern of adherence, in which medication use alternates between fully adherent (usually when symptomatic) and under-use or total non-use (when asymptomatic). Patients with erratic adherence may present for treatment of acute asthma although they apparently adhere completely to their prescribed regimen. Some patients relying solely on inhaled beta-agonists for symptom relief may be prone to over-use during acute bronchospasm. This may cause a patient to delay seeking care, or lead to complications associated with excessive use of beta-agonists (2).

Patients may exhibit a different pattern of adherence to each of the various medications prescribed for the management of their asthma. For example, a patient may under-use the prescribed prophylactic anti-inflammatory ("controller" or "preventer") medications while remaining appropriately adherent to the regular taking of the beta-agonist. Adherence to an asthma action plan that outlines how and when both controller and reliever medications should be taken and when to seek urgent care has been shown to be one of the most effective forms of asthma self-management (3). Finally, in order for medications delivered by metered dose inhaler (MDI) to control asthma optimally, the patient must adhere to the instructions for correct MDI use, or use an MDI spacer. Although MDI adherence has rarely been assessed in clinical or research settings, those studies that have examined patterns of MDI use by patients have suggested that poor technique is widespread (resulting both from inadequate instruction and patients' forgetfulness), and that improved MDI adherence can influence asthma management (4).

2. Rates of adherence to inhaled corticosteroids and other drugs for the prevention of asthma

Extensive research conducted in Australia, Canada, the United Kingdom, the United States and elsewhere has found that nonadherence with asthma therapy is widespread, and is a significant risk factor for asthma morbidity and mortality. Because of the limited sensitivity and specificity of self-reported measures of adherence (5), some of the most convincing studies have used objective measures, such as pharmacy databases, medication measurement and electronic medication monitors to assess adherence behaviour.

Conservative estimates indicate that almost half of the prescription medications dispensed yearly are not taken as prescribed (6). The real-life response to a clinician's prescription of preventive therapy will include a range of undesirable patient behaviours, including a failure to fill the initial prescription, erratic use or under-use of therapy, and premature discontinuation of therapy. Studies indicate that primary nonadherence (not filling initial prescriptions) ranges from 6–44% (7–12).

Even when patients fill prescriptions for asthma medications, studies of secondary nonadherence (rates of medication use) suggest that long-term rates of adherence to preventive therapies (e.g. controller or preventer medications) among adult patients are often poor. Spector et al. (13), one of the first investigative teams to use an electronic medication monitor to examine adherence to MDI-delivered medications, followed 19 adult asthmatic patients using an anti-inflammatory drug for 12 weeks. Patients adhered to the four-times-daily regimen for a mean of 47% of the days, with a range of 4.3% to 95%. Patients were also asked to maintain asthma diaries as part of this study, and a comparative analysis of electronic data and diary data found that subjects over-reported their appropriate use of medication in their diaries more than 50% of the time. In a similar study, Mawhinney et al. *(14)* studied adherence in adult asthmatic patients over a 3–4 week period. Adherence to the medication as prescribed was observed, on average, for 37% of the days, and under-use on more than 38% of the days monitored. Yeung et al. *(15)* used an electronic monitor to follow patients' use of inhaled corticosteroids over a period of 2–3 weeks. When patients were aware that they were being monitored, 60% of them were fully adherent, 20% were partially adherent (taking just 70% of the prescribed dose) and 20% were totally nonadherent. However, when patients were unaware of the monitoring, 6 out of 11 took between 30% and 51% of the prescribed doses.

Several studies have suggested that patients from low-income, ethnic-minority groups (primarily African American) in developed countries may have lower rates of adherence to asthma therapy. Celano et al. *(16)* examined adherence to anti-inflammatory medication delivered by MDI in low-income, urban, primarily African American children with asthma. Adherence to treatment administered by MDI was estimated by weighing canisters and calculating the ratio of the number of puffs used over the study period to the number of puffs prescribed. Estimated MDI adherence in this study was 44% for all participants and only12% of the children had rates above 75%. In a group of 80 asthma patients, treated under the Medicaid scheme, who were repeat users of the emergency department or overnight hospitalization, only 46% had been prescribed ICSs and only 43% had a written action plan *(17)*. Less than half of children with asthma living in Tennessee, receiving treatment funded by Medicaid, had a prescription for oral corticosteroids filled following an emergency department visit or a period of hospitalization for asthma *(18)*.

Low rates have also been reported from studies that used different measurement systems. Coutts, Gibson and Paton *(19)* in the United Kingdom published the first study to examine children's adherence to anti-inflammatory therapy using an electronic medication monitor that recorded and stored the date and time of each use. Children (aged 9–16 years) were monitored for 2–6 months and asked to maintain asthma diaries as well as to use the monitored inhaler. Despite symptomatic asthma, underuse of the inhaled corticosteroids was observed on 55% of the study days. In a second study from the United Kingdom, Gibson et al. *(20)* used electronic monitoring to evaluate the adherence of preschool children to inhaled prophylactic medication. Median adherence was 100% on 50% of study days, and an overall median of 77% of the prescribed doses were taken during the average 2-month monitoring period. It is important to realize that the poor adherence observed occurred in the children of a group of parents who had a clear understanding that adherence was being monitored, and who had been provided with careful explanations of the importance of adherence to prophylactic medications. The authors noted that this poor adherence might reflect persistent misunderstandings or concerns about the side-effects of the medications.

Jonasson et al. *(21)* reported from Sweden on adherence to inhaled budesonide administered with a breath-driven asthma inhaler in 163 children (aged 7–16 years) with mild asthma who were participating in a randomized, double-blind clinical trial. Mean daily diary-card adherence was 93% over the 12-week study, whereas inhaler dose-counting recorded only 77% adherence. Milgrom et al. *(22)*, in the United States used electronic monitors to study the adherence of school-aged children to inhaled corticosteroids. The participants were unaware of the function of the electronic device. Diary-card data showed that patients reported taking all doses on a median of 54% of study days and at least one dose on 97% of study days. However, electronic records of inhaled corticosteroid use showed a median of only 5% of study days on which all inhaled corticosteroid doses were taken and a median of 58% of days on which at least one dose was taken. The participants skipped all inhaled corticosteroid doses on a median of 42% of days and almost half of them missed their inhaled corticosteroids completely for more than a week at a time.

3. Forms of nonadherence

Understanding patient nonadherence to ICS therapy requires the recognition that there are different forms of nonadherent behaviour with diverse contributory factors. Careful clinical interviewing can reveal these problems and set the stage for identifying appropriate strategies for ameliorating them.

Erratic nonadherence. Perhaps the form of nonadherence that is most common and most acknowledged by patients and providers is doses missed because of forgetfulness, changing schedules or busy lifestyles. Patients who exhibit erratic nonadherence understand their prescribed regimen and would often like to adhere appropriately. However, they find it difficult to comply because the complexity of their lives interferes with adherence, or because they have not prioritized asthma management. Patients who have changing work schedules or chaotic lifestyles may have difficulty establishing the habit of a new medication regimen. For some patients Monday–Friday adherence presents no problem, but weekends or holidays disrupt medication routines. Strategies to improve erratic adherence centre on simplification of the regimen (e.g. once-a-day dosing), establishing new habits through linking (e.g. keeping the MDI next to the toothbrush) and cues and memory aids (e.g. pill organizers).

Unwitting nonadherence. Many patients may be inadvertently nonadherent to the prescribed therapy because they have failed to understand fully either the specifics of the regimen or the necessity for adherence. Studies have found that patients frequently forget instructions given to them by a physician during a clinic visit (23). MDIs, unlike pill bottles, do not usually have attached labels with dosing instructions. In asthma management it is common for patients to misunderstand the difference between PRN medication and daily medication. Or, they may interpret the prescription for "ICS twice every day" as meaning "ICS twice every day – when you have symptoms".

Patients may overuse their inhaled beta-agonist because they have never been given clear guidelines for when and how to adjust controller medications or seek medical assistance when asthma control worsens. The ubiquity of unwitting nonadherence is illustrated by the findings of a study by Donnelly et al. (24). The investigators interviewed 128 Australian parents of children with asthma about their knowledge about the disease, attitudes, beliefs and knowledge of asthma medications. Only 42% of parents had a basic understanding of the mode of action of beta-agonists, 12% for methylxanthines, 12% for cromoglycate and 0% for inhaled corticosteroids. Approximately half of the parents reported that sodium cromoglycate and inhaled corticosteroids were used to prevent asthma attacks, while 40–50% were unsure of the mode of usage. Most of the parents reported using antibiotics, antihistamines and decongestants in treating their child's asthma. The authors suggested that this poor parental understanding of asthma medications may result from inadequate communication between doctor and patient and this misunderstanding may contribute to the high prevalence of nonadherence to asthma treatments.

In a study in the Netherlands of adult patients with asthma and patients with chronic obstructive pulmonary disease, Dekker et al. (25) found that 20% of the patients using pulmonary medications admitted that they did not know the prescribed daily dosage. Twenty-nine per cent thought that their regular daily medication was actually to be used "short-term" or "as needed". Only 51% correctly perceived that their medications were to be taken regularly.

Intelligent nonadherence. Sometimes patients purposely alter, discontinue, or even fail to initiate ICS therapy. This deliberate nonadherence is called intelligent nonadherence, reflecting a reasoned choice, rather than necessarily a wise one (26). Patients who feel better may decide that they no longer need to take prescribed medications. Fear of perceived short- or long-term side-effects of ICS may cause some patients to reduce or discontinue dosing. Patients may abandon a therapy because bad taste, complexity or interference with daily life may convince them that the disadvantages of therapy outweigh the ben-efits. Patients may find that some variation of the prescribed therapy works better than the prescribed by the doctor. Given the well-documented underuse of ICS, the fact that ICS therapy is as successful in the management of asthma as it is, suggests that many patients manage quite well with altered or reduced doses. This deliberate nonadherence, like any other pattern of nonadherence does not necessarily result in worsening asthma. In every clinical practice there are patients who have knowingly altered their prescribed therapy, yet their health professional may never discover this modification. Regardless of the reason for nonadherence to medication, the necessary first step towards addressing the problem is identifying it through effective, open-ended communication between patient and provider. Only careful interviewing and active listening will equip the provider of asthma care with the information necessary to establish and reinforce adherence to appropriate medication. The time constraints placed on clinicians by managed care represent a serious barrier to carrying out this recommendation.

4. Factors associated with adherence to asthma treatment

Severity of asthma. Because of the significant burden of symptoms and the risk associated with severe asthma it would seem logical that patients with severe disease would have a greater incentive for, and hence a greater likelihood of adhering to prescribed therapy. Conversely, it could be argued that for some asthmatic patients more symptomatic disease is the consequence of inadequate adherence to treatment. For example, Milgrom et al. (22) demonstrated in a study of paediatric asthmatic patients that prednisone bursts were more common in those patients who were found by electronic monitoring to be the least adherent to therapy with inhaled anti-inflammatory medication.

It has also been suggested that the immediate awareness of active asthma symptoms should serve as a cue for improved adherence to medication. Mann et al. (27) tested this hypothesis by measuring the relationship between patient adherence to four-times-daily beclomethasone and periods of increased severity of asthma. Ten adult patients with moderate-to-severe asthma were monitored over a 9-week period using an electronic device attached to the MDI to measure adherence to inhaled medication, and peak flow monitoring to measure airflow obstruction. The authors concluded that compliance with inhaled corticosteroids was not modulated by asthma severity (as measured by peak expiratory flow), or by patient-reported symptoms.

Patients' beliefs about inhaled corticosteroids and asthma. The relationship between beliefs about asthma and adherence to preventive therapy was clearly illustrated in a study by Adams et al. (28). The investigators interviewed adult patients in Wales, United Kingdom, using qualitative interviewing strategies and identified three common self-perspectives among this group: asthma deniers/distancers, asthma accepters, and pragmatics. Each of these perspectives was associated with very different beliefs held by the patients about the nature of asthma and the use of preventive medication. This analysis suggested that an asthmatic patient's self-perception of his or her disease may influence his or her adherence to preventive asthma therapy.

Parents and patients who are concerned about using corticosteroids may under-dose or discontinue long-term use in an effort to be "steroid-sparing". Boulet (29) conducted a telephone survey of over 600 adult asthmatic patients in Canada to find out about patients' perceptions about the role of ICS in the treatment of asthma and the potential side-effects of this therapy. The investigators found that patients frequently had misperceptions about the role of ICSs, even if they had recently used them. For example, over 40% of patients believed that ICS opened up the airways to relieve bronchoconstriction, while less than a quarter of the patients reported that ICS reduced airway inflammation. This fundamental misunderstanding of the mechanism of ICS suggests that these patients may also have failed to understand the underlying chronic inflammation that characterizes asthma and the need for preventive therapy. Forty-six per cent of the patients interviewed indicated that they were reluctant to take ICS regularly and only 25% of patients reported that they had discussed their fears and concerns about ICS with their primary care provider. Misconceptions about the side-effects and long-term consequences of ICS use were also common. However, when the true side-effects of inhaled corticosteroids were explained, most of the patients reported being reassured. Boulet (29) concluded that information about the safety and usefulness of ICS does not seem to have reached many patients with asthma. This study also suggests that health care providers should discuss with patients any possible concerns about ICS therapy that might interfere with adherence.

In a similar study conducted in the United States, Chambers et al. (30) surveyed 694 largely symptomatic asthmatic patients aged 18–49 years who had been prescribed ICS in 1995–1996. The most notable finding in this survey was the low level of self-reported adherence with therapy. Sixty-two per cent of patients reported less than regular twice-daily ICS use. Thirty-six per cent of the patients endorsed the option "some days I use it at least twice, but on other days I don't use it at all", and 22% reported that they no longer used ICS. Four per cent of patients claimed that they had never used ICS. Those who were less than fully adherent were asked to state their reasons for not using ICS, and the reason most frequently cited was that they used therapy only when they believed they needed it. This study suggests that many patients with asthma believe that their asthma is an episodic rather than a chronic disease, and that therapy is necessary only when there is disease exacerbation.

Psychological models of disease management have suggested that adherence to medication may be related to the patient's perceived vulnerability to the negative consequences of illness, with an increased sense of risk being associated with better adherence. In paediatric research, several studies have suggested that parents who consider their children's health to be fragile or vulnerable (whether based on real events or not) will be vigilant and will adhere to health care recommendations. Spurrier et al. (31) examined the relationship between the asthma management strategies used by 101 parents of children with asthma and the perceptions of these parents of their child's vulnerability to illness. The study found that after controlling for the frequency and severity of asthma symptoms, those parents who felt their child had greater vulnerability to illness were more likely to use regular preventive medications, take the child to the doctor and keep him or her home from school. The authors suggested that one possible explanation of this finding is that "parents who do not perceive their child to be medically vulnerable may discontinue administering regular medication…" (31).

Regimen factors in asthma therapy. A number of studies across a range of chronic diseases have found that certain characteristics of the prescribed treatment regimen are strongly associated with patient adherence. In general, the longer the duration of therapy, the more frequent the dosing, and the more complex the regimen (e.g. multiple devices or tasks), the poorer the adherence of the patient (32). Actual or perceived side-effects of treatment and the cost of therapy can also reduce adherence levels.

In recent years considerable effort has been directed towards developing an effective and safe once-a-day therapy for asthma because of its presumed advantage in promoting patient compliance. However, although there is convincing evidence that doses that must be administered more than twice a day lead to decreased adherence (19), the data are equivocal on the superiority of once-a-day dosing over twice-a-day dosing (33–35). Adherence considerations apart, once-daily asthma therapy appears to be preferable for most patients. Venables et al. (36) studied patient preferences in asthma therapy and found that 61% of patients expressed a preference for once-a-day treatment, 12% preferred twice-a-day treatment and 27% expressed no preference. While preference may not necessarily lead to improved compliance, it may well reduce the burden of therapy and enhance the quality of life of the patients.

5. Adherence in special populations

Children. There can be great diversity among families in how medication is managed. The responsibility for administration of medication generally shifts as a child grows, from total parental management for a young child, to shared medication management for a school-aged child, to complete self-management for an adolescent. Day-care providers, grandparents and siblings may assume the responsibility for the regular delivery of asthma medication in some households. In chaotic, troubled families there may be confusion as to who has the primary responsibility for the medication monitoring. The age at which a child is capable of assuming responsibility for remembering to take daily medication is highly variable, and is more a reflection of the child's maturity and personality than his or her chronological age. In some families children may be expected to manage their own medication early, less because the child has demonstrated sufficient responsibility, than because the parent believes the child is old enough to do it. For older children and adolescents, asthma management has the potential for turning into a battle in the war of independence. Research on juvenile diabetes, haemophilia and rheumatoid arthritis has emphasized the particular vulnerability of adolescents to problems with adherence to medication *(37,38)*. Family conflict and a denial of disease severity in an adolescent with severe asthma should therefore suggest a patient at a high risk for nonadherence to therapy.

Elderly patients. Some barriers to adherence to therapy are more common in older patients and warrant particular attention in clinical management. For example, although patients of any age may forget to take their medication, for some older patients memory difficulties may be exacerbated by other medications or early dementia. In addition, older patients are often receiving treatment for several other chronic health conditions simultaneously. The resulting polypharmacy is a well-recognized problem for many elderly patients, presenting both pharmacological and adherence risks *(39)*. The treatment of multiple ailments can result in complicated and burdensome medication regimens that require medications to be taken many times per day. Clinicians treating older patients for asthma should carefully review all prescribed medications, be attentive to potential memory difficulties, and assist the patient in integrating ICS therapy into his or her existing regimens.

Cultural differences. Culture and lay beliefs about illness and treatment can also influence the acceptance of asthma therapies by patients and their families. Diverse cultural beliefs can affect health care through competing therapies, fear of the health care system or distrust of prescribed therapies.

Income. While income per se does not predict adherence, the co-variates of poverty and inner-city living may make adherence to asthma self-management more difficult. Barriers to adherence related to low income can include inconsistent primary health care, inability to pay for asthma medications, lack of transport, family dysfunction and substance abuse *(40–43)*.

In some countries, patients may not be able to afford preventive asthma therapies. Research suggests that these cost barriers may lead some patients to treat their disease only during periods of exacerbation, or to reduce their dosage to "stretch" their medication.

6. Interventions to improve adherence to asthma therapy

Haynes et al. *(44)* recently reviewed the results of randomized controlled trials of interventions to promote adherence to pharmacological regimens across a range of chronic diseases, including asthma, where both adherence and clinical outcome were measured. This rigorous analysis found that over half (10/19) of the interventions for long-term treatments reviewed were associated with significant improvements in adherence; however, the magnitude of the improvements in adherence or clinical outcome was generally not large. The authors concluded that successful interventions to promote adherence were complex and multi-faceted and included combinations of counselling, education, more convenient care, self-monitoring, reinforcement, reminders, and other forms of additional attention or supervision. Specific intervention strategies that can be used for promoting adherence to therapy are outlined below (see also Table 1).

Educational strategies. Asthma is a complex disease and requires education of the patient and his or her family if it is to be managed successfully. Knowledge of the regimen is necessary, but not sufficient in itself, to ensure patient adherence. Several studies have emphasized the central role of effective communication between patients and health care providers in promoting adherence *(45,46)*.

Written instructions about the asthma regimen that are culturally appropriate and adapted to suit the patient's level of literacy should be a core part of every interaction with the patient. For older patients, comprehension and recall of information on how to take medication was shown to be significantly improved when medication-taking instructions were clear, presented as lists rather than paragraphs, used pictures or icons in combination with written medication instructions and were consistent with patients' mental representations of medication taking *(47)*.

Self-management programmes that include both educational and behavioural components have been developed *(48)*. The educational formats use basic learning principles to promote adherence to asthma therapy. Key points in the most recent set of treatment guidelines have included the following:

- education of the patient beginning at the time of diagnosis and integrated into every step of asthma care;

- patient education provided by all members of the team;

- teaching skills for the self-management of asthma by tailoring the information and the treatment approach to fit the needs of each patient;

- teaching and reinforcing behavioural skills such as inhaler use, self-monitoring and environmental control;

- joint development of treatment plans by team members and patients;

- encouragement of an active partnership by providing written self-management and individualized asthma action plans to patients; and

- encouraging adherence to the treatment plan jointly developed by the interdisciplinary team and the patients.

These self-management programmes have demonstrated their effectiveness in decreasing symptoms, school absence and emergency care as well as improving asthma knowledge. However, little is known about the direct effects of these programmes on adherence. Future educational programmes will need to include objective monitoring of adherence in order to examine their effectiveness in promoting it.

Behavioural strategies. Behavioural strategies are those procedures that attempt to promote adherence behaviours directly by using techniques such as reminders, contracting and reinforcement *(49)*. The use of reminders has been shown to be helpful in maintaining adherence both in asthmatic children followed in an asthma clinic and asthmatic children followed as outpatients after inpatient asthma rehabilitation *(50,51)*. Providing feedback to patients regarding adherence to medication is an important behavioural clinical strategy. Informing patients that they will be objectively monitored for adherence has been shown to be effective in improving adherence in outpatient clinics *(15)*, at follow-up visits after inpatient rehabilitation *(52)* and in clinical trials *(53)*. Reinforcement is an essential component of all behavioural strategies. Reinforcement refers to any consequences that increase the probability of the behaviour being repeated. Dunbar et al. suggested that a clinician's time and attention to the patient may be the most powerful available reinforcer *(49)*. The length of time a patient spends with the clinician is positively related to adherence *(54)*. Investigators have used contracts to include the families of asthmatic children. In this setting patients receive reinforcement from those people who are most significant to them and most readily available at the time the health behaviour occurs *(55)*.

Tailoring of therapy. Tailoring the therapy to the patient is a strategy that is sometimes overlooked by health care providers. Tailoring refers to fitting the prescribed regimen and intervention strategies to specific characteristics of the patient. It is another effective behavioural method used to improve adherence *(55)*. Whenever possible, negotiating a therapy that the patient is able to follow should be a first priority. Some examples of ways in which the therapy may be tailored include exploring the patient's schedule, beliefs, and preferences *(56)*; simplifying the dosing regimen *(57)*; altering the route of administration *(58)*, and using adherence aids *(59)*.

Maintenance interventions to achieve adherence. Achieving and maintaining adherence over long periods of time is difficult for both patients and clinicians. Investigators in the management of childhood and adult asthma have developed self-management programmes to enable a patient and his or her family to manage asthma efficiently and effectively over time in conjunction with their health professional. Self-management programmes for adult and childhood asthma have been shown to reduce asthma morbidity and costs, and may be useful in promoting and sustaining long-term adherence to therapy *(60–63)*.

Table 1 Factors affecting adherence to asthma treatment and interventions for improving it, listed according to the five dimensions and the interventions used to improve adherence

Asthma	Factors affecting adherence	Interventions to improve adherence
Socioeconomic-related factors	(–) Vulnerability of the adolescent to not taking medications; family conflict and denial of severity of disease in adolescents *(37)*; memory difficulties in older patients; polypharmacy in older patients *(39)*; cultural and lay beliefs about illness and treatment; alternative medicines; fear of the health care system; poverty; inner-city living; lack of transport; family dysfunction *(40)*	List-organized instructions; clear instructions about treatment for older patients *(47)*
Health care team/health system-related factors	(–) Health care providers' lack of knowledge and training in treatment management and/or an inadequate understanding of the disease; short consultations; lack of training in changing behaviour of nonadherent patients	Education on use of medicines; management of disease and treatment in conjunction with patients *(48)*; adherence education *(58)*; multidisciplinary care *(48)*; training in monitoring adherence; more intensive intervention by increasing the number and duration of contacts *(49)*
Condition-related factors	(–) Inadequate understanding of the disease *(29)*	Patient education beginning at the time of diagnosis and integrated into every step of asthma care *(48)*
Therapy-related factors	(–) Complex treatment regimens; long duration of therapy; frequent doses *(32)*; adverse effects of treatment	Simplification of regimens *(57)*; education on use of medicines *(48)*; adaptation of prescribed medications *(55,56,58)*; continuous monitoring and reassessment of treatment *(15, 52,53)*
Patient-related factors	(–) Forgetfulness; misunderstanding of instructions about medications; poor parental understanding of children's asthma medications; patients' lack of perception of his or her own vulnerability to illness *(31)*. Patients' lack of information about the prescribed daily dosage/ misconceptions about the disease and treatments *(29)*; persistent misunderstandings about side-effects *(29)*; drug abuse *(40)*	(+) Perceiving that they are vunerable to illness *(31)*. Self-managment programmes that include both educational and behaviour components *(58, 60)*; memory aids and reminders *(50)*; incentives and/or reinforcements *(49)*; multi-faceted interventions, including combinations of counselling, education, more convenient care, self-monitoring, reinforcement, remindres and other forms of additional attention or supervision *(44, 65–67)*.

(+) Factors having a positive effect on adherence; (–) factors having a negative effect on adherence.

A group of investigators developed and tested the effectiveness of a psycho-educational self-management programme for severely asthmatic children that was delivered in an inpatient setting *(64)*. Patients were admitted to the programme if they met morbidity criteria in the year prior to admission that included a minimum of three hospitalizations, four emergency visits, four corticosteroid bursts and agreement of the families to participate in self-management meetings. The rehabilitation intervention included medical assessment and management, physical activity training, education about asthma for the child and family, and a sequence of family interviews designed to facilitate home-management of the illness and promote adherence to medication. These individuals were followed as outpatients for 4 years; they received three to four medications concurrently and achieved a marked reduction in hospitalization, emergency care, oral corticosteroid use and total costs of asthma by maintaining adherence, as measured by monitoring theophylline levels at outpatient visits.

7. Discussion

Because adherence to therapy is an integral part of the effective management of asthma, all international public health efforts to improve asthma outcomes should include educational strategies for both patients and health care providers that target the promotion of adherence. Regular adherence to ICS therapy is dependent on the patient's acceptance that asthma is a chronic disease requiring preventive treatment. Patients must also feel that the prescribed therapy is effective in achieving the desired treatment goals and is safe for long-term use. Several studies have confirmed that the beliefs that patients hold about their asthma and the therapy prescribed for it are closely associated with the likelihood of adherence. When patients do not perceive that their asthma is chronic or that it requires preventive treatment, adherence with therapy is generally episodic.

Effective communication between patients and providers has been identified as having an important influence on patients' adherence. Most health professionals lack the training to change the behaviour of nonadherent patients. Educational efforts sponsored by both public and private sources are needed to improve the communication skills of health professionals so as to promote adherence to the treatments recommended for asthma.

Limited evidence from studies of adherence to asthma therapy among immigrant populations in developed countries suggests that use of alternative medicine and lay beliefs may significantly reduce adherence to therapy. Watson and Lewis *(68)* reported that inhaled corticosteroids were available in only 15 of 24 countries surveyed in Africa and Asia, and when available the median (range) cost of a 50 µg beclomethasone inhaler was 20% (6.8–100%) of the average local monthly income. Additional research is needed on the rates of adherence and barriers to adherence in developing countries.

Guidelines on the management of patients with asthma may be modified in the future following the development of accurate and affordable systems for monitoring anti-inflammatory medication. By objectively evaluating the adherence of symptomatic patients, those who are nonadherent may be identified, appropriately treated and counselled in an accurate, efficient and cost-effective manner *(69)*.

8. Conclusions

Nonadherence to regimens for asthma treatment may have several causes including inadequate knowledge and skill on the part of the patient, and inadequate awareness of the problem, or lack of skill to address it, on the part of the health professional. Patients must have a basic understanding of their illness and its treatment if we are to expect even minimal adherence. Achievement of adherence requires considerable effort from both the patient and caregiver. To perform the daily tasks necessary for successful control of their asthma, patients must be well motivated and convinced that their own behaviour will result in improved health, a concept referred to as self-efficacy. Simply giving information to patients is unlikely to change behaviour; health care providers must understand the psychological principles that underlie self-management training and comprehend that motivating patients requires more than informing them briefly about the prescription that has just been written. At the core of these principles is the need to establish treatment goals that can be embraced both by health professionals and patients in a partnership that requires regular and reciprocal communication. Patients will not perform the work necessary to achieve goals they do not understand or do not view as necessary and important. Once appropriate goals have been established, most patients require assistance in determining how to evaluate their changing symptoms and how to use their written action plan to make effective decisions about daily self-management behaviour.

9. References

1. Baena-Cagnani CE. The global burden of asthma and allergic diseases: the challenge for the new century. *Current Allergy & Asthma Reports*, 2001, 1:297–298.

2. Spitzer WO et al. The use of beta-agonists and the risk of death and near death from asthma. *New England Journal of Medicine*, 1992, 326:501–506.

3. Gibson PG et al. Self-management education and regular practitioner review for adults with asthma. *Cochrane Database of Systematic Reviews*, 2000, CD001117.

4. Wilson SR et al. A controlled trial of two forms of self-management education for adults with asthma. *American Journal of Medicine*, 1993, 94:564–576.

5. Rand C. I took the medicine like you told me, Doctor. Self-Report of adherence with medical regimens. In: Stone A et al. eds. *The science of self-report*. New Jersey, USA, Lawrence Erlbaum Associates, 1999:257–276.

6. Clepper I. Noncompliance, the invisible epidemic. *Drug Topics*, 1992, 17:44–65.

7. Waters WH, Gould NV, Lunn JE. Undispensed prescriptions in a mining general practice. *British Medical Journal*, 1976, 1:1062–1063.

8. Rashid A. Do patients cash prescriptions?, *British Medical Journal – Clinical Research*. 284:24–26.

9. Saunders CE. Patient compliance in filling prescriptions after discharge from the emergency department. *American Journal of Emergency Medicine*, 1987, 5:283–286.

10. Krogh C, Wallner L. Prescription-filling patterns of patients in a family practice. *Journal of Family Practice*, 1987, 24:301–302.

11. Beardon PH et al. Primary non-compliance with prescribed medication in primary care. *British Medical Journal*, 1993, 307:846–848.

12. Cerveri I et al. International variations in asthma treatment compliance: the results of the European Community Respiratory Health Survey (ECRHS). *European Respiratory Journal*, 1999, 14:288–294.

13. Spector SL et al. Compliance of patient with asthma with an experimental aerosolized medication: Implications for controlled clinical trials. *Journal of Allergy and Clinical Immunology*, 1986, 77:65–70

14. Mawhinney H et al. As-needed medication use in asthma usage patterns and patient characteristics. *Journal of Asthma*, 1993, 30:61–71.

15. Yeung M et al. Compliance with prescribed drug therapy in asthma. *Respiratory Medicine*, 1994, 88:31–35.

16. Celano M et al. Treatment adherence among low-income children with asthma. *Journal of Pediatric Psychology*, 1998, 23:345–349.

17. Apter AJ et al. Adherence with twice-daily dosing of inhaled steroids. Socioeconomic and health-belief differences. *American Journal of Respiratory & Critical Care Medicine*, 1998, 157:1810–1817.

18. Cooper WO, Hickson GB. Corticosteroid prescription filling for children covered by Medicaid following an emergency department visit or a hospitalization for asthma. *Archives of Pediatrics & Adolescent Medicine*, 2001, 155:1111–1115.

19. Coutts JA, Gibson NA, Paton JY. Measuring compliance with inhaled medication in asthma. *Archives of Disease in Childhood*, 1992, 67:332–333.

20. Gibson NA et al. Compliance with inhaled asthma medication in preschool children. *Thorax*, 1995, 50:1274–1279.

21. Jonasson G, Carrlsen K, Sodaal A. Patient compliance in a clinical trial with inhaled budesonide in children with mild asthma. *European Respiratory Journal*, 1999, 14:150–154.

22. Milgrom H et al. Noncompliance and treatment failure in children with asthma. *Journal of Allergy & Clinical Immunology*, 1996, 98:1051–1057.

23. DiMatteo MR. Enhancing patient adherence to medical recommendations. *Journal of the American Medical Association*, 1983, 271:79–83.

24. Donnelly JE, Donnelly WJ, Thong YH. Inadequate parental understanding of asthma medications. *Annals of Allergy*, 1989, 62:337–341.

25. Dekker FW et al. Compliance with pulmonary medication in general practice. *European Respiratory Journal*, 1993, 6:886–890.

26. Hindi-Alexander M. Compliance or noncompliance: that is the question! *American Journal of Health Promotion*, 1987, 1:5–11.

27. Mann MC et al. An evaluation of severity-modulated compliance with q.i.d. dosing of inhaled beclomethasone. *Chest*, 1992, 102:1342–1346.

28. Adams S, Pill R, Jones A. Medication, chronic illness and identity: the perspective of people with asthma. *Social Science & Medicine*, 1997, 45:189–201.

29. Boulet LP. Perception of the role and potential side effects of inhaled corticosteroids among asthmatic patients. *Chest*, 1998, 113:587–592.

30. Chambers CV et al. Health beliefs and compliance with inhaled corticosteroids by asthmatic patients in primary care practices. *Respiratory Medicine*, 1999, 93:88–94.

31. Spurrier NJ et al. Association between parental perception of children's vulnerability to illness and management of children's asthma. *Pediatric Pulmonology*, 2000, 29:88–93.

32. Sackett DL, Haynes RB. *Compliance with therapeutic regimens*. Baltimore, Johns Hopkins University Press, 1976.

33. Lan AJ, Colford JM, Colford JM, Jr. The impact of dosing frequency on the efficacy of 10-day penicillin or amoxicillin therapy for streptococcal tonsillopharyngitis: A meta-analysis. *Pediatrics*, 2000, 105:E19.

34. Mason BJ, Matsuyama JR, Jue SG. Assessment of sulfonylurea adherence and metabolic control. *Diabetes Educator*, 1995, 21:52–57.

35. Weiner P, Weiner M, Azgad Y. Long term clinical comparison of single versus twice daily administration of inhaled budesonide in moderate asthma. *Thorax*, 1995, 50:1270–1273.

36. Venables T et al. A comparison of the efficacy and patient acceptability of once daily budesonide via Turbohaler and twice daily fluticasone propionate via disc-inhaler at an equal daily dose of 400μg in adult asthmatics. *British Journal of Clinical Research,* 1996, 7:15–32.

37. Jay S, Litt IF, Durant RH. Compliance with therapeutic regimens. *Journal of Adolescent Health Care,* 1984, 5:124–136.

38. Varni J, Wallander J. Adherence to health-related regimens in pediatric chronic disorders. *Clinical Psychology Review,* 1984, 4:585–596.

39. Kazis LE, Friedman RH. Improving medication compliance in the elderly. Strategies for the health care provider. *Journal of the American Geriatrics Society,* 1988, 36:1161–1162.

40. Lanier B. Who is dying of asthma and why? *Journal of Pediatrics,* 1989, 115:838–840.

41. Levenson T et al. Asthma deaths confounded by substance abuse. An assessment of fatal asthma. *Chest,* 1996, 110:604–610.

42. Wamboldt M, Wamboldt F. Psychosocial aspects of severe asthma in children. In: Szefler S, Leung D, eds. Severe asthma: pathogenesis and clinical management. *Lung biology in health and disease.* New York, Marcel Dekker, 1996:465–496.

43. Weitzman M, Gortmaker S, Sobol A. Racial, social, and environmental risks for childhood asthma. *American journal of diseases of Childhood,* 1990, 144:1189–1194.

44. Haynes RB et al. Interventions for helping patients to follow prescriptions for medications. *Cochrane Database of Systematic Reviews,* 2000.

45. Hall JA et al. Patients' health as a predictor of physician and patient behavior in medical visits. A synthesis of four studies. *Medical Care,* 1996, 34:1205–1218.

46. Roter DL et al. Communication patterns of primary care physicians. *Journal of the American Medical Association,* 1997, 277:350–356.

47. Morrow DG et al. The influence of list format and category headers on age differences in understanding medication instructions. *Experimental Aging Research,* 1998, 24:231–256.

48. Lewis C, Rachelefsky G, Lewis MA. ACT for kids. In: *Self-management educational programs for childhood asthma.* Washington, DC, National Institute of Allergy and Infectious Diseases, 1981:21–52.

49. Dunbar J, Marshall G, Hovell M. Behavioral strategies for improving compliance. In: Haynes RB. ed. *Compliance in health care.* Baltimore, John Hopkins University Press, 1979:174–190.

50. Walker NM, Mandell KL, Tsevat J. Use of chart reminders for physicians to promote discussion of advance directives in patients with AIDS. *AIDS Care,* 1999, 11:345-353.

51. Weinstein AG. Clinical management strategies to maintain drug compliance in asthmatic children. *Annals of Allergy, Asthma, & Immunology,* 1995, 74:304–310.

52. Weinstein AG et al. Outcome of short-term hospitalization for children with severe asthma. *Journal of Allergy & Clinical Immunology,* 1992, 90:66–75.

53. Nides MA et al. Improving inhaler adherence in a clinical trial through the use of the nebulizer chronolog. *Chest,* 1993, 104:501–507.

54. Korsch BM, Negrete VF. Doctor–patient communication. *Scientific American,* 1972, 227:66–74.

55. Hukla B. *Patient–clinician interaction and compliance.* Baltimore, John Hopkins University Press, 1979.

56. Dunbar-Jacob J et al. Predictors of patient adherence: Patient characteristics. In: Shumaker S et al., eds. *Handbook of health behavior change.* New York, Springer, 1998.

57. Feldman R et al. Adherence to pharmacologic management of hypertension. *Canadian Journal of Public Health,* 1998, 89:16–18.

58. Heyscue BE, Levin GM, Merrick JP. Compliance with depot antipsychotic medication by patients attending outpatient clinics. *Psychiatric Services,* 1998, 49:1232–1234.

59. Cramer JA. Enhancing patient compliance in the elderly. Role of packaging aids and monitoring. *Drugs & Aging,* 1998, 12:7–15.

60. Clark NM et al. Developing education for children with asthma through study of self-management behavior. *Health Education Quarterly,* 1980, 7:278–297.

61. Bailey WC et al. A randomized trial to improve self-management practices of adults with asthma. *Archives of Internal Medicine,* 1990, 150:1664–1668.

62. Windsor RA et al. Evaluation of the efficacy and cost effectiveness of health education methods to increase medication adherence among adults with asthma. *American Journal of Public Health,* 1990, 80:1519–1521.

63. Taitel MS et al. A self-management program for adult asthma. Part II: Cost-benefit analysis. *Journal of Allergy & Clinical Immunology,* 1995, 95:672–676.

64. Weinstein AG et al. An economic evaluation of short-term inpatient rehabilitation for children with severe asthma. *Journal of Allergy & Clinical Immunology,* 1996, 98:264–273.

65. Ward S et al. Patient education in pain control. *Supportive Care in Cancer,* 2001, 9:148–155.

66. de Wit R et al. Improving the quality of pain treatment by a tailored pain education programme for cancer patients in chronic pain. *European Journal of Pain,* 2001, 5:241–256.

67. Rimer B et al. Enhancing cancer pain control regimens through patient education. *Patient Education & Counseling,* 1987, 10:267–277.

68. Watson JP, Lewis RA. Is asthma treatment affordable in developing countries? *Thorax,* 1997, 52:605–607.

69. Weinstein AG, Feldstein J, Esterly K. Final Report of the Medication Adherence Task Force (Medical Society of Delaware). *Delaware Medical Journal,* 2001, 73:413–345.

Chapter VIII

Cancer (Palliative care)

1. Definitions and epidemiology of adherence   61
2. Factors and interventions affecting adherence   61
3. Conclusions   63
4. References   63

In most parts of the world, the majority of cancer patients suffer an advanced stage of the disease, which unfortunately is not responsive to curative treatment. Nearly 75% of patients with advanced cancer experience pain, very often in conjunction with many other symptoms, such as asthenia, anorexia and malnutrition, skin problems, dry mouth or thirst, constipation, nausea or vomiting, anxiety, low mood, depression, confusion and sleeplessness *(1,2)*. For such patients, the only available management is palliative care, which focuses mainly on pain relief *(3)*.

Palliative care is an approach that improves the quality of life of patients through the prevention and relief of suffering. To meet the multiple and varying needs of the patients, it is believed that the care should be holistic, multidisciplinary, and family – as well as patient – centred. The aims of palliative care are achieved by:

- providing relief from pain and other distressing symptoms;

- affirming life and regarding dying as a normal process;

- intending neither to hasten nor to postpone death;

- integrating the psychological and spiritual aspects of patient care;

- offering a support system to help patients live as actively as possible until death;

- offering a support system to help the family to cope during the patient's illness and during bereavement;

- using a team approach to address the needs of patients and their families, including bereavement counselling, if indicated;

- enhancing quality of life, and possibly also positively influencing the course of illness; and

- starting palliative care early in the course of illness, in conjunction with other therapies that are intended to prolong life, such as chemotherapy or radiation therapy, and including those investigations needed to better understand and manage distressing clinical complications (4).

Palliative care is still a neglected area worldwide and several million cancer patients suffer needlessly every day as a result (5). Most cancer patients in developing countries receive inadequate palliative care and less than 10% of the resources committed to cancer control in these countries are available to them (1). Palliative care remains far from satisfactory, mainly because of:

- an absence of national policies on cancer pain relief and other aspects of palliative care;

- the lack of education for health care providers, policy-makers, administrators and the general public;

- the concern that the medical use of morphine and related drugs will fuel the problem of drug abuse in a community and result in increased restrictions on prescription and supply;

- limitations on the supply and distribution of the drugs needed for the relief of pain and other symptoms, particularly in developing countries;

- restrictions imposed by the adoption of regional, district or hospital formularies, which contain insufficient drugs for the control of pain and other symptoms;

- the shortage of professional health care workers empowered to prescribe analgesics and other drugs for palliative care; and

- the lack of financial resources for research and development in palliative care (1).

Pain relief is a key component of a comprehensive palliative care programme. Relief from cancer pain can be achieved in about 90% of patients, but unfortunately pain is often poorly managed. Pain relief may be achieved by drug use, but may also include various other means: psychological approaches, pathological processes (e.g. nerve degeneration) and modification of daily activities. The pharmacological approach to the palliative care of cancer patients uses a variety of drugs for managing symptoms. These include non-opioid analgesics (mild analgesics and nonsteroidal anti-inflammatory drugs), opioids for moderate to severe pain, ulcer-healing drugs, antispasmodics, corticosteroids, bronchodilators, laxatives, antiemetics, antifungals, antidepressants and hypnotics among others.

Data from studies by Miaskowski, Du pen and Ward et al. (6–8) indicate that one of the main factors contributing to the undertreatment of cancer pain is the patients' lack of adherence to the therapeutic regimen. The study by Ward et al. (8) showed that a third of the patients they monitored delayed or omitted many prescribed doses. This reflects the fact that patients often take their doses at intervals longer than those prescribed, commonly longer by hours, but sometimes by days and occasionally by weeks. The clinical and economic consequences of these lapses in dosing are uniquely difficult to measure due to the complexity of treatment and the severity of disease.

Because more than 90% of palliative care is provided on an outpatient basis, it is critically important for clinicians to know how their patients adhere to their regimen for analgesics or other palliative therapies, and if possible, they should also know which effective interventions are available for improving adherence. The aim of this chapter is to summarize the available literature on adherence to palliative care and provide answers to some of these questions.

1. Definitions and epidemiology of adherence

Published studies were considered for inclusion here if they reported relevant epidemiological or economic data on adherence to one of the therapies usually used in palliative care. A search on adherence to cancer palliative care was made using Medline (1990–2002). Some reviews and reports from international and national organizations were also included. The search retrieved only studies that evaluated adherence to pain relief in palliative care.

Adherence was usually not explicitly defined in the articles retrieved, but referred to generally as "patients following medical recommendations". In operational terms, the variables of adherence were defined as: "not filling a prescription", "not taking medication", "errors in dosage", "reducing medication", "taking extra medication" and "taking additional nonprescribed medication" *(6,7,9,10)*.

The studies reviewed here used several different methods to estimate the adherence of patients to their medication. These methods, which can be used either separately or in combination, include review of medical records, patient self-report, family report, residual pill counting, electronic measurement devices, prescription refill rates, biological markers in serum or urine, assays to quantify medications or their metabolites and therapeutic outcome *(6,9)*.

Few studies have provided data on the level of adherence of oncology patients to their pain relief, and the methods used to calculate adherence rates were not always described. Zeppetella et al., reported that 40% of patients with cancer adhered to pain relief drugs *(9)*. Miaskowski et al. reported adherence rates for opioid analgesics. Cancer patients prescribed relief on an around-the-clock basis took an average of 88.9%, whereas those who were prescribed relief on an as-needed basis had an adherence rate of about 24.7% *(6)*. Du Pen et al. reported that adherence of oncology patients to their prescribed opioid therapy was between 62% and 72% *(7)* and Ferrell et al. reported a mean adherence rate of 80% *(10)*.

2. Factors and interventions affecting adherence

Nonadherence is a problem that has many determinants; the responsibility for adherence has to be shared by health professionals, the health care system, the community and the patients. Many studies have identified the factors affecting adherence, and these were grouped into five dimensions: socioeconomic-related factors, health care team-/health system-related factors, condition-related factors, treatment-related factors and patient-related factors, as shown in Table 2.

Many factors, such as lack of knowledge about pain management *(5,11)*, misunderstanding instructions about how to take drugs *(9)*, complex treatment regimens *(9)*, anxiety about adverse effects *(12)*, inadequate understanding by health professionals of drug dependence *(13)* and long distance from the treatment setting, among many others, have been shown to be significant barriers to adherence, and should be taken into account when developing interventions.

Several interventions have been designed to improve adherence to medications for the relief of cancer pain. Some of them target specific factors as described below:

- *Patient cooperation.* This is achieved by educating the patient about pain and the management of side-effects, and encouraging the active participation of the patient in his or her own pain treatment *(9)*.

- *Therapeutic relationship.* Good relationships between health professionals and patients should be encouraged *(14)*.

- *Simplification of regimens.* The use of once-daily, or at most twice-daily, preparations is desirable wherever possible *(9)*.

- *Adaptations of prescribed medications.* The patient should agree on a medication formulation and medication should be chosen not only for the clinical indication, but also to suit the patient, taking into account his or her lifestyle and preferences *(15)*.

- *The role of home care nurses.* Home care nurses can play an important role in educating patients and their families about pain management, in administering medications and providing support and counselling *(16–18)*.

Failure to address the barriers affecting pain management may lead to therapeutic failure and poor quality of life for the patient.

Table 2 Factors affecting adherence to palliative care for cancer and interventions for improving it, listed by the five dimensions and the interventions used to improve adherence

Cancer	Factors affecting adherence	Interventions to improve adherence
Socioeconomic-related factors	(–) Long distance from treatment setting	Optimizing the cooperation between services; assessment of social needs *(3)*; family preparedness *(3)*; mobilization of community-based organizations
Health care team/health system-related factors	(–) Lack of knowledge of health professionals about pain management; inadequate understanding of drug dependence by health professionals *(5)*; health professionals' fears of investigation or sanction *(19)*; poor delivery of care education to the patient *(20)*; poor delivery of care education to family and caregivers *(20)*; reluctance of health professionals to prescribe opioids for use at home *(20)* (+) Good relationship between patient and physician *(14)*	Training of health professionals on adherence *(20)*; pain education component in training programmes *(13)*; support to caregivers; multidisciplinary care; follow-up consultation by community nurses *(20)*; supervision in home pain management *(20)*; identification of the treatment goals and development of strategies to meet them
Condition-related factors	(–) Nature of the patient's illness; poor understanding of the disease and its symptoms	Education on use of medicine *(11)*
Therapy-related factors	(–) Complex treatment regimens; taking too many tablets *(9)*; frequency of dose; having no treatment instructions *(9)*; misunderstanding instructions about how to take the drugs *(9)*; bad tasting medication; adverse effects of treatment *(9)*; inadequate treatment doses; perceived ineffectiveness *(9)* unnecessary duplicate prescribing *(9)* (+) Monotherapy with simple dosing schedules *(9)*	Simplification of regimens *(15)*; education on use of medications *(9)*; giving clear instructions *(9)*; clarifying misunderstandings about the recommendation of opioids; patient-tailored prescriptions *(9,15)*; continuous monitoring and reassessment of treatment; assessment and management of side-effects; coordination of prescribing *(9)*
Patient-related factors	(–) Forgetfulness *(9)*; misconceptions about pain *(11,12)*; difficulty in taking the preparation as prescribed *(9)*; fear of injections *(11)*; anxieties about possible adverse effects *(12)*; no self-perceived need for treatment *(9,21)*; feeling that it is not important to take medications *(9,21)*; undue anxiety about medication dependence *(11)*; fear of dependence *(14)*; psychological stress	Interventions to redress misconceptions about pain treatment and to encourage dialogue about pain control between patient and oncologist *(9,11)*; exploration of fears (e.g. about dependence) *(9,11)*; assessment of psychological needs *(3)*; education on use of medications *(11)*; behavioural and motivational intervention *(11)*; good patient–provider relationship *(14)*; self-management of disease and treatment *(11,16–18)*; self-management of side-effects *(16–18)*

(+) Factors having a positive effect on adherence; (–) factors having a negative effect on adherence.

3. Conclusions

Definitions and measurements of adherence vary widely; this prevents comparisons being made between studies and populations. There is little information on the adherence to palliative treatment of patients with cancer, and it covers only treatments for relief of pain. The available information reports adherence rates ranging from 24.7% to 88.9%. A general programme of palliative care must include the management of adherence in order to improve the effectiveness of the interventions and ensure an acceptable quality of life for this group of patients.

More research on adherence to palliative care is required in the following areas:

– epidemiology of adherence, especially to medicines other than those for pain relief;

– determination of the most appropriate methods and definitions for the measurement of adherence to analgesic medications;

– determining the additional factors that contribute to a patient's level of adherence to all required therapies; and

– studies evaluating interventions to improve adherence to all required therapies.

4. References

1. *Cancer pain relief and palliative care. Report of a WHO Expert Committee.* Geneva, World Health Organization, 1990 (WHO Technical Report Series, No. 804).
2. Addington-Hall J, McCarthy M. Dying from cancer: results of a national population-based investigation. *Pall Medicine*, 1995, 9:295–305.
3. Jordhoy MS et al. Quality of life in palliative cancer care: results from a cluster randomized trial. *Journal of Clinical Oncology*, 2001, 19:3884–3894.
4. *National cancer control programmes: policies and managerial guidelines.* Geneva, World Health Organization, 2002.
5. *Cancer pain relief,* 2nd ed. *With a guide to opioid availability.* Geneva, World Health Organization, 1996.
6. Miaskowski C et al. Lack of adherence with the analgesic regimen: a significant barrier to effective cancer pain management. *Journal of Clinical Oncology*, 2001, 19:4275–4279.
7. Du Pen SL et al. Implementing guidelines for cancer pain management: results of a randomized controlled clinical trial. *Journal of Clinical Oncology*, 1999, 17:361–370.
8. Ward SE et al. Patient-related barriers to management of cancer pain. *Pain*, 1993, 52:319–324.
9. Zeppetella G. How do terminally ill patients at home take their medication? *Palliative Medicine*, 1999, 13:469–475.
10. Ferrell BR, Juarez G, Borneman T. Use of routine and breakthrough analgesia in home care. *Oncology Nursing Forum*, 1999, 26:1655–1661.
11. Ward S et al. Patient education in pain control. *Supportive Care in Cancer*, 2001, 9:148–155.
12. Horne R, Weinman J. Patients' beliefs about prescribed medicines and their role in adherence to treatment in chronic physical illness. *Journal of Psychosomatic Research*, 1999, 47:555–567.
13. MacDonald N et al. A Canadian survey of issues in cancer pain management. *Journal of Pain & Symptom Management*, 1997, 14:332–342.
14. Ferrell BR, Dean GE. Ethical issues in pain management at home. *Journal of Palliative Care*, 1994, 10:67–72.
15. Mullen PD. Compliance becomes concordance. *British Medical Journal*, 1997, 314:691–692.
16. Chelf JH et al. Cancer-related patient education: an overview of the last decade of evaluation and research. *Oncology Nursing Forum*, 2001, 28:1139–1147.
17. de Wit R et al. Improving the quality of pain treatment by a tailored pain education programme for cancer patients in chronic pain. *European Journal of Pain*, 2001, 5:241–256.
18. Rimer B et al. Enhancing cancer pain control regimens through patient education. *Patient Education & Counseling*, 1987, 10:267–277.
19. Jones WL et al. Cancer patients' knowledge, beliefs, and behavior regarding pain control regimens: implications for education programs. *Patient Education & Counseling*, 1984, 5:159–164.
20. Barriers and benefits of managing cancer pain at home. Geneva, World Health Organization, *Cancer Pain Release 10,* 1997.
21. Horne R, Weinman J. Patient's beliefs about prescribed medicines and their role in adherence to treatment in chronic physical illness. *Journal psychosomatic research.* 1999, 47:555–67.

CHAPTER IX

Depression

1. Research methods: measurement of adherence and sampling   66
2. Rates of adherence   66
3. Predictors of adherence   67
4. Interventions to improve adherence   68
5. Clinical implications and need for further research   69
6. References   70

Depressive disorder is one of the most prevalent forms of mental illness, and is of major public health importance (1). It is characterized by abnormal and persistent low mood, accompanied by other symptoms including sleep disturbance, loss of appetite, suicidal thoughts, impaired concentration and attention, guilt and pessimism. Symptoms vary in severity, and the pattern of illness can range from an isolated and relatively mild episode, through recurrent episodes of moderate severity, to chronic and persistent severe illness. Owing to its prevalence, and to health system factors, primary care practitioners see most of the patients with depression and few are referred to specialist psychiatric services, even when they are readily available.

Although psychological treatments of proven efficacy are available for the management of depression, the most common form of treatment worldwide is antidepressant medication. For patients with a definitive diagnosis of depression, pharmacotherapy guidelines advocate that treatment should continue for at least 6 months following remission of symptoms. Furthermore, for patients who have suffered two or more episodes of significant depression within 5 years, long-term preventive treatment is suggested (2).

The clinical effectiveness of drug therapies for depression is limited by two groups of factors; patient adherence to the recommended protocol, and under-diagnosis and/or suboptimal treatment by primary care doctors. Both groups of factors appear to be relatively common, but the focus here is on adherence. However, the diagnosis and treatment cannot be ignored as they are likely to interact with, or to mediate, adherence.

This chapter discusses research methods, the overall prevalence of adherence, predictors of adherence and the efficacy of interventions designed to improve adherence. A literature search was made using Medline (1990–2001). A total of 287 publications were identified and evaluated.

1. Research methods: measurement of adherence and sampling

As is the case when attempting to measure patient behaviour in many other contexts, it is difficult to derive accurate estimates of patient adherence to medication for depression. Across studies, several techniques have been used including clinician estimation or patient self-report, pill-counting, estimation of blood levels of drug, metabolite or tracer substance, and the use of electronic monitoring systems that record pill dispensing. Two studies directly compared methods of measurement. In 1990 Kroll et al., using a small sample of patients with mixed diagnoses, demonstrated that levels of medication in the blood correlated with clinical outcome, and that many patients who claimed to be taking a medication regularly had low levels of it in their blood (3). In 2000, George et al. compared four methods of assessment in depressed patients treated by primary care practitioners, and were able to show that an event monitoring system (EMS) that electronically counted the amount of medication dispensed from its container was the most sensitive method of measuring adherence, although the specificity of a patient report of nonadherence was also high (4). Estimations of plasma levels of drugs and their metabolites were less useful. Although these types of measure overcome some of the bias associated with either physician observation or patient self-report, they still lack some of the features required of a "gold-standard" measure (i.e. being direct, objective and unobtrusive).

The second important methodological issue is the nature of the patient samples studied. Much research has been conducted on hospital outpatients or inpatients, or patients recruited into randomized trials to test the efficacy of medications. This pre-selection bias makes it very unlikely that the patients in these studies represent the true population of depressed patients receiving treatment in primary care settings. This makes it hard to generalize from the results of these studies.

2. Rates of adherence

Many studies have attempted to estimate the prevalence of adherence using different methods in a variety of patient samples. Early studies in primary care settings in the United Kingdom indicated that up to two-thirds of depressed patients who started courses of tricyclic drugs stopped taking them within a month (29). Peveler et al. assessed a large population of patients receiving tricyclic medication in primary care settings in the United Kingdom using EMS, and found that around 40% had discontinued treatment within 12 weeks (5). In 1990, McCombs et al. attempted to assess adherence in a large sample of depressed Medicaid-funded patients in California, United States, but found it difficult to separate patient's adherence to therapies from physician's adherence to treatment guidelines (6). Katon et al. assessed the extent to which patients of an HMO, on receiving prescriptions for antidepressant drugs, actually obtained supplies of medication. They reported that only 20% of patients who had been prescribed tricyclic drugs filled four or more prescriptions within 6 months, while 34% of patients who had been prescribed newer antidepressants did so (7). Lin et al. assessed a very large sample of HMO patients 6–8 weeks after starting treatment and found that 32–42% had not filled their prescriptions (8).

In a sample of patients with psychiatric disorders receiving prophylactic lithium treatment for unipolar and bipolar affective illness, Schumann et al. found that 43% of patients had discontinued their medication within 6 months (9). Ramana et al. interviewed patients discharged from hospital following admission for depression and found that at 18 months about 70% were "compliant", although this study also noted problems with physicians under-prescribing according to guidelines (10).

Gasquet et al. conducted a large telephone survey of the general population in France (11). He reported that 15% of the subjects admitted to early termination of their treatment, and 22% admitted to reducing their dose.

3. Predictors of adherence

Frequency of dosing. In an early study in a psychiatric outpatient practice in the United Kingdom, Myers & Branthwaite randomized patients into groups that received their treatment once daily or three times daily, or chose one of the two schedules. Adherence was assessed by pill count and interview (12). There was no overall difference in reported adherence between patients receiving once-daily or three-times-daily doses, but those who elected to take their medication three times daily reported better adherence than the others. This suggests that the element of personal control over choice of dose, rather than the frequency of dosing itself was influential. A recent study has suggested that prescribing a once-weekly dose of enteric-coated fluoxetine may lead to better adherence than a once-daily dose (13); thus substantial gains in convenience may also improve adherence.

Education. Lin et al. reported that patients were more likely to continue to take their medication during the first month of treatment if they had received specific educational messages, namely that they should take their medication daily, that they might notice no benefit for the first 2–4 weeks, that they should continue even if they felt better and that they should not stop medication without consulting their doctor. They also received advice about how to seek answers to questions about medication (14). The impact of such advice has not been evaluated prospectively.

Drug type. There has been considerable interest in the question of whether or not different antidepressant drugs are associated with better or worse adherence. A naturalistic study of claims data of 2000 patients suggested that adherence may be poorer in patients treated with tricyclic antidepressants, and that the provision of family, group or individual psychotherapy may improve adherence (15).

Several meta-analyses of randomized trials have also addressed this question. Montgomery & Kasper reviewed 67 trials and reported that the number of patients who discontinued their treatment because of side-effects was 5% lower in patients treated with selective serotonin reuptake inhibitors (SSRIs) than in patients treated with tricyclics (16). Anderson & Tomenson reviewed 62 trials and also found a marginally lower discontinuation rate in patients treated with SSRIs, but commented that the difference was probably too small to be of clinical significance (17). Hotopf et al. reporting the results of another meta-analysis suggested that even this small difference might be due to the preponderance of older tricyclic drugs used in most of the early trials, and that it would disappear if the comparison were made with newer tricyclic and heterocyclic medicines (18). Although the generalizability of meta-analysis may be limited by the characteristics of the patient samples in the trials reviewed, these results suggest that drug type may not be a particularly influential variable.

Co-medication. Furukawa et al. conducted a meta-analysis of trials comparing combinations of antidepressants and benzodiazepines with antidepressants prescribed alone for periods of up to 8 weeks and reported a marginal benefit of co-prescribing benzodiazepines. Any potential benefit must be offset against the possible clinical disadvantages such as the development of dependence on benzodiazepines (19).

Psychiatric co-morbidity and personality traits. Keeley et al. reported from a small study in family practice, that patients with more frequent somatoform symptoms were more likely to be nonadherent to drug treatment (20). Ekselius et al. reported that sensation-seeking personality traits were associated with lower blood-levels of antidepressant drug, though not with lower self-reported adherence, in patients participating in a randomized trial (21).

4. Interventions to improve adherence

As mentioned above, one difficulty in the study of depression therapy is that unsatisfactory treatment may reflect a combination of poor patient adherence and medical advice that is inconsistent with expert guidelines. To be clinically effective, interventions should ideally deal with both aspects of quality improvement. In 1999, Peveler et al. were able to show that two brief sessions of counselling provided by a primary care nurse could greatly reduce rates of discontinuation of treatment at 12 weeks (from 61% to 37%), but clinical benefit was only seen in a post hoc analysis of the subgroup of patients receiving adequate doses of medication (5). A small feasibility study also suggested that similar benefits could be obtained by telephone counselling (22). Information alone, provided by leaflet (5) or by repeated mailings (23), did not appear to be effective in improving rates of adherence (see also Table 3).

Most other studies have tested complex, multi-faceted, interventions designed to improve the overall quality of care. For example, Katon et al. (24–27) evaluated the impact of increased involvement of secondary care specialist staff and closer surveillance of patients receiving treatment in primary care. They reported improved adherence, boosting the proportion of patients receiving an adequate dose of their medication at 90 days to 75%, but although this group initially had better clinical outcomes, these benefits were no longer evident at 19-month follow-up. Subsequent work has shown that a relapse prevention programme can also improve longer-term outcome (28).

Table 3 Factors affecting adherence to treatment for depression and interventions for improving it, listed by the five dimensions and the interventions used to improve adherence

Depression	Factors affecting adherence	Interventions to improve adherence
Socioeconomic-related factors	No information was found	No information was found
Health care team/health system-related factors	(–) Poor health education of the patient (+) Multi-faceted intervention for primary care	Multidisciplinary care (24–27); training of health professionals on adherence; counselling provided by a primary care nurse (5); telephone consultation/counselling (22); improved assessment and monitoring of patients (24)
Condition-related factors	(–) Psychiatric co-morbidity (+) Clear instructions on management of disease (14); nature of the patient's illness; poor understanding of the disease and its symptoms	Education of patient on use of medicines (14)
Therapy-related factors	(–) High frequency of dose (13); co-prescribing of benzodiazepines (19); adequate doses of medication (5,24–27) (+) Low frequency of dose (13); clear instructions on management of treatment (14)	Education on use of medicines (14); patient-tailored prescriptions (13); continuous monitoring and reassessment of treatment (28)
Patient-related factors	(–) Personality traits (20,21)	Counselling (24); relapse-prevention counselling; psychotherapy (15); family psychotherapy (15); frequent follow-up interviews (28); specific advice targeted at the needs and concerns of individual patients (24)

(+) Factors having a positive effect on adherence; (–) factors having a negative effect on adherence.

5. Clinical implications and need for further research

Ten years ago research in this field was limited, but considerable progress has since been made. Although by no means complete, we now have data for estimating the extent of the problem, and there is an increasing awareness of its clinical and social impact and of the fact that high levels of patient adherence to treatment and physician adherence to best-practice protocols are important co-determinants of treatment outcome. There is broader recognition that, at least for those patients with severe and recurrent illness, a chronic disease model should be adopted.

Furthermore, practitioners treating patients with depression can be guided by several recent findings that are summarized below.

- If the problem of poor adherence is not addressed, 30–40% of patients will discontinue their medication early (after 12 weeks), regardless of perceived benefits or side-effects.

- Simple to follow advice and education such as that tested by Lin et al. *(14)* is beneficial, and such advice should be given both in the early phase of treatment *(5)* and repeated at later stages *(28)*.

- If patients admit to poor adherence, then it is highly likely that they are not taking their medication as prescribed; if they report good adherence, but lack of clinical progress suggests that adherence may nevertheless be a problem, the most sensitive method of detection is electronic monitoring.

- There is at best only weak evidence that treatment with the newer antidepressants leads directly to better rates of adherence and this is therefore probably not a material factor in choice of medication.

- Improved patient outcomes in primary care are probably best achieved through complex interventions such as those used by Katon et al. comprising improved assessment and monitoring of patients and relapse prevention counselling, together with specific advice targeted at the needs and concerns of individual patients.

A considerable research agenda still remains. More accurate estimations of the prevalence of adherence are needed in addition to research to address and measure the different forms that poor adherence may take, e.g. patients missing doses, taking "drug holidays", substituting agents, changing dosing, not filling prescriptions or discontinuing treatment early. The ways in which primary care physicians assess depression and deliver treatment should be further explored to identify determinants that explain adherence (and nonadherence) behaviours. Electronic event monitoring systems offer a useful approach to measuring some forms of adherence. An improved understanding of the relationships between health beliefs and medication-taking behaviour should lead to more robust theoretical frameworks, and to more effective methods of improving adherence, that can be added to existing techniques. Depression management programmes of the type pioneered by Katon and others in the United States require evaluation in other health care systems to ascertain whether their apparent benefits are transferable to other situations.

6. References

1. Murray C, Lopez A. *The global burden of disease: a comprehensive assessment of mortality and disability from diseases, injuries and risk factors in 1990.* Cambridge, MA, Harvard University Press, 1996.

2. Peveler R, Kendrick A. Treatment delivery and guidelines in primary care. *British Medical Bulletin,* 2001, 57:193–206.

3. Kroll J et al. Medication compliance, antidepressant blood levels, and side effects in Southeast Asian patients. *Journal of Clinical Psychopharmacology,* 1990, 10:279–283.

4. George CF et al. Compliance with tricyclic antidepressants: the value of four different methods of assessment. *British Journal of Clinical Pharmacology,* 2000, 50:166–171.

5. Peveler R et al. Effect of antidepressant drug counselling and information leaflets on adherence to drug treatment in primary care: randomised controlled trial. *British Medical Journal,* 1999, 319:612–615.

6. McCombs JS et al. The cost of antidepressant drug therapy failure: a study of antidepressant use patterns in a Medicaid population. *Journal of Clinical Psychiatry,* 1990, 51 (Suppl):60–69.

7. Katon W et al. Adequacy and duration of antidepressant treatment in primary care. *Medical Care,* 1992, 30:67–76.

8. Lin EH et al. Low-intensity treatment of depression in primary care: is it problematic? *General Hospital Psychiatry,* 2000, 22:78–83.

9. Schumann C et al. ;Nonadherence with long-term prophylaxis: a 6-year naturalistic follow-up study of affectively ill patients. *Psychiatry Research,* 1999, 89:247–257.

10. Ramana R et al. Medication received by patients with depression following the acute episode: adequacy and relation to outcome. *British Journal of Psychiatry,* 1999, 174:128–134.

11. Gasquet I et al. [Determinants of compliance with antidepressive drugs.] [French] *Encephale,* 2001, 27:83–91.

12. Myers ED, Branthwaite A. Out-patient compliance with antidepressant medication. *British Journal of Psychiatry,* 1992, 160:83–86.

13. Claxton A et al. Patient compliance to a new enteric-coated weekly formulation of fluoxetine during continuation treatment of major depressive disorder. *Journal of Clinical Psychiatry,* 2000, 61:928–932.

14. Lin EH et al. The role of the primary care physician in patients' adherence to antidepressant therapy. *Medical Care,* 1995, 33:67–74.

15. Tai-Seale M, Croghan TW, Obenchain R. Determinants of antidepressant treatment compliance: implications for policy. *Medical Care Research & Review,* 2000, 57:491–512.

16. Montgomery SA, Kasper S. Comparison of compliance between serotonin reuptake inhibitors and tricyclic antidepressants: a meta-analysis. *International Clinical Psychopharmacology,* 1995, 9 (Suppl 4):33–40.

17. Anderson IM, Tomenson BM. Treatment discontinuation with selective serotonin reuptake inhibitors compared with tricyclic antidepressants: a meta-analysis. *British Medical Journal,* 1995, 310:1433–1438.

18. Hotopf M, Hardy R, Lewis G. Discontinuation rates of SSRIs and tricyclic antidepressants: a meta-analysis and investigation of heterogeneity. *British Journal of Psychiatry,* 1997, 170:120–127.

19. Furukawa TA, Streiner DL, Young LT. Is antidepressant-benzodiazepine combination therapy clinically more useful? A meta-analytic study. *Journal of Affective Disorders,* 2001, 65:173–177.

20. Keeley R, Smith M, Miller J. Somatoform symptoms and treatment nonadherence in depressed family medicine outpatients. *Archives of Family Medicine,* 2000, 9:46–54.

21. Ekselius L, Bengtsson F, von Knorring L. Non-compliance with pharmacotherapy of depression is associated with a sensation seeking personality. *International Clinical Psychopharmacology,* 2000, 15:273–278.

22. Tutty S, Simon G, Ludman E. Telephone counseling as an adjunct to antidepressant treatment in the primary care system. A pilot study. *Effective Clinical Practice,* 2000, 3:170–178.

23. Mundt JC et al. Effectiveness of antidepressant pharmacotherapy: the impact of medication compliance and patient education. *Depression & Anxiety,* 2001, 13:1–10.

24. Katon W et al. Collaborative management to achieve treatment guidelines. Impact on depression in primary care. *Journal of the American Medical Association,* 1995, 273:1026–1031.

25. Katon W et al. A multifaceted intervention to improve treatment of depression in primary care. *Archives of General Psychiatry,* 1996, 53:924–932.

26. Lin EH et al. Can enhanced acute-phase treatment of depression improve long-term outcomes? A report of randomized trials in primary care. *American Journal of Psychiatry,* 1999, 156:643–645.

27. Katon W et al. Stepped collaborative care for primary care patients with persistent symptoms of depression: a randomized trial. *Archives of General Psychiatry,* 1999, 56:1109–1115.

28. Katon W et al. A randomized trial of relapse prevention of depression in primary care. *Archives of General Psychiatry,* 2001, 58:241–247.

29. Johnson, DA. Treatment of depression in general practice. 1973, *British Medical Journal.* 266:18–20.

CHAPTER X

Diabetes

1. Introduction 71

2. Treatment of diabetes 72

3. Definition of adherence 72

4. Prevalence of adherence to recommendations for diabetes treatment 73

5. Correlates of adherence 75

6. Interventions 79

7. Methodological and conceptual issues in research on adherence to treatment for diabetes 81

8. Conclusions 81

9. References 82

1. Introduction

Diabetes mellitus is a group of diseases characterized by high levels of blood glucose resulting from defects in insulin secretion, insulin action or both (1). Diabetes is highly prevalent, afflicting approximately 150 million people worldwide (2), and this number is expected to rise to 300 million in the year 2025 (3). Much of this increase will occur in developing countries and will result from population ageing, unhealthy diet, obesity and a sedentary lifestyle (4). In developed countries, such as the United States, diabetes has been reported as the seventh leading cause of death (5), and the leading cause of lower extremity amputation, end-stage renal disease and blindness among persons aged 18–65 years (6–9). It has been estimated that diabetes costs the United States economy more than 98 billion dollars per year in direct and indirect costs (5,10). It has also been estimated that low-income families in the United States supporting an adult member with diabetes devote 10% of their income to his or her care, and that this figure rises to 25% in India (11).

There are four known subtypes of diabetes mellitus (1).

- Type 1 diabetes, previously called insulin-dependent diabetes mellitus (IDDM) or juvenile onset diabetes, accounts for 5 to 10% of all diagnosed cases of diabetes (12). Type 1 diabetes, caused by failure of pancreatic beta-cells to produce insulin, can afflict both children and adults who will require daily injections of insulin. Inadequate use of insulin results in ketoacidosis and this inevitable consequence limits the extent to which patients can ignore recommendations to take exogenous insulin and still survive. Ketoacidosis is a significant cause of mortality in young persons with type 1 diabetes (13,14). Patients with diabetic ketoacidosis often require hospitalization and, in most instances, poor adherence to insulin therapy is the suspected cause (15,16).

- Type 2 diabetes, previously called non-insulin-dependent diabetes mellitus (NIDDM) or adult-onset diabetes, may account for about 90% of all diagnosed cases of the disease. It is typically associated with being overweight and is caused by insulin resistance. For patients with type 2 diabetes, weight control, by means of dietary and physical activity regimens, is the cornerstone of the treatment. However, pancreatic beta-cell function decreases over time, so many patients will eventually require treatment with oral medications or exogenous insulin.

- Gestational diabetes develops in 2 to 5% of all pregnancies, but disappears postpartum (17). Risk factors include race/ethnicity and a family history of diabetes and obesity.

- Other specific types of diabetes result from specific genetic syndromes, surgery, drugs, malnutrition, infections and other illness, and account for 1 to 2% of all diagnosed cases of diabetes.

2. Treatment of diabetes

The goals of diabetes treatment are to keep blood glucose levels as near normal as possible while avoiding acute and chronic complications (7,18). Because the normal homeostatic control mechanisms are disrupted in patients with diabetes, food intake, emotional stress and changes in physical activity can cause blood glucose to become too low or too high leading to the acute complications of hypoglycaemia or hyperglycaemia. In addition, inappropriate nutrition and insufficient physical activity increase the risk of developing the long-term complications of diabetes, especially heart disease. Keeping blood glucose within a target range requires feedback in the form of self-monitoring of blood glucose. Patients with type 1 diabetes must carefully balance food intake, insulin and physical activity. Patients with type 2 diabetes are often prescribed oral medications that increase insulin production, decrease insulin resistance, or block carbohydrate absorption and may have to take exogenous insulin to achieve adequate metabolic control. Because improved metabolic control ends the spilling of glucose in the urine, patients who do not reduce their food intake will gain weight thus increasing insulin resistance, risk for heart disease and other obesity-related complications (19,20).

3. Definition of adherence

Contemporary perspectives on diabetes care accord a central role to patient self-care, or self-management. Self-care implies that the patient actively monitors and responds to changing environmental and biological conditions by making adaptive adjustments in the different aspects of diabetes treatment in order to maintain adequate metabolic control and reduce the probability of complications (21). The self-care behaviours involved in achieving adequate metabolic control and avoiding long-term complications are: home glucose monitoring (in blood or urine); adjustment of food intake, especially of carbohydrates, to meet daily needs and match available insulin; administration of medication (insulin or oral hypoglycaemic agents); regular physical activity; foot care; regular medical monitoring visits, and other behaviours (i.e. dental care, appropriate clothing, etc.) that may vary depending on the type of diabetes (18).

Against this background of illness-related demands, adherence is conceptualized as the active, voluntary involvement of the patient in the management of his or her disease, by following a mutually agreed course of treatment and sharing responsibility between the patient and health care providers (22). Hentinen (23) described adherence to self-care as an active, responsible and flexible process of self-management, in which the patient strives to achieve good health by working in close collaboration with health care staff, instead of simply following rigidly prescribed rules. Other terms have been proposed such as "collaborative diabetes management" *(24)*, "patient empowerment" *(25)* or "self-care behaviour management" *(23,26–28)*. Another important concept is "inadvertent nonadherence" which occurs when a patient believes he or she is adhering to the recommended treatment but, through errors in knowledge or skill, is not doing so *(29)*.

4. Prevalence of adherence to recommendations for diabetes treatment

From the study of adherence to treatments for diabetes, it is apparently important to assess the level of adherence to each component of the treatment regimen independently (i.e. self-monitoring of blood glucose, administration of insulin or oral hypoglycaemic agents, diet, physical activity, foot care and other self-care practices) instead of using a single measure to assess adherence to the overall treatment. This is because there appears to be little correlation between adherence to the separate self-care behaviours, suggesting that adherence is not a unidimensional construct *(21,30)*. This finding has been reported for both type 1 and type 2 diabetes *(31)*. Furthermore, there appear to be different relationships between adherence and metabolic control for persons with different types of diabetes *(32)*. Consequently, the following section on adherence rates has been organized to reflect these two issues. First there is a discussion of adherence to each element of the regimen; this is followed by an analysis of adherence by diabetes type.

A. Adherence to treatment for type 1 diabetes

Self-monitoring of glucose. The extent of adherence to prescribed self-monitoring of glucose levels in blood varies widely, depending on the frequency or aspect assessed in the study. For example, in a sample of children and adolescents with type 1 diabetes *(33)*, only 26% of study participants reported monitoring glucose levels as recommended (3–4 times daily), compared to approximately 40% of the adults with type 1 diabetes *(34)*. Similar findings were reported in a Finnish study ($n = 213$; patients aged 17–65 years), in which 20% of the study participants monitored their blood glucose as recommended, and 21% of respondents made daily or almost daily adjustments to their insulin dosage according to the results of self-monitoring of blood glucose. Only 6% reported never performing the prescribed blood glucose tests *(35)*. A study conducted in the United States replicated the latter result in patients with type 1 diabetes (mean age = 30 years), of whom 7% reported *never* testing their glucose levels *(21)*.

Other studies have assessed adherence based on incorrect performance (intentional or unintentional) of the component behaviours involved in glucose monitoring in urine or blood. One study reported that up to 80% of adolescents made significant mistakes when estimating glucose concentrations in urine *(36)*. Between 30% and 60% made errors in the timing procedures involved in self-monitoring of blood glucose *(37)*. Others inaccurately reported concentrations; up to 75% may under-report actual mean concentrations of blood glucose, and up to 40% have been found to over-report or to invent phantom values *(38)*. Other studies have found that between 40% and 60% of patients fabricated results *(39,40)* and 18% failed to record their results *(40)*. In recent years, the development of blood glucose meters with electronic memory has made it more difficult, though not impossible, for patients to fabricate the results of blood-glucose monitoring.

Administration of insulin. The prevalence of adherence to insulin administration varies widely. In a study conducted in Finland *(35)* most of the respondents reported adhering to insulin injections as scheduled either daily (84%) or almost daily (15%). Other studies have framed the adherence question differently. Rates for "never missing a shot" varied from 92% in a sample of young adults *(21)* to 53% in a sample of children *(41)*; while 25% of adolescents reported "missing insulin shots within 10 days before a clinic visit" *(42)*.

A study conducted by Wing et al. *(37)* assessed the quality of performance of insulin administration (intentional or unintentional errors). The use of unhygienic injections was noted in 80% of patients and the administration of incorrect doses of insulin in 58%. In studies assessing the intentional omission of insulin to control weight, Polonsky et al. *(43)* reported that 31% of study participants (n = 341; female patients aged 13–60 years) admitted to intentional omission of insulin, but only 9% reported frequent omission to control weight. More recently, Bryden et al. *(44)* reported that 30% of female adolescents (but none of the males in the sample) admitted under-using insulin to control weight.

Diet. The results of research on adherence to prescribed dietary recommendations have been inconsistent. In studies by Carvajal et al. *(45)* in Cuba, and Wing et al. *(37)* in the United States, 70–75% of study participants reported not adhering to dietary recommendations, but in a study in Finland by Toljamo et al. *(35)*, adherence to dietary recommendations was high: 70% of participants reported always or often having a regular main meal, while only 8% reported always having irregular mealtimes. In answer to questions regarding the foods prescribed, over half of the participants reported assessing both the content and amount of food that they ate daily (48%) while 14% of the respondents did not evaluate their food at all. Christensen et al. reported similar findings *(46)*: 60% of study participants (n = 97) adhered to the number and timing of planned meals, while only 10% of patients adhered to planned exchanges, 90% of the time.

Physical activity and other self-care measures. Literature on the extent of adherence to prescribed recommendations for physical activity among patients with type 1 diabetes is scarce. One study conducted in Finland indicated that two-thirds of study participants (n = 213) took regular daily exercise (35%) or almost daily exercise (30%), while 10% took no exercise at all *(35)*. In the same study, only 25% of study participants reported taking care of their feet daily or almost daily, while 16% reported never taking care of their feet as recommended *(35)*.

B. Adherence rates for type 2 diabetes

Glucose monitoring. In a study conducted to assess patterns of self-monitoring of blood glucose in northern California, United States, 67% of patients with type 2 diabetes reported *not* performing self-monitoring of blood glucose as frequently as recommended (i.e. once daily for type 2 diabetes treated pharmacologically) *(34)*. Similar findings were reported in a study conducted in India, in which only 23% of study participants reported performing glucose monitoring at home *(47)*.

Administration of medication. Among patients receiving their medication from community pharmacies (n = 91), adherence to oral hypoglycaemic agents was 75%. Dose omissions represented the most prevalent form of nonadherence; however, more than one-third of the patients took more doses than prescribed. This over-medication was observed more frequently in those patients prescribed a once-daily dose *(48)*. Similar adherence rates of between 70 and 80% were reported from the United States in a study of oral hypoglycaemic agents in a sample of patients whose health insurance paid for prescribed drugs *(49)*. Dailey et al. *(50)* studied 37 431 Medicaid-funded patients in the United States, and used pharmacy records to show that patients with type 2 diabetes averaged about 130 days per year of continuous drug therapy, and that at the end of 1 year, only 15% of the patients who had been prescribed a single oral medication were still taking it regularly.

Diet. In a study conducted in India, dietary prescriptions were followed regularly by only 37% of patients *(47)*, while in a study in the United States about half (52%) followed a meal plan *(51)*. Anderson & Gustafson *(52)* reported good-to-excellent adherence in 70% of patients who had been prescribed a high-carbohydrate, high-fibre diet. Wing et al. *(53)* showed that patients with type 2 diabetes lost less weight than their nondiabetic spouses and that the difference was mainly due to poor adherence to the prescribed diet by the diabetic patients. Adherence to dietary protocols may depend upon the nature of the treatment objective (e.g. weight loss, reduction of dietary fat or increased fibre intake).

Physical activity. Several studies have reported on adherence to prescribed physical activity. For example, in a study in Canada of a sample of patients with type 2 diabetes randomly selected from provincial health records, few respondents participated in informal (37%) or organized (7.7%) physical activity programmes *(54)*. A survey in the United States found that only 26% of respondents followed a physical activity plan *(51)*. A study assessing the attitudes and adherence of patients who had completed outpatient diabetes counselling observed that only 52% exercised on three or more days per week after the counselling programme was completed *(55)*.

C. Adherence to treatment for gestational diabetes

One study was found that had assessed adherence to treatment for gestational diabetes. Forty-nine pregnant women with pre-existing (overt) diabetes (68% with type 1 and 32% with type 2 diabetes) were assessed, using self-report, on their adherence to a number of self-care tasks on three occasions during pregnancy (mid-second, early third and late third trimester) *(56)*. In general, the participants reported being adherent. However, there was considerable variation across different regimen components: 74-79% of women reported always following dietary recommendations, compared to 86-88% who followed the recommendations for insulin administration, 85-89% who followed the recommendations for managing insulin reactions and 94-96% who followed those for glucose testing.

5. Correlates of adherence

Variables that have been considered to be correlates of various adherence behaviours in diabetes can be organized into four clusters:

– treatment and disease characteristics;

– intra-personal factors;

– inter-personal factors; and

– environmental factors.

A. Treatment and disease characteristics

Three elements of treatment and of the disease itself have been associated with adherence: complexity of treatment, duration of disease and delivery of care (see also Table 4).

In general, the *more complex the treatment regimen*, the less likely the patient will be to follow it. Indicators of treatment complexity include frequency of the self-care behaviour – i.e. the number of times per day a behaviour needs to be performed by the patient. Adherence to oral hypoglycaemic agents has been associated with frequency of dosing. Higher adherence levels were reported by patients required to take less frequent doses (a once-daily dose), compared to those prescribed more frequent doses (three times daily) *(48)*. Dailey et al. *(50)* showed that patients prescribed a single medication had better short-term and long-term adherence rates than patients prescribed two or more medications.

Duration of disease appears to have a negative relationship with adherence: the longer a patient has had diabetes, the less likely he or she is to be adherent to treatment. Glasgow et al. *(21)* studied a sample of patients with type 1 diabetes (mean age = 28 years), and found that level of physical activity was associated with duration of disease. Patients who had had diabetes for 10 years or less reported greater energy expenditure in recreational physical activities, and exercising on more days per week, than those with a longer history of diabetes. Patients with a longer history of diabetes also reported eating more inappropriate foods, consuming a greater proportion of saturated fats and following their diets plans less well. More recently, in a study conducted in both Polish and American children with type 1 diabetes

(41), duration of disease was also associated with adherence to insulin administration, as children with a longer history of diabetes were more likely to forget their insulin injections than children who had been diagnosed more recently.

Delivery of care for diabetes can vary from intensive treatment delivered by a multidisciplinary diabetes team, to outpatient care delivered by a primary care provider. Yawn et al. (57) observed interactions between patients and providers in a family practice setting and reported that patients with diabetes seen specifically for their diabetes received more counselling on diet and adherence than patients with diabetes seen for an acute illness. Kern & Mainous *(58)* found that although physicians preferred to follow a planned, systematic strategy for treating diabetes, acute illness and failure of patients to adhere forced them to spend less time on diabetes care.

Adherence can also be affected by the setting in which care is received. Piette *(59)* examined the problems experienced by patients in accessing care in two public health settings in the United States and found that the cost of care was a major barrier to access, especially for patients in a community treatment setting. Perceived barriers to access to care were also associated with poor metabolic control.

B. Intra-personal factors

Seven important variables have been associated with adherence: age, gender, self-esteem, self-efficacy, stress, depression and alcohol abuse.

Age of the patient has been associated with adherence to physical activity regimens in a sample of patients with type 1 diabetes *(21)*. Compared to younger participants, patients over 25 years of age reported exercising on fewer days per week, and spending less time (and expending fewer calories) in recreational physical activities. There were no associations reported between age and adherence to other self-care measures.

Age has also been associated with adherence to insulin administration in a study of adolescents with type 1 diabetes. The investigators found that older adolescents were more likely to mismanage their insulin (missing injections) than their younger counterparts *(42)*. In a study assessing adherence to self-monitoring of blood glucose, younger adolescents reported monitoring their blood glucose concentrations more frequently than did the older ones *(60)*. Older adults may also practice better self-management than younger adults *(61)*.

Gender has also been associated with adherence. The men in a sample of patients with type 1 diabetes *(21)* were found to be more physically active than the women, but they also consumed more calories, ate more inappropriate foods and had lower levels of adherence as assessed using a composite measure of diet.

Self-esteem has been associated with adherence to self-management of diabetes among patients with type 1 diabetes. High levels of self-esteem were related to high levels of adherence to physical activity regimens, adjustment of insulin doses and dental self-care *(62)*. Murphy-Bennett, Thompson & Morris *(63)* found that lower self-esteem in adolescents with type 1 diabetes was associated with less frequent testing of blood glucose.

Self-efficacy has been studied in relation to adherence to prescribed treatments for diabetes. In a combined sample of patients with type 1 and type 2 diabetes in Canada *(64)*, a measure of diabetes-specific self-efficacy beliefs was found to be the strongest predictor of energy expenditure suggesting a positive relationship between self-efficacy and adherence to prescribed physical activity. Senecal, Nouwen & White *(65)* reported that beliefs in self-efficacy were a strong predictor of adherence and that both self-efficacy and autonomy predicted life satisfaction. Ott et al. *(66)* found that self-efficacy was a predictor of adherence to diabetes care behaviours in adolescents with type 1 diabetes. Aljasem et al. *(67)* showed that self-efficacy beliefs predicted adherence to a prescribed regimen in 309 adults with type 2 diabetes after controlling for health beliefs and perceptions of barriers.

Stress and emotional problems are also correlated with adherence. Fewer minor stressors were associated with higher levels of adherence to insulin administration and diet in women with gestational diabetes *(56,68)*. In a study using a diabetes-specific stress scale in a combined sample of adults with type 1 and type 2 diabetes *(69)*, stress was found to be significantly associated with two aspects of the diet regimen (diet amount and diet type). However, no associations were found between stress and adherence to physical activity regimens or glucose testing in this sample. Peyrot et al. *(70)* reported that psychosocial stress was associated with poor adherence to a prescribed regimen and poor metabolic control in a mixed group of patients with type 1 and type 2 diabetes. Mollema et al. *(71)* reported that patients who had an extreme fear of insulin injections or self-monitoring of blood glucose had lower levels of adherence and higher levels of emotional distress. Schlundt, Stetson & Plant *(72)* grouped patients with type 1 diabetes according to the problems they encountered in adhering to prescribed diets and found that two of the groups of patients – emotional eaters and diet-bingers – had adherence problems related to negative emotions such as stress and depression.

Depression. The incidence of *depression* has been observed to be twice as high among persons with diabetes than in the general population *(73)*. Patients with depression are more likely to experience complications of diabetes *(74)*, have worse glycaemic control *(75)*, and be less adherent to self-care behaviours than patients who are not depressed. Depression is also associated with higher costs of medical care in patients with diabetes *(76)*.

Alcohol abuse. Patterns of alcohol use have been related to the quality of diabetes self-management. Johnson, Bazargan & Bing *(77)*, studied 392 patients with type 2 diabetes from ethnic minority groups in Los Angeles, CA, and found that alcohol consumption within the previous 30 days was associated with poor adherence to diet, self-monitoring of blood glucose, oral medications and appointment-keeping. Cox et al. *(78)* examined alcohol use in 154 older men with diabetes and found that greater alcohol use was associated with poorer adherence to insulin injections.

C. Inter-personal factors

Two important inter-personal factors: the quality of the relationship between patients and providers of care, and social support, have been found to correlate with adherence. Good communication between patient and provider has been related to improved adherence. Among patients with type 2 diabetes, adherence to administration of oral hypoglycaemic agents and glucose monitoring were significantly worse in patients who rated their communication with their care provider as poor *(79)*.

Social support has been the subject of much research. Greater social support was found to be associated with better levels of adherence to dietary recommendations and insulin administration in women with gestational diabetes *(68)*. Parental involvement, as a measure of social support, has also been associated with adherence to blood glucose monitoring. Adolescents and children with type 1 diabetes, who experienced greater parental involvement with their blood glucose monitoring, reported higher levels of daily checks of blood sugar concentrations *(60)*. McCaul et al. *(21)* followed a sample of adolescents and adults with type 1 diabetes. For both adults and adolescents disease-specific social support was associated with better adherence to insulin administration and glucose testing. For the adolescent group only, general family support was associated with adherence to insulin administration and glucose testing. The study found no association between any of the social support measures and adherence to diet and physical activity regimens. Other studies have shown a relationship between poor social support and inadequate self-management of diabetes *(80–84)*.

D. Environmental factors

Two environmental factors – *high-risk situations and environmental systems* – have been linked to poor adherence in patients with diabetes. Self-care behaviours occur in the context of a continually changing series of environmental situations at home, at work, in public, etc., which are associated with different demands and priorities. As their circumstances change, patients are challenged to adjust and maintain their self-care behaviours. Patients are frequently called upon to choose between giving attention to diabetes self-management or to some other life priority. Situations associated with poor adherence have been called "high-risk" situations *(85)*.

Schlundt, Stetson & Plant *(72)* created a taxonomy of high-risk situations that posed difficulties for patients following diet prescriptions. The situations included: overeating in response to people, place and emotions; situations associated with under-eating, and difficulty in integrating food intake according to social context, time of day and place. Schlundt et al. *(82)* described 10 high-risk situations for poor dietary adherence that included social pressure to eat; being alone and feeling bored; interpersonal conflicts, and eating at school, social events or holidays. Schlundt et al. *(83)* identified 12 categories of high-risk dietary situations in adults with type 1 and type 2 diabetes: these included resisting temptation, eating out, time pressure, competing priorities and social events. Other studies have also shown that environmental barriers are predictive of adherence to various aspects of diabetes self-care *(34,67,86)*.

Many environmental factors that influence behaviour operate on a larger scale than the immediate situation confronting a person *(87)*. These environmental systems include economic, agricultural, political, health care, geographical, ecological and cultural systems *(88)*. The large-scale environmental changes that occurred in the twentieth century created the current epidemics of obesity and type 2 diabetes *(89–91)*. These changes included increased availability of inexpensive fast foods high in fat, salt and calories *(92)*, and the mechanization of transport systems *(93,94)*. Changes in economic and political systems have allowed women to move into the workforce, but these same changes have altered the composition of families and the way in which families deal with food selection and preparation *(95,96)*. Large corporations spend billions of dollars each year on marketing foods high in fat and calories *(97)*. Increasing segments of the population spend many hours per day in sedentary activities. These activities have been linked to obesity in both children and adults *(98–101)* and to the risk of developing type 2 diabetes *(102)*.

Some authors have described the current environment as "toxic" to healthy lifestyles *(103,104)*. The incidences of both obesity and diabetes are rapidly increasing in developing nations and are likely to be associated with urbanization, mechanized transportation and widespread changes in food supply. The same factors that encourage sedentary lifestyles and the over-consumption of food, and lead to obesity and diabetes, probably also make it difficult for people who do develop diabetes to adhere to best-practice protocols.

Many people in developed nations, including the poor and members of ethnic minority groups, have to some degree been bypassed by the economic prosperity of the twentieth century. It is these groups that have been most adversely affected by the environmental changes that lead to disparities in health status *(105,106)*. Even living in a poor community can contribute to poor health outcomes *(107)*.

Given the powerful influence of these larger social factors, it is important to avoid over-attributing the responsibility for adherence to patient-related factors or to health care providers *(108)*. A patient's ability to manage his or her behaviour, achieve tight metabolic control and prevent the long-term complications of diabetes is determined by a host of intra-personal, inter-personal and environmental factors that interact in ways that are not yet understood *(27,109)*.

6. Interventions

Almost any intervention that is designed to improve metabolic control in diabetes or to reduce the probability of acute or chronic complications does so by influencing patient self-care or self-management behaviours. Early efforts focused on patient education *(110)*, but more recently, the importance of psychological and behavioural interventions has been stressed as a result of the growing recognition that knowledge alone is insufficient to produce significant changes in behaviour *(111)*.

Elasy et al. *(112)* developed a taxonomy for describing educational interventions for patients with diabetes based on a thorough review and analysis of the literature published between 1990 and 1999 which revealed the great diversity of interventions employed to improve self-management of diabetes.

Brown conducted a meta-analysis of studies that had tested interventions to improve self-management of diabetes, and found a recent trend towards combining patient education with behavioural intervention strategies. Combining behavioural techniques with the provision of information was found to be more effective than interventions that provided only information. In general, the literature supports the conclusion that diabetes education results in at least short-term improvements in adherence and metabolic control *(113)*, but more research is needed to learn which interventions work best with different types of patient and for specific behaviours *(111, 112)*.

Beyond interventions that focus on individual patients, two other approaches can be used to improve the self-management of diabetes – interventions that target health providers and interventions at the community or systems level. Several studies have reported that physicians and other health care providers deliver less-than-optimal care to patients with diabetes. There have been several corresponding studies of attempts to modify professional behaviours and attitudes in ways that might lead to improved patient outcomes. Kinmonth et al. *(114)* trained nurses to provide patient-centred diabetes care, and showed that patient satisfaction was improved although metabolic parameters were not. Olivarius et al. *(115)* in a study of physicians in Denmark used goal-setting, feedback and continuing education and found that the patients of the physicians who had received this intervention had improved metabolic parameters when compared to the patients of the physicians in the control group. In a series of studies, Pichert and colleagues showed that a training programme for nurses and dieticians improved their education and problem-solving skills *(116–118)*. Other studies of training for health care providers have not documented any changes in patient behaviour or metabolic control *(119)*.

Systems interventions can change the way in which environmental determinants influence the self-management behaviour of patients with diabetes. Systems interventions can focus on economic determinants, such as changing Medicare policy to pay for medical nutrition therapy *(120)*. Health care delivery systems are also a target for intervention by means of changing programmes, policies or procedures to improve quality of care and outcomes for patients. For example, Hardy et al. *(121)* used telephone reminders to patients to improve appointment-keeping behaviour.

The chronic care model is a systems approach to improving the quality of care for patients with chronic diseases such as diabetes *(122)*. Feifer *(123)* conducted a cross-sectional analysis of nine community-based primary care practices and showed that providing system supports to health providers resulted in better care of patients with diabetes. Wagner et al. *(124)* modified the way in which care was provided to patients with diabetes in primary care clinics and showed that these systemic changes resulted in better achievement of treatment goals, improved metabolic control, more time spent on diabetes education and enhanced patient satisfaction. Wagner et al. *(125)* intervened using a continuous quality care approach combined with the chronic care model in 23 health care organizations and documented improvements in diabetes care and patient outcomes in many of them.

Clearly, the solution to the problem of poor adherence must involve a combination of approaches that include intensive efforts to modify the behaviour of individuals with diabetes together with intelligent efforts to make changes in the larger environmental systems that shape and modify behaviours *(126)*.

Table 4 Factors affecting adherence to therapy for the control of diabetes and interventions for improving it, listed by the five dimensions and the interventions used to improve adherence

Diabetes	Factors affecting adherence	Interventions to improve adherence
Socioeconomic-related factors	(–) Cost of care *(59)*; patients aged over 25 years *(21)* (adherence to physical activity); older adolescents (insulin administration) *(42)*; older adolescents (SMBG) *(60)*; male (adherence to diet) *(21)*; female (adherence to physical activity) *(21)*; environmental high-risk situations *(72,82,83,85–89,92,93,95,98,102,103,105)* (+) Patients aged less than 25 years *(21)* (adherence to physical activity); younger adolescents (insulin administration) *(42)*; younger adolescents (SMBG) *(60)*; male (adherence to physical activity) *(21)*; female (adherence to diet) *(21)*; social support *(21,68)*; family support *(21)*	Mobilization of community-based organizations; assessment of social needs *(21,68)*; family preparedness *(21)*
Health care team/health system-related factors	(–) Poor relationship between patient and physician *(79)*	Multidisciplinary care; training of health professionals on adherence *(114,116)*; identification of the treatment goals and development of strategies to meet them; continuing education; continuous monitoring and reassessment of treatment *(115)*; systems interventions: health insurance for nutrition therapy *(120)*, telephone reminders to patients *(121)*, chronic care models *(122–125)*
Condition-related factors	(–) Depression *(73)*; duration of disease *(21,41)*	Education on use of medicines *(110,113)*
Therapy-related factors	(–) Complexity of treatment *(48,50)* (+) Less frequent dose *(48)*; monotherapy with simple dosing schedules *(50)*; frequency of the self-care behaviour *(48,50)*	Patient self-management *(112)*; simplification of regimens *(48,50)*; education on use of medicines *(110,112,113)*
Patient-related factors	(–) Depression *(75)*; stress and emotional problems *(70–72)*; alcohol abuse *(77)* (+) Positive self-esteem *(62,63)* /self-efficacy *(64–67,78)*	Behavioural and motivational interventions *(111,112)*; assessment of psychological needs *(111)*

SMBG, Self-monitoring of blood glucose; (+) factors having a positive effect on adherence; (–) factors having a negative effect on adherence.

7. Methodological and conceptual issues in research on adherence to treatment for diabetes

In a review of methodological and conceptual issues relevant to measuring adherence in patients with diabetes, Johnson *(127)* suggested that the prevalence of adherence may vary across the different components of the diabetes regimen and the patient's lifespan, during the course of the disease, as well as between populations of patients with diabetes (i.e. type 1 and type 2). Johnson also noted the conceptual problems encountered in defining and measuring adherence including:

- the absence of explicit adherence standards against which a patient's behaviour can be compared;

- inadvertent nonadherence attributable to miscommunication between patient and provider and deficits in the knowledge or skills of the patient;

- the behavioural complexity of the diabetes regimen; and

- the confounding of compliance with diabetes control.

Furthermore, the multiplicity of measurements used to assess adherence (i.e. health status indicators; provider ratings; behavioural observations; permanent products, and patient self-reports, including behaviour ratings, diaries and 24-hour recall interviews) also makes comparison of studies troublesome. Johnson concluded that a measurement method should be selected on the basis of reliability, validity, non-reactivity, sensitivity to the complexity of the diabetes regimen behaviours and measurement-independence from the indicators of health status. Glasgow et al. *(30)* also noted the methodological shortcomings of studies on diabetes self-care correlates, the lack of clear conceptualizations and the failure to differentiate between regimen adherence, self-care behaviour and metabolic control, as well as the empirical–atheoretical nature of many studies that lacked a comprehensive model or theory.

The present review of studies reported from 1980 to 2001, has revealed that research on adherence to treatment for diabetes yields some inconsistent findings. These inconsistent results may have several causes including variability in:

- research designs (e.g. longitudinal as opposed to cross-sectional studies) and study instruments;

- sampling frames employed for study recruitment;

- the use of general measures (e.g. general stress) as opposed to more specific ones (e.g. diabetes-specific stress);

- sample sizes (in some studies the small samples used decreased the likelihood of detecting significant associations between the variables); and

- lack of control of potentially confounding variables.

8. Conclusions

Poor adherence to treatment is very prevalent in patients with diabetes, and varies according to the type of nonadherence being measured, and across the range of self-care behaviours that are components of treatment. Thus prevalence rates should be assessed by type of behaviour. In addition, prevalence rates may vary by diabetes subtype (i.e. type 1, type 2 or gestational), and also appear to be influenced by other factors such as age, gender and level of complexity of the treatment regimen. The rate of adherence, or the variables affecting adherence, may vary according to nationality, culture or subculture. Therefore, these factors should also be taken into account when assessing the prevalence of adherence in populations of patients with diabetes.

The lack of standard measurements prevents comparison being made between studies and across populations. Much work needs to be done to develop standardized, reliable and valid measurement tools.

Data from developing countries concerning the prevalence and correlates of adherence in patients with diabetes are particularly scarce. The pressing need to undertake more research in developing countries is emphasized by the WHO estimates indicating that by 2025 the largest absolute increase in prevalence rates of diabetes worldwide will occur in developing countries. Patients and providers of care in developing nations face additional barriers to achieving adequate diabetes self-care because of poverty, inadequate systems for delivering health care, and a host of other priorities that compete for national and individual attention.

More research is needed on adherence in women with gestational diabetes, and in study populations that include minorities and ethnic groups. Also, cross-cultural comparison studies should be encouraged. However, when making comparisons between different ethnic groups or countries, a number of aspects should be taken into account and controlled for, including types of health care system, health care coverage and socioeconomic macro- and micro-factors, as well as language and cultural differences. Adequate translation and validation of study measurements are required when using questionnaires developed in another country.

It is also important to point out not only the large number of factors that affect adherence behaviours in patients with diabetes, but also that the complex interactions that take place between them affect both adherence and metabolic control. Multivariate approaches to data are required to obtain more accurate representations of the relevant predictors and correlates.

9. References

1. The Centers for Disease Control and Prevention. *National diabetes fact sheet: National estimates and general information on diabetes in the United States.* Revised edition. Atlanta, GA, US Department of Health and Human Services, Centers for Disease Control and Prevention, 1998.

2. King H. WHO and the International Diabetes Federation: Regional Partners. *Bulletin of the World Health Organization*, 1999, 77:954.

3. King H, Aubert RE, Herman WH. Global burden of diabetes 1995–2025: Prevalence, numerical estimates and projections. *Diabetes Care*, 1998, 21:1414–1431.

4. Diabetes fact sheet. Geneva, World Health Organization, 1999 (available on the Internet at http://www.who.int/inf-fs/en/fact138.html).

5. Chronic disease prevention: The impact of diabetes. Centers for Disease Control and Prevention, 2000 (available on the Internet at http://www.cdc.gov/nccdph/diabetes).

6. Okhubo Y et al. Intensive insulin therapy prevents the progression of diabetes microvascular complications in Japanese patients with non-insulin dependent diabetes mellitus: A randomized prospective six year study. *Diabetes Research & Clinical Practice*, 1995, 28:103–117.

7. The Diabetes Control and Complications Trial Research Group. The effect of intensive treatment of diabetes on the development and progression of long-term complications in insulin-dependent diabetes mellitus. *New England Journal of Medicine*, 1993, 329:977–986.

8. Litzelman DK, Slemenda CW, Langefel CD. Reduction of lower clinical abnormalities in patients with non-insulin-dependent diabetes mellitus. *Annals of Internal Medicine*, 1993, 119:36–41.

9. Ferris FL. How effective are treatments for diabetic retinopathy. *Journal of the American Medical Association*, 1993, 269:1290–1291.

10. American Diabetes Association. Economic consequences of diabetes mellitus in the U.S.– 1997. *Diabetes Care*, 1998, 21:296–309.

11. Diabetes fact sheet. Geneva, World Health Organization, 1999 (available on the Internet at http://www.who.int/inf-fs/en/fact236.html).

12. American Diabetes Association. Report of the Expert Committee on the Diagnosis and Classification of Diabetes Mellitus. *Diabetes Care*, 2002, 25:5–20.

13. Laron-Kenet T et al. Mortality of patients with childhood onset (0–17 years) Type I diabetes in Israel: a population-based study. *Diabetologia*, 2001, 44:B81–B86.

14. Podar T et al. Mortality in patients with childhood-onset type 1 diabetes in Finland, Estonia, and Lithuania: follow-up of nationwide cohorts. *Diabetes Care*, 2000, 23:290–294.

15. Flood RG, Chiang VW. Rate and prediction of infection in children with diabetic ketoacidosis. *American Journal of Emergency Medicine*, 2001, 19:270–273.

16. Morris AD et al. Adherence to insulin treatment, glycaemic control, and ketoacidosis in insulin-dependent diabetes mellitus. The DARTS/MEMO Collaboration. Diabetes Audit and Research in Tayside Scotland. Medicines Monitoring Unit. *Lancet*, 1997, 350:1505–1510.

17. American Diabetes Association. Gestational diabetes mellitus. *Diabetes Care*, 2002, 25:94–96.

18. American Diabetes Association. Standards of medical care for patients with diabetes mellitus. *Diabetes Care*, 2002, 25:213–229.

19. Zinman B. Glucose control in type 1 diabetes: from conventional to intensive therapy. *Clinical Cornerstone*, 1998, 1:29–38.

20. Gaster B, Hirsch IB. The effects of improved glycemic control on complications in type 2 diabetes. *Archives of Internal Medicine*, 1998, 158:134–140.

21. Glasgow RE, McCaul KD, Schafer LC. Self care behaviors and glycemic control in Type 1 diabetes. *Journal of Chronic Diseases*, 1987, 40:399–412.

22. Barofsky I. Compliance, adherence and the therapeutic alliance: Steps in the development of self care. *Social Science and Medicine*, 1978, 12:369–376.

23. Hentinen M. Hoitoon sitoutuminen. [Adherence to treatment.] *Pro Nursing Vuosikirja [Pro Nursing Annual Book]*, 1987, Julkaisusarja A 1 [Publication Series A 1]:78–82.

24. Von Korff M et al. Collaborative management of chronic illness. *Annals of Internal Medicine*, 1997, 127:1097–1102.

25. Anold M et al. Guidelines for facilitating a patient empowerment program. *Diabetes Education*, 1995, 21:308–312.

26. Glasgow RE, Wilson W, McCaul KD. Regimen adherence: A problematic construct in diabetes research. *Diabetes Care*, 1985, 8:300–301.

27. Glasgow RE, Anderson RA. In diabetes care, moving from compliance to adherence is not enough. Something entirely different is needed. *Diabetes Care*, 1999, 22:2090–2092.

28. Anderson RM, Funnell MM. Compliance and adherence are dysfunctional concepts in diabetes care. *Diabetes Educator*, 2000, 26:597–604.

29. Johnson SB. Knowledge, attitudes and behavior: Correlates of health in childhood diabetes. *Clinical Psychology Review*, 1984, 4:503–524.

30. Glasgow RE et al. Diabetes-specific social learning variables and self care behaviors among persons with type II diabetes. *Health Psychology*, 1989, 8:285–303.

31. Orme CM, Binik YM. Consistency of adherence across regimen demands. *Health Psychology*, 1989, 8:27–43.

32. Wilson W et al. Psychosocial predictors of self care behaviours (compliance) and glycemic control in non insulin dependent diabetes mellitus. *Diabetes Care*, 1986, 9:614–622.

33. Wing RR et al. Frequency and accuracy of self-monitoring of blood glucose in children: relationship to glycemic control. *Diabetes Care*, 1985, 8:214–218.

34. Karter AJ et al. Self-monitoring of blood glucose: language and financial barriers in a managed care population with diabetes. *Diabetes Care*, 2000, 23:477–483.

35. Toljamo M, Hentinen M. Adherence to self care and glycaemic control among people with insulin dependent diabetes mellitus. *Journal of Advanced Nursing*, 2001, 34:780–786.

36. Epstein LH et al. Measurement and modification of the accuracy of the determinations of urine glucose concentration. *Diabetes Care*, 1980, 3:535–536.

37. Wing RR et al. Behavioral skills in self-monitoring of blood glucose: relationship to accuracy. *Diabetes Care*, 1986, 9:330–333.

38. Mazze RS et al. Reliability of blood glucose monitoring by patients with diabetes mellitus. *American Journal of Medicine*, 1984, 77:211–217.

39. Dorchy H, Roggemans M. Improvement of the compliance with blood glucose monitoring in young insulin-dependent diabetes mellitus patients by the Sensorlink system. *Diabetes Research and Clinical Practice*, 1997, 36:77–82.

40. Wilson DP, Endres RK. Compliance with blood glucose monitoring in children with type 1 diabetes mellitus. *Journal of Pediatrics*, 1986, 108:1022–1024.

41. Jarosz-Chobot P et al. Self care of young diabetics in practice. *Medical Science Monitor*, 2000, 6:129–132.

42. Weissberg-Benchell J et al. Adolescent diabetes management and mismanagement. *Diabetes Care*, 1995, 18:77–82.

43. Polonsky WH et al. Insulin omission in women with IDDM. *Diabetes Care*, 1994, 17:1178–1185.

44. Bryden K et al. Eating habits, body weight and insulin misuse. *Diabetes Care*, 1999, 22:1959–1960.

45. Carvajal F et al. [Compliance with diet of 45 children and adolescents with insulin-dependent diabetes mellitus.] [Spanish] *Revista de la Asociación Latinoamericana de Diabetes*, 1998, 6:84.

46. Christensen NK et al. Quantitative assessment of dietary adherence in patients with insulin-dependent diabetes mellitus. *Diabetes Care*, 1983, 6:245–250.

47. Shobhana R et al. Patient adherence to diabetes treatment. *Journal of the Association of Physicians of India*, 1999, 47:1173–1175.

48. Paes AH, Bakker A, Soe-Agnie CJ. Impact of dosage frequency on patient compliance. *Diabetes Care*, 1997, 20:1512–1517.

49. Boccuzzi SJ et al. Utilization of oral hypoglycemic agents in a drug-insured U.S. population. *Diabetes Care*, 2001, 24:1411–1415.

50. Dailey G, Kim MS, Lian JF. Patient compliance and persistence with antihyperglycemic drug regimens: Evaluation of a Medicaid patient population with type 2 diabetes mellitus. *Clinical Therapeutics*, 2001, 23:1311–1320.

51. Schultz J et al. A comparison of views of individuals with type 2 diabetes mellitus and diabetes educators about barriers to diet and exercise. *Journal of Health Communication*, 2001, 6:99–115.

52. Anderson JW, Gustafson NJ. Adherence to high-carbohydrate, high-fiber diets. *Diabetes Educator*, 1998, 15:429–434.

53. Wing RR et al. Type II diabetic subjects lose less weight than their overweight nondiabetic spouses. *Diabetes Care*, 1987, 10:563–566.

54. Searle MS, Ready AE. Survey of exercise and dietary knowledge and behaviour in persons with type II diabetes. *Canadian Journal of Public Health*, 1991, 82:344–348.

55. Swift CS et al. Attitudes and beliefs about exercise among persons with non-insulin dependent diabetes. *Diabetes Educator*, 1995, 21:533–540.

56. Ruggieron L et al. Self reported compliance with diabetes self management during pregnancy. *International Journal of Psychiatry in Medicine*, 1993, 23:195–207.

57. Yawn B et al. Is diabetes treated as an acute or chronic illness in community family practice? *Diabetes Care*, 2001, 24:1390–1396.

58. Kern DH, Mainous AG. Disease management for diabetes among family physicians and general internists. Opportunism or planned care? *Family Medicine*, 2001, 33:621–625.

59. Piette JD. Perceived access problems among patients with diabetes in two public systems of care. *Journal of General Internal Medicine*, 2000, 15:797–804.

60. Anderson B et al. Parental involvement in diabetes management tasks: Relationships to blood glucose monitoring adherence and metabolic control in young adolescents with insulin dependent diabetes mellitus. *Journal of Pediatrics*, 1997, 130:257–265.

61. Stetson B et al. Barriers to diet and exercise differ by age in adults with type 2 diabetes. *Annals of Behavioral Medicine*, 2000, 22:S197.

62. Kneckt MC et al. Self esteem adherence to diabetes and dental self care regimens. *Journal of Clinical Periodontology*, 2001, 28:175–180.

63. Murphy-Bennett LM, Thompson RJ, Morris MA. Adherence behavior among adolescents with type I insulin dependent diabetes mellitus: The role of cognitive appraisal processes. *Journal of Pediatric Psychology*, 1997, 22:811–825.

64. Plotnikoff RC, Brez S, Hotz S. Exercise behavior in a community sample with diabetes: Understanding the determinants of exercise behavioral change. *Diabetes Educator*, 2000, 26:450–459.

65. Senecal C, Nouwen A, White D. Motivation and dietary self-care in adults with diabetes: Are self-efficacy and autonomous self-regulation complementary or competing constructs? *Health Psychology*, 2000, 19:452–457.

66. Ott J et al. Self-efficacy as a mediator variable for adolescents' adherence to treatment for insulin dependent diabetes mellitus. *Children's Health Care*, 2000, 29:47–63.

67. Aljasem LI et al. The impact of barriers and self-efficacy on self-care behaviors in type 2 diabetes. *Diabetes Educator,* 2001, 27:393–404.

68. Ruggieron L et al. Impact of social support and stress on compliance in women with gestational diabetes. *Diabetes Care,* 1990, 13:441–443.

69. Karkashian C. A model of stress, resistance factors, and disease-related health outcomes in patients with diabetes mellitus. *Dissertation Abstracts International,* 2000, 60:6413.

70. Peyrot M, McMurry JF, Kruger DF. A biopsychosocial model of glycemic control in diabetes; stress, coping and regimen adherence. *Journal of Health and Social Behavior,* 1999, 40:141–158.

71. Mollema ED et al. Insulin treated diabetes patients with fear of self-injecting or fear of self-testing – psychological comorbidity and general well being. *Journal of Psychosomatic Research,* 2001, 51:665–672.

72. Schlundt DG, Stetson BA, Plant DD. Situation taxonomy and behavioral diagnosis using prospective self-monitoring data: Application to dietary adherence in patients with type 1 diabetes. *Journal of Psychopathology and Behavioral Assessment,* 1999, 21:19–36.

73. Anderson RJ et al. The prevalence of comorbid depression in adults with diabetes: a meta-analysis. *Diabetes Care,* 2001, 24:1069–1078.

74. De Groot M et al. Association of depression and diabetes complications: a meta-analysis. *Psychosomatic Medicine,* 2001, 63:619–630.

75. Lustman PJ et al. Depression and poor glycemic control: A meta-analytic review of the literature. *Diabetes Care,* 2000, 23:934–942.

76. Ciechanowski PS, Katon WJ, Russo JE. Depression and diabetes: impact of depressive symptoms on adherence, function, and costs. *Archives of Internal Medicine,* 2000, 27:3278–3285.

77. Johnson KH, Bazargan M, Bing EG. Alcohol consumption and compliance among inner-city minority patients with type 2 diabetes mellitus. *Archives of Family Medicine,* 2000, 9:964–970.

78. Cox WM et al. Diabetic patients' alcohol use and quality of life: Relationships with prescribed treatment compliance among older males. *Alcoholism: Clinical and Experimental Research,* 1996, 20:327–331.

79. Ciechanowski PS et al. The patient provider relationship: Attachment theory and adherence to treatment in diabetes. *American Journal of Psychiatry,* 2001, 158:29–35.

80. Lloyd CE et al. Psychosocial correlates of glycemic control: the Pittsburgh epidemiology of diabetes complications (EDC) study. *Diabetes Research and Clinical Practice,* 1993, 21:187–195.

81. Albright TL, Parchman M, Burge SK. Predictors of self-care behaviors in adults with type 2 diabetes: An RRNest study. *Family Medicine,* 2001, 33:354–360.

82. Schlundt DG et al. Situational obstacles to adherence for adolescents with diabetes. *Diabetes Educator,* 1994, 20:207–211.

83. Schlundt DG et al. Situational obstacles to dietary adherence for adults with diabetes. *Journal of the American Dietetic Association,* 1994, 94:874–876.

84. Belgrave F, Moorman D. The role of social support in compliance and other health behaviors for African Americans with chronic illness. *Journal of Health and Social Policy,* 1994, 5:55–68.

85. Schlundt DG, Sbrocco T, Bell C. Identification of high risk situations in a behavioral weight loss program: Application of the relapse prevention model. *International Journal of Obesity,* 1989, 13:223–234.

86. Glasgow RE et al. Personal-model beliefs and social-environmental barriers related to diabetes self-management. *Diabetes Care,* 1997, 20:556–561.

87. Ramlogan R. Environment and human health: A threat to all. *Environmental Management and Health,* 1997, 8:51–56.

88. Miller S et al. Shaping environments for reductions in type 2 risk behaviors: A look at CVD and cancer interventions. *Diabetes Spectrum,* 2002, 15:176-186.

89. French SA, Story M, Jeffery RW. Environmental influences on eating and physical activity. *Annual Review of Public Health,* 2001, 22:309–335.

90. Sorensen TI. The changing lifestyle in the world. Body weight and what else? *Diabetes Care,* 2000, 23:B1–B4.

91. Hill JO, Peters JC. Environmental contributions to the obesity epidemic. *Science,* 1998, 280:1371–1374.

92. Frazao E. High costs of poor eating patterns in the United States. In Frazao E. ed. America's eating habits: Changes and consequences. *Agriculture Information Bulletin – US Department of Agriculture,* 1999, 750:5–32.

93. Stahl T et al. The importance of the social environment for physically active lifestyle – results from an international study. *Social Science and Medicine,* 2001, 52:1–10.

94. U.S.Department of Transportation Bureau of Transportation Statistics. *Transportation Statistics Annual Report 1999.* Washington, DC, 2000, No. BTS99-03.

95. Curtis LJ et al. The role of permanent income and family structure in the determination of child health in Canada. *Health Economics,* 2001, 10:287–302.

96. Auslander WF et al. Disparity in glycemic control and adherence between African Americans and Caucasian youths with diabetes. Family and community contexts. *Diabetes Care,* 1997, 20:1569–1575.

97. Galo AE. Food Advertising in the United States. In Frazao E. ed. America's eating habits: Changes and consequences. *Agriculture Information Bulletin – US Department of Agriculture,* 1999, 750:173–180.

98. Dietz W, Gortmaker S. Preventing obesity in children and adolescents. *Annual Review of Public Health,* 2001, 22:337–353.

99. Sidney S et al. Television viewing and cardiovascular risk factors in young adults: the CARDIA study. *Annals of Epidemiology,* 1996, 6:154–159.

100. Salmon J et al. The association between television viewing and overweight among Australian adults participating in varying levels of leisure-time physical activity. *International Journal of Obesity and Related Metabolic Disorders,* 2000, 24:600–606.

101. Jeffery R, French SA. Epidemic obesity in the United States: are fast foods and television viewing contributing? *American Journal of Public Health,* 1998, 88:277–280.

102. Hu F et al. Physical activity and television watching in relation to risk for type 2 diabetes mellitus in men. *Archives of Internal Medicine,* 2001, 161:1543–1548.

103. Poston WS, Foreyt JP. Obesity is an environmental issue. *Atherosclerosis,* 1999, 146:201–209.

104. Rogers PJ. Eating habits and appetite control: A psychobiological perspective. *Proceedings of the Nutrition Society,* 1999, 58:59–67.

105. Mueller KJ et al. Health status and access to care among rural minorities. *Journal of Health Care for the Poor and Underserved,* 1999, 10:230–249.

106. Mayberry RM, Mili F, Ofili E. Racial and ethnic differences in access to medical care. *Medical Care Research Reviews,* 2000, 57:108–145.

107. Robert SA. Socioeconomic position and health: the independent contribution of community socioeconomic context. *Annual Review of Sociology,* 1999, 25:489–516.

108. Glasgow RE. A practical model of diabetes management and education. *Diabetes Care,* 1995, 18:117–126.

109. Marmot MG. Improvement of social environment to improve health. *Lancet,* 1998, 351:57–60.

110. Fain JA et al. Diabetes patient education research: An integrative literature review. *Diabetes Educator,* 1999, 25:7–15.

111. Peyrot M. Behavior change in diabetes education. *Diabetes Educator,* 1999, 25:62–73.

112. Elasy TA et al. A taxonomy for diabetes educational interventions. *Patient Education and Counseling,* 2001, 43:121–127.

113. Brown SA. Interventions to promote diabetes self-management: state of the science. *Diabetes Education,* 1999, 25:52–61.

114. Kinmonth AL et al. Randomized controlled trial of patient centred care of diabetes in general practice: Impact on current wellbeing and future disease risk. The Diabetes Care from Diagnosis Research Team. *British Medical Journal*, 1998, 317:1202–1208.

115. Olivarius NF et al. Randomized controlled trial of structured personal care of type 2 diabetes mellitus. *British Medical Journal*, 2001, 323:970–975.

116. Pichert JW et al. Adherence-related questioning by fourth-year medical students interviewing ambulatory diabetic patients. *Teaching and Learning in Medicine*, 1989, 1:146–150.

117. Lorenz RA et al. Teaching skills training for health professionals: Effects on immediate recall by surrogate patients. *Teaching and Learning in Medicine*, 1989, 1:26–30.

118. Schlundt DG et al. Evaluation of a training program for improving adherence promotion skills. *Patient Education and Counseling*, 1994, 24:165–173.

119. Pill R et al. A randomized controlled trial of an intervention designed to improve the care given in general practice to type II diabetic patients: patient outcomes and professional ability to change behaviour. *Family Practice*, 1998, 15:229–235.

120. Michael P. Impact and components of the Medicare MNT benefit. *Journal of the American Dietetic Association*, 2001, 101:1140–1141.

121. Hardy KJ, O'Brien SV, Furlong NJ. Quality improvement report: Information given to patients before appointments and its effect on non-attendance rates. *British Medical Journal*, 2001, 323:1298–1300.

122. McCulloch DK et al. A population-based approach to diabetes management in a primary care setting: Early results and lessons learned. *Effective Clinical Practice*, 1998, 1:12–22.

123. Feifer C et al. System supports for chronic illness care and their relationship to clinical outcomes. *Topics in Health Information Management*, 2001, 22:65–72.

124. Wagner EH et al. Chronic care clinics for diabetes in primary care: A system-wide randomized trial. *Diabetes Care*, 2001, 24:695–700.

125. Wagner EH et al. Quality improvement in chronic illness care: A collaborative approach. *Journal on Quality Improvement*, 2001, 27:63–80.

126. Glasgow RE et al. Behavioral science in diabetes. *Diabetes Care*, 1999, 22:832–843.

127. Johnson SB. Methodological issues in diabetes research: Measuring adherence. *Diabetes Care*, 1992, 15:1658–1667.

Chapter XI

Epilepsy

1. Introduction 87

2. Adherence to epilepsy therapy 88

3. Epidemiology of adherence 89

4. Factors affecting adherence and interventions used to improve it 89

5. Conclusions 92

6. References 92

1. Introduction

Epilepsy is a common neurological disease affecting almost 50 million people worldwide *(1,2)* 5 million of whom have seizures more than once per month *(3)*. Approximately 85% of people afflicted with epilepsy live in developing countries. Two million new cases occur in the world each year. The results of studies suggest that the annual incidence in developed countries is approximately 50 per 100 000 of the general population whereas in developing countries this figure is nearly doubled to 100 per 100 000 *(1)*.

In developing countries few patients with epilepsy receive adequate medical treatment, and an estimated 75 to 90% receive no treatment at all *(4)*. The treatment of epilepsy in developing countries remains far from satisfactory, mainly because of:

– the general lack of medical personnel;

– non-availability of medications; and

– lack of information and/or education on epilepsy for both patients and medical staff (1,4,5).

Epilepsy is characterized by a tendency to recurrent seizures and it is defined by two or more unprovoked seizures (generally within 2 years). Seizures may vary from the briefest lapses or muscle jerks to severe and prolonged convulsions. They may also vary in frequency, from less than one a year to several per day *(1)*. The risks of recurrent seizures include intractable epilepsy, cognitive impairment, physical injury, psychosocial problems and death *(6)*. Children suffer mainly from idiopathic generalized epilepsy and absence, myoclonus and generalized tonic–clonic seizures are the most common forms of seizure seen in children. In adults, symptomatic partial epilepsy is the most common form, and it may cause simple partial, complex partial, or secondarily generalized tonic–clonic seizures *(3)*. Convulsive or tonic–clonic status epilepsy is of major concern as it is associated with a mortality rate of 5–15% *(7)*.

The aim of antiepileptic drug (AED) therapy is to achieve freedom from seizures. The treatment goals for patients with epilepsy are to prevent the occurrence of seizures, prevent or reduce drug side-effects and drug interactions, improve the patient's quality of life, provide cost-effective care and ensure patient satisfaction *(6,8)*. Much of the treatment of epilepsy is aimed at creating a balance between prevention of seizures and minimization of side-effects to a level that the patient can tolerate *(6,9)*. Although AED therapy does not offer a permanent cure, successful therapy can eliminate or reduce symptoms. The most commonly used AEDs are (in aphabetical order): carbamazepine, ethosuximide, phenobarbital, phenytoin and valproic acid. New AEDs such as gabapentin, lamotrigine, leviteracetam, felbamate, oxcarbazepine, tiagabine, topiramate, vigabatrin and zonisamide have a role in the management of the 20–30% of patients with epilepsy who remain refractory to conventional drug therapy *(9)*. About 25% of patients with epilepsy have intractable seizure disorders, of those between 12 and 25% are candidates for surgery *(3)*.

The direct costs attributable to epilepsy include physician visits, laboratory tests, emergency department visits, antiepileptic drugs and hospitalizations. Indirect costs include working days lost, lost income, decreased quality of life, the cost of failed therapy and side-effects of drugs *(6)*. Garnett et al., referring to the "Epilepsy Foundation of America data", reported that the annual direct and indirect costs of epilepsy exceeded $12.5 billion. The direct costs of epilepsy are significantly lower for patients whose epilepsy is controlled than for those whose disease is not controlled *(6)*.

Recent studies in both developed and developing countries have shown that up to 70% of children and adults newly diagnosed with epilepsy can be successfully treated (i.e. their seizures can be completely controlled for several years) with antiepileptic drugs. After 2–5 years of successful treatment, drugs can be withdrawn in about 70% of children and about 60% of adults without relapse occurring *(1)*. In the case of treatment failure it is crucial to establish whether the failure is a result of inappropriate drug selection, inappropriate dosing, refractory disease or poor adherence to the therapeutic regimen *(3,6)*.

Good adherence to treatment and proper health education are fundamental to the successful management of epilepsy *(10,11)*. Poor adherence to prescribed medication is considered to be the main cause of unsuccessful drug treatment for epilepsy *(2,3,12–18)*. Nonadherent patients experience an increase in the number and severity of seizures, which leads to more ambulance rides, emergency department visits and hospitalizations *(12,19)*. Nonadherence therefore results directly in an increase in health care costs, and reduced quality of life *(19)*.

The aim of this chapter is to describe the prevalence of adherence (or nonadherence), to treatment for epilepsy, to identify the factors affecting adherence to anti-epilepsy treatment, and to discuss the interventions that have proven effective for improving adherence.

A search on adherence to anti-epilepsy therapies was made using Medline (1990–2002). Reviews and reports from international and national organizations were also included. Publications were considered for inclusion if they reported on one of the following: prevalence data on rates of adherence (or nonadherence), factors affecting adherence, interventions for improving adherence, and information on how poor adherence rates affect illness, costs and treatment effectiveness. Of the 99 studies retrieved by the search, 36 were reviewed for this report.

2. Adherence to epilepsy therapy

Adherence was not usually defined in the published studies, but referred to generally as patients following medical recommendations. Authors generally considered adherence in behavioural terms, whereby the patient had an active and informed role to play in a therapeutic situation *(13,20)*. In this sense, adherence to prescribed medication was seen as a health-promoting behaviour (21).

The types of nonadherence were described as follows: reduced or increased amount of single dose; decreased or increased number of daily doses; extra dosing; incorrect dosing intervals; being unaware of the need for life-long regular medication; taking duplicate medication; taking discontinued medication; discontinuing prescribed medication; regularly forgetting to take medication, and incorrect use of medication (18,20,22).

Medication use was assessed by review of medical records; patient self-report; family report; pill counts; prescription refill rates, and biological markers, including serum, urine and saliva assays to quantify medications or their metabolites (2,11,12,14,23–26). The best indicator of adherence is believed to be serum levels of anticonvulsant drugs (18,27). Other methods of monitoring adherence, such as electronic measures are not discussed further here because of the lack of published studies in this area. In several studies, patients whose serum levels were outside the therapeutic range were classified as nonadherent (19,23,28). However, serum levels are not a perfect measure. Although blood levels of anticonvulsant medications can be measured, it is difficult to translate them into comparable measures of adherence for patients on different medications and doses. Furthermore, sub-therapeutic levels of a drug in the serum can be due either to poor compliance or the need for a higher dosage (2). Patients with impaired absorption or rapid or ultra-rapid metabolism can have low serum levels even if their intake of AEDs is regular and according to prescription (11,26,29).

Dowse et al. and Leppik et al. reported that indirect measures such as patient interview, tablet counts and prescription refill records gave no indication of the true amount of the drug present in the body and could be inaccurate or biased (18,19). However, using the measurement of drug concentration in blood alone, except in cases of extremely low adherence and variability of drug intake, is not sufficient to detect incorrect drug intake. Therefore, the use of clinical markers and self-reported adherence should also be considered (11).

3. Epidemiology of adherence

Adherence can vary from an occasional missed dose to chronic defaulting on medication regimens (21). Adherence to antiepileptic drugs in patients with epilepsy generally ranges from 20 to 80% (12,19–21). Some studies reported different ranges of adherence for adult patients (40–60%) and children (25–75%) (3,12).

4. Factors affecting adherence and interventions used to improve it

Nonadherence is a problem that has many determinants and the responsibility for adherence must be shared by health professionals, the health care system, the community and the patients. Many studies have identified factors affecting adherence, and these have been grouped into the five dimensions described in section II (see Table 5).

– socioeconomic-related factors;

– health care team/health system-related factors;

– condition-related factors;

– treatment-related factors, and

– patient-related factors.

Many factors, such as misunderstanding instructions about how to take the drugs (6,12,20,23,26), combined antiepileptic medication, complex medication regimens (3,12,26,30), forgetfulness (6), duration and previous treatment failures (14), fear of dependence (20), feeling stigmatized by the epilepsy (20), inadequate or nonexistent reimbursement by health insurance plans *(19)* and poverty *(6)*, among many others, have been shown to be significant barriers to adherence, and should be taken into account when developing interventions.

Contrary to expectations, a study by Mitchell et al. *(14)* found that frequency and duration of seizures and previous treatment failure, which are usually thought to be valid prognostic indicators of low adherence, did not affect adherence to treatment. Also, the severity of seizures was not significantly associated with any adherence outcome. However, families reporting less parental education, illiteracy, lower income and high levels of stressful life events were more likely to adhere to treatment.

Some interventions have been designed to improve adherence to anti-epilepsy medications. Some of them target specific factors, such as:

– the therapeutic relationship (increasing communication between patient and health professional) *(2,15,16,18,19,23)*;

– giving full instructions about the treatment and discussing the pros and cons of treatment with the patient *(19)*;

– reducing the number of medications and the frequency of doses *(3)*;

– suggesting memory aids, linking doses to events in the patient's daily schedule, and using alarmed watches or pill cases *(3,14,16,31)*;

– motivating patients to incorporate drug adherence into their lifestyles *(6,32)*; and

– providing a regular, uninterrupted supply of medicines in developing countries *(33)*.

Education in the diagnosis and management of epilepsy was found to be effective in improving recruitment of patients into treatment programmes and in improving drug adherence, or markedly reducing nonadherence *(5)*. The use of educational materials, regular interviews, instructions from nurses and physicians about methods of incorporating drug administration into patients' daily lives, a real partnership between physician and patient, and patient self-management of epilepsy treatment, have all been found to improve adherence to AED therapies *(6,11,14,16,18)*. Other helpful measures were: clear information about the treatment, including giving full instructions; discussing the pros and cons of treatment; reinforcing the value of treatment; explaining and repeating the rationale for the regimen; involving the patients in planning their regimens, and explaining the results of medical tests.

Good adherence education may be based on:

– stressing the importance of adherence at the time the therapy is initiated;

– emphasizing the consequences of nonadherence;

– spending adequate time with the patient;

– enquiring about adherence at each visit;

– motivating patients to incorporate drug adherence into their lifestyles; and

– designing and implementing intervention strategies to improve adherence to self-medication.

These latter strategies include simplifying the regimen with careful explanation of the dosing schedule; reducing the number of medications and the frequency of doses; improving the medication routine through cognitive cueing and through structuring the task and the environment; providing the patients with control and choices; suggesting memory aids; linking doses to events in the patient's daily schedule, or using alarm watches, calendar packs, pill cases, or specialized dose dispensers.

Encouraging patients to develop their own methods to improve maintenance, after educating them about the nature of epilepsy and the need for long-term therapy, may help them to incorporate drug administration into their daily lives. It is important to note that patients from different cultures require different educational approaches to improve adherence *(15)*. In developing countries it is necessary to maintain a regular, uninterrupted supply of medicines *(33)*, to provide drugs at subsidized costs and to organize effective distribution systems *(27)*.

Table 5 Factors affecting adherence to treatment for epilepsy and interventions for improving it, listed by the five dimensions and the interventions used to improve adherence

Epilepsy	Factors affecting adherence	Interventions to improve adherence
Socioeconomic-related factors	(–) Long distance from treatment setting *(27)*; under 60 years old *(12,20)*; teenagers *(20)*; poverty *(6)*; illiteracy *(6)*; unwillingness to pay the cost of medicines *(6,23,27)*; high cost of medication *(21,34)*; local beliefs or beliefs about the origin of illness *(6,27)*. (+) Elderly patients (over 60 years old) *(20)*; children from family reporting less parental education *(14)*; non-English speaking in an English-speaking community *(14)*; lower income *(14)*; recent immigrants *(14)*.	Assessment of social and career needs *(3)*
Health care team/health system-related factors	(–) Inadequate or non-existent reimbursement by health insurance plans *(19)*; irregular or poor drug supply *(27)*; lack of free medicine supplies *(33)*; poorly developed health services *(27)*; lack of education about AEDs *(21,26,34,35)*. (+) Good relationship between patient and physician *(20)*	A regular, uninterrupted supply of medicines in developing countries *(33)*; good patient–physician relationship *(6,11,14,16,18)*; instruction by nurses and physicians about methods of incorporating drug administration into patient's daily life; training health professionals on adherence; adherence education *(11,14,16,19,31)*
Condition-related factors	(–) Forgetfulness *(6)*; memory deficits *(12)*; duration, and previous treatment failures *(14)*; high frequency of seizures *(14)*.	Education on use of medicines *(5,14,31)*; suggesting memory aids *(3,14,16,19,26,31)*
Therapy-related factors	(–) Complex treatment regimens *(3)*; misunderstanding instructions about how to take the drugs *(6,12,20,23,26)*; adverse effects of treatment *(6,9,16,20–23,27)*. (+) Monotherapy with simple dosing schedules *(2)*	Simplification of regimens; single antiepileptic therapy (monotherapy) *(3,16,19,30)*; education on use of medicines; patient-tailored prescriptions *(36)*; clear instructions; use of educational materials; monitoring and reassessment of treatment *(6,11,14,16,18)*
Patient-related factors	(–) Disbelief of the diagnosis *(16,22)*; refusal to take medication *(34)*; delusional thinking *(16,31)*; inconvenience of treatment *(21,34)*; denial of diagnosis *(21,34)*; lifestyle and health beliefs; parental worry about child's health *(29)*; behavioural restrictions placed on child to protect his/her health *(29)*; fear of addiction *(20)*; doubting the diagnosis *(20)*; uncertainty about the necessity for drugs *(20)*; anxiety over the complexity of the drug regimen *(20)*; feeling stigmatized by the epilepsy *(20)*; not feeling that it is important to take medications *(20)*. (+) Parent and child satisfaction with medical care *(29)*; not feeling stigmatized by the epilepsy *(20)*; feeling that it is important to take medications *(20)*; high levels of stressful life events *(14)*.	Self-management of side-effects *(6,11,14,16,18)*; behavioural and motivational intervention; education on adherence *(6,32)*; providing the patients with control and choices; assessment of psychological needs *(3)*; frequent follow-up interviews *(11,16)*

AEDs, Anti-epileptic drugs; (+) factors having a positive effect on adherence; (–) factors having a negative effect on adherence.

5. Conclusions

Poor adherence to drug therapy is one of the primary causes of treatment failure.

Forgetfulness of patients that may or may not be linked to memory difficulties, refusal to take medication and side-effects are the factors most commonly associated with decreased adherence. The impact of epilepsy and the side-effects of its treatment on cognition and of limited or compromised cognition on adherence deserve more attention.

The use of memory aids, linking doses to events in the patient's daily schedule or watch alarms, calendar packs, pill cases or specialized dose dispensers may be helpful tools to increase adherence to treatment in patients who regularly forget to take their AEDs. However, no studies demonstrating this were found in the literature search.

Communication with the patient about medication regimens and the value of treatment is extremely important. It can facilitate the identification of problems and barriers to adequate adherence, and help with treatment planning. Also a real partnership between the physician and the patient is needed to set and achieve goals related to treatment outcomes and adherence.

More research on adherence to anti-epileptic therapies is required to:

– deepen our understanding of the epidemiology of adherence;

– provide clear and consistent definitions of adherence;

– evaluate interventions to improve adherence; and

– collect data on adherence in developing countries.

6. References

1. Epilepsy: epidemiology, etiology and prognosis. Geneva, World Health Organization, 2001 (WHO Fact Sheet No 165; available on the Internet at http://www.who.int/inf-fs/en/fact165.html).

2. Chandra RS et al. Compliance monitoring in epileptic patients. *Journal of the Association of Physicians of India*, 1993, 41:431–432.

3. French J. The long-term therapeutic management of epilepsy. *Annals of Internal Medicine*, 1994, 120:411–422.

4. Kaiser C et al. Antiepileptic drug treatment in rural Africa: involving the community. *Tropical Doctor*, 1998, 28:73–77.

5. Adamolekun B, Mielke JK, Ball DE. An evaluation of the impact of health worker and patient education on the care and compliance of patients with epilepsy in Zimbabwe. *Epilepsia*, 1999, 40:507–511.

6. Garnett WR. Antiepileptic drug treatment: outcomes and adherence. *Pharmacotherapy*, 2000, 20:191S–199S.

7. Khurana DS. Treatment of status epilepticus. *Indian Journal of Pediatrics*, 2000, 67:S80–S87.

8. Ogunniyi A, Oluwole OS, Osuntokun BO. Two-year remission in Nigerian epileptics. *East African Medical Journal*, 1998, 75:392–395.

9. Lhatoo SD et al. Long-term retention rates of lamotrigine, gabapentin, and topiramate in chronic epilepsy. *Epilepsia*, 2000, 41:1592–1596.

10. Sureka RK. Clinical profile and spectrum of epilepsy in rural Rajasthan. *Journal of the Association of Physicians of India*, 1999, 47:608–610.

11. Gomes M, Maia FH, Noe RA. Anti-epileptic drug intake adherence. The value of the blood drug level measurement and the clinical approach. *Arquivos de Neuro-Psiquiatria*, 1998, 56:708–713.

12. Hargrave R, Remler MP. Noncompliance. *Journal of the National Medical Association*, 1996, 88:7.

13. Gomes M, Maia FH. Medication-taking behavior and drug self regulation in people with epilepsy. *Arquivos de Neuro-Psiquiatria*, 1998, 56:714–719.

14. Mitchell WG, Scheier LM, Baker SA. Adherence to treatment in children with epilepsy: who follows "doctor's orders"? *Epilepsia*, 2000, 41:1616–1625.

15. Snodgrass SR, Parks BR. Anticonvulsant blood levels: historical review with a pediatric focus. *Journal of Child Neurology*, 2000, 15:734–746.

16. Yuen HK. Increasing medication compliance in a woman with anoxic brain damage and partial epilepsy. *American Journal of Occupational Therapy*, 1993, 47:30–33.

17. Gledhill RF. In the shadow of epilepsy. *Lancet*, 1997, 350:811.

18. Dowse R, Futter WT. Outpatient compliance with theophylline and phenytoin therapy. *South African Medical Journal*, 1991, 80:550–553.

19. Leppik IE. How to get patients with epilepsy to take their medication. The problem of noncompliance. *Postgraduate Medicine*, 1990, 88:253–256.

20. Buck D et al. Factors influencing compliance with antiepileptic drug regimes. *Seizure*, 1997, 6:87–93.

21. Lannon SL. Using a health promotion model to enhance medication compliance. *Journal of Neuroscience Nursing*, 1997, 29:170–178.

22. Cramer JA et al. How often is medication taken as prescribed? A novel assessment technique. *Journal of the American Medical Association*, 1989, 261:3273–3277 [erratum published in *Journal of the American Medical Association*, 1989, 262:1472].

23. Alonso NB, Da Silva DF, de Campos CJ. [Compliance in epilepsy. I. Concept factors and influence factors.] [Portuguese] *Arquivos de Neuro-Psiquiatria*, 1991, 49:147–149.

24. Anonymous. Clobazam has equivalent efficacy to carbamazepine and phenytoin as monotherapy for childhood epilepsy. Canadian Study Group for Childhood Epilepsy. *Epilepsia*, 1998, 39:952–959.

25. Valodia P et al. Benefits of a clinical pharmacokinetic service in optimising phenytoin use in the western Cape. *South African Medical Journal*, 1998, 88:873–875.

26. DiIorio C, Henry M. Self-management in persons with epilepsy. *Journal of Neuroscience Nursing*, 1995, 27:338–343.

27. Elechi CA. Default and non-compliance among adult epileptics in Zaria, Nigeria. The need to restructure continued care. *Tropical & Geographical Medicine*, 1991, 43:242–245.

28. Snodgrass SR et al. Pediatric patients with undetectable anticonvulsant blood levels: comparison with compliant patients. *Journal of Child Neurology*, 2001, 16:164–168.

29. Hazzard A, Hutchinson SJ, Krawiecki N. Factors related to adherence to medication regimens in pediatric seizure patients. *Journal of Pediatric Psychology*, 1990, 15:543–555.

30. Cloyd JC et al. Comparison of sprinkle versus syrup formulations of valproate for bioavailability, tolerance, and preference. *Journal of Pediatrics*, 1992, 120:634–638.

31. Alonso NB et al. [Compliance in epilepsy. II. Practical aspects.] [Portuguese] *Arquivos de Neuro-Psiquiatria*, 1991, 49:150–154.

32. Cramer JA. Medication compliance in epilepsy. *Archives of Internal Medicine*, 1991, 151:1236–1237.

33. Desai P et al. Knowledge, attitudes and practice of epilepsy: experience at a comprehensive rural health services project. *Seizure*, 1998, 7:133–138.

34. Buchanan N. Noncompliance with medication amongst persons attending a tertiary referral epilepsy clinic: implications, management and outcome. *Seizure*, 1993, 2:79–82.

35. Abduljabbar M et al. Epilepsy classification and factors associated with control in Saudi adult patients. *Seizure*, 1998, 7:501–504.

36. Mullen PD. Compliance becomes concordance. *British Medical Journal*, 1997, 314:691–692.

CHAPTER XII

Human immunodeficiency virus and acquired immunodeficiency syndrome

1. Types of nonadherence 96

2. Challenges in assessing adherence 96

3. Predictors of adherence 96

4. A framework for interventions to increase adherence 101

5. Conclusions 104

6. References 104

Of those patients suffering from HIV/AIDS, approximately one-third take their medication as prescribed *(1)*. Even when patients fully comprehend the consequences of nonadherence to medications, adherence rates are suboptimal *(2,3)*. Good adherence is a decisive factor in treatment success.

Unlike other chronic diseases, the rapid replication and mutation rate of HIV means that very high levels of adherence (e.g. ≥ 95%) are required to achieve durable suppression of viral load (4–6). Recent studies of patients with HIV/AIDS have reported low adherence rates, similar to those seen for other chronic diseases. Suboptimal adherence may rapidly lead to resistance, which can then be transmitted to other people (7–10). The potent and effective new combinations of antiretroviral agents, known as highly active antiretroviral therapy (HAART), have proven efficacious in reducing viral load and improving clinical outcomes. However, the large number of medications involved, the complicated dosing requirements, and the suboptimal tolerability make adherence difficult. Because of the great importance of adherence to antiretroviral treatment of HIV, good strategies for maximizing adherence are essential.

There is no doubt that HAART is one of the most celebrated treatment advances in recent medical history. Nucleoside reverse transcriptase inhibitors (usually two) when combined with non-nucleoside reverse transcriptase inhibitors, protease inhibitors, or both, are highly effective in reducing viral replication and improving clinical outcomes *(11,12)*. In patients with HIV/AIDS, these multidrug regimens, although remarkably efficacious, result in HIV treatment having the most complicated regimens that have ever been prescribed for conditions requiring continuous open-ended treatment *(13)*.

Many researchers believed initially that HAART would completely eradicate the virus from the host (14,15). However, low levels of viral replication persist in small reservoirs even when viral loads are undetectable. Resting memory T-cells, which harbour proviral DNA, survive for far longer than originally thought (5,6,16–18). Therefore, adherence to HAART must be almost perfect to achieve lasting viral suppression. Paterson and colleagues (6) found that adherence at levels less than 95% independently predicted viral resistance, hospital admissions and opportunistic infections. Even among patients who reported adherence rates of ≥ 95%, 22% experienced virologic failure during the study period. In another study, Bangsberg and colleagues (4) found that none of the individuals with adherence greater than 90% progressed to AIDS, whereas 38% and 8% of those with adherence rates ≥ 50% and 51–89%, respectively, progressed to AIDS. Missing even a single dose in a 28-day reporting period has been shown to predict treatment failure (5).

Nonadherence to HAART can have important public health implications. Drug resistance can be transmitted to other persons during high-risk activity, which can then limit therapeutic options (7–10). Some studies have reported that as many as 80% of isolates from newly infected people are resistant to at least one class of currently approved antiretroviral medications, and that 26% of isolates are resistant to several classes of medication (18). Although these estimates are at the higher end of the spectrum, they nonetheless suggest that transmission of drug-resistant strains is increasing (10).

Because adherence of patients with HIV to antiretroviral medications is essential for both clinical effectiveness and public health, research in this area has burgeoned over the past few years.

1. Types of nonadherence

Nonadherence can take many different forms (19). The patient may simply fail to fill the prescription. If the prescription is filled, the patient may incorrectly time the medication or take the wrong dose because he or she misunderstood, or forgot, the health professional's instructions. Patients may also forget a dose completely or prematurely terminate the medication. Moreover, patients may self-adjust their regimen because of side-effects and toxicity or personal beliefs.

2. Challenges in assessing adherence

It is easy for health professionals to miss adherence problems because patient self-reports of adherence tend to be exaggerated (20,21) due perhaps both to a recall bias and a desire to please the provider and avoid criticism. Some patients have been known to dispose of their medication before a scheduled check on their adherence to it so as to appear to have adhered (22). Inadequate adherence coupled with biased reporting is ubiquitous across medicine (23). Conversely, patients who report problems with adherence are rarely trying to mislead their providers (24).

In addition to the misreporting of adherence by patients, estimates of adherence made by health care providers are also usually over-optimistic (25,26). Moreover, providers of health care are not able to predict very accurately which patients will adhere. Many providers believe that factors associated with socioeconomic status, such as lack of education and poverty are good predictors of nonadherence. However, predictors of adherence vary greatly across populations and settings and no one factor has been consistently associated with nonadherence across all studies (27).

3. Predictors of adherence

Four types of factor have generally been found to predict problems with adherence to medication: regimen characteristics, various patient factors, the relationship between provider and patient and the system of care. The following section focuses on the first three factors; a discussion of factors associated with the system of care is beyond the scope of this report.

A. Regimen-related factors

Complexity of regimen. For many chronic diseases, research has shown that adherence decreases as the complexity of the medication regimen increases (i.e. the number of pills per dose and number of doses per day; the necessity to observe strict requirements related to the intake of food, and the existence of special requirements regarding fluid intake). Adherence to HIV medications is an extremely complicated process that includes both the drugs themselves and the adjustments to daily life necessary to provide the prerequisite conditions for effective drug therapy *(13)*. Some regimens require several doses of medication per day together with various requirements or restrictions on food intake and other activities. These complexities, in addition to the problems of toxicity and side-effects, can greatly influence an individual's willingness and ability to adhere to the therapy *(28–31)*.

Many health professionals believe that pill burden strongly influences adherence. However, the effect of pill burden on adherence is closely associated with disease stage. Symptomatic individuals perceive a higher risk for complications of nonadherence to medication, than do asymptomatic patients *(32)*. Dosing schedules and food restrictions or requirements appear to have a more pervasive influence on adherence than pill burden. In the treatment of many diseases, once-daily or twice-daily doses are preferred *(33,34)*. For instance, Eldred and colleagues *(33)* found that patients on twice-daily doses or less reported better adherence (>80%) and were more likely to take their medications when away from home. Paterson and colleagues *(6)* also found that a twice-daily dose was associated with better adherence than a three-times-daily dose. However, other studies have failed to confirm this association, including the large Health Care Services Utilization Study with more than 1900 participants *(35)*. Wenger and colleagues demonstrated that the "fit" of the regimen to an individual's lifestyle and schedule, and the individual's attitude towards treatment were better predictors of adherence than dosing schedule *(35)*. It is likely, however, that fewer doses do allow for easier "fitting" of medications into an individual's schedule.

Regimens that involve close monitoring and severe lifestyle alterations together with side-effects may lead not only to frustration and treatment fatigue, but also ultimately to noncompliance *(36)*. Regimens requiring fewer alterations in lifestyle patterns (e.g. fewer pills per day and fewer dietary restrictions) are likely to have a positive influence on adherence to medication.

To the extent possible, regimens should be simplified by reducing the number of pills and frequency of therapy, and by minimizing drug interactions and side-effects. This is particularly important for patients with strong biases against many pills and frequent dosing. There is evidence that simplified regimens that require fewer pills and lower dose frequencies improve adherence *(37)*. When choosing appropriate regimens, the patient's eating habits should be reviewed and the specific food requirements of the regimen discussed so that the patient understands what is required before his or her agreement to such restrictions is sought. Regimens requiring an empty stomach several times per day may be difficult for patients suffering from wasting, just as regimens requiring a high fat intake may be difficult for patients with lactose intolerance or fat aversion.

Side-effects. Side-effects have also been consistently associated with decreased adherence and patients who experience more than two aversive reactions are less likely to continue their treatment *(38)*. HAART regimens usually have temporary side-effects including transient reactions (diarrhoea and nausea) as well as longer-lasting effects (i.e. lipodystrophy and neuropathy). The extent to which side-effects alter a patient's motivation to adhere to a treatment regimen depends greatly on the specific contextual issues surrounding the individual. The literature on side-effects clearly shows that optimal adherence occurs with medications that remove symptoms, whereas adherence is reduced by medications that produce side-effects *(13,27)*. Although HAART may greatly increase quality of life in symptomatic individuals, it probably has a negative effect on quality of life in asymptomatic individuals *(39)*.

Patients quickly discontinue therapy or request changes of medication if they experience side-effects *(40)*. Whether real or perceived, side-effects account for more regimen changes than does treatment failure *(30,40,41)*. One large study of more than 860 HIV-positive patients in Italy reported that more than 25% of treatment-naive patients discontinued their treatment within the first year because of toxicity and other side-effects *(30)*. Another study in France found that the patients' subjective experience of side-effects within the first 4 months of treatment predicted nonadherence more than any other predictors, including sociodemographic variables, number of medications or doses per day *(42)*. The symptoms that cause the most distress are fatigue, diarrhoea, nausea and stomach pain, most of which can be successfully treated *(30,42)*.

One serious side-effect that may affect adherence to HIV medications is lipodystrophy. Kasper and colleagues *(43)* found that 37% of their respondents either stopped or changed their medications because they developed lipodystrophy. Of those who were adherent, 57% stated that they had seriously considered discontinuation of therapy, while 46% stated that they would change medications if symptoms worsened.

Lipodystrophy affects between 30% and 60% of persons on HAART *(44,45)*. Physical manifestations vary greatly but can include fat accumulation on the upper back and neck (buffalo hump), under the muscles of the abdomen (crix belly or protease paunch), lipomas and breast enlargement; it may also cause peripheral wasting of fat in the face, legs, arms and buttocks *(46–48)*. Physiologically, these physical deformities are usually preceded by hyperglycaemia, insulin resistance, hypercholesterolaemia and hypertriglyceridaemia. The exact relationship of these physiological changes to lipodystrophy is unclear. Nonetheless, lipid abnormalities must be treated and this can increase the complexity and side-effects of already complex regimens. Selecting regimens that do not contribute to dyslipidaemia or lipodystrophy may allay fears of disfigurement and support adherence.

In the light of these findings, simplified regimens with fewer pills and fewer doses, and that minimize side-effects, are desirable for achieving maximum adherence *(38)*.

B. Patient-related factors

A patient's behaviour is the critical link between a prescribed regimen and treatment outcome. The most effective regimen will fail if the patient does not take the medication as prescribed or refuses to take it. Consequently, all things being equal, the most important factors influencing adherence are patient-related *(27)*.

Psychosocial issues. Perhaps more than anything else, life stress can interfere with proper dosing of protease medication regimens *(49,50)*, and such stress is experienced more often and to a greater degree by individuals of low socioeconomic status. Although studies of most demographic characteristics of patients have generally failed to establish consistent links with adherence to medication, some recent studies have described several variables that have a possible association. Adherence is apparently most difficult for patients with lower levels of education and literacy, and a few studies have reported lower adherence among blacks and women, although this finding has not been consistent *(38)*. Women have cited the stress of childcare as being related to missed doses *(36)*. The abuse of alcohol and intravenous drugs and the presence of depressive symptoms have also been linked with poor adherence to medication.

Although some studies have demonstrated that a history of substance abuse is unrelated to adherence *(51,52)*, active substance abuse is one of the stronger predictors of nonadherence *(53,54)*. Nevertheless, even active substance abusers can achieve good adherence if the provider takes the time to address the patient's concerns about the medications, including anticipation of, and management of, side-effects. Mocroft and colleagues *(52)* demonstrated that intravenous drug abusers were significantly less likely to begin antiretroviral therapy, but among those who did, the response to therapy was similar to that of other exposed groups.

Psychological distress has also been shown to affect adherence. Depression, stress, and the manner in which individuals manage stress, are among the most significant predictors of adherence, but correlations with other psychiatric comorbidities are weaker *(6,53–57)*. Hopelessness and negative feelings can reduce motivation to care for oneself and may also influence a patient's ability to follow complex instructions. Adolescents with HIV who reported high levels of depression demonstrated lower adherence than did their peers who were not depressed *(56)*. These findings are similar to those of studies on other chronic conditions that have demonstrated a relationship between adherence and depression *(58)*.

Just as social support acts as a buffer for many psychosocial problems, it also affects adherence behaviour. Patients with supportive friends and families tend to adhere to HAART better than those without these supports *(6,59,60)*. In addition to the support that can be provided by clinic staff in the form of a good relationship between providers and patients, recommendations for improving adherence often include providing a telephone-counselling line where messages can be left for nurses, and enlisting the support of pharmacists *(61)*. It is important to encourage patients to involve family and friends in their care, and to follow up on referrals to support groups, peer-counselling and community-based organizations.

Several psychosocial predictors of acceptable levels of adherence to HIV medications have been identified in a large-scale, multisite investigation of HAART *(62)*. These include:

– availability of emotional and practical life support;

– the ability of patients to fit the medications into their daily routines;

– the understanding that poor adherence leads to resistance;

– the recognition that taking every dose of the medications is important; and

– feeling comfortable taking medications in front of other people.

Such psychosocial aspects of treatment may be easily overlooked yet have been documented as being crucial to consistent adherence to HIV medication regimens.

Patient-belief system. A patient's knowledge and beliefs about disease and medicine can influence adherence. Understanding the relationship between adherence and viral load and between viral load and disease progression is integral to good adherence behaviour *(53)*. Wenger and colleagues *(35)* found better adherence in patients who believed antiretroviral medication to be effective. Negative beliefs regarding the efficacy of HAART may also affect adherence behaviour. For example, many African Americans were found to be reluctant to take zidovudine because they believed that it was toxic. Siegel and colleagues *(63)* showed that African American men were more likely than Caucasian men to report scepticism about medications and their ability to adhere to those medications. Other beliefs such as those regarding interference with the actions of HAART by alcohol and drugs can also affect adherence *(64)*.

The list below, adapted from the NIH Antiretroviral Guidelines *(62)*, lists additional patient- and medication-related strategies to improve adherence.

• Inform patient, anticipate, and treat side-effects.

• Simplify food requirements.

• Avoid adverse drug interactions.

• If possible, reduce dose frequency and number of pills.

- Negotiate a treatment plan, which the patient understands and to which he or she is committed.

- Take time, and use several encounters, to educate the patient and explain the goals of therapy and the need for adherence.

- Establish the patient's readiness to take medication before the first prescription is written.

- Recruit family and friends to support the treatment plan.

- Develop a concrete plan for a specific regimen including dealing with side-effects and relate it to meals and the patient's daily schedule.

- Provide a written schedule with pictures of medications, daily or weekly pill boxes, alarm clocks, pagers or other mechanical aids to adherence.

- Set up adherence support groups, or add adherence issues to the regular agenda of support groups.

- Develop links with local community-based organizations to help explain the need for adherence using educational sessions and practical strategies.

- Consider "pill trials" with jelly beans.

Confusion and forgetfulness are major obstacles in achieving adherence to HIV medication regimens. Difficulty in understanding instructions has also been reported to affect adherence. Requirements and/or restrictions on the intake of food and water, or the temporal sequences of dosing can be confusing. Misunderstandings may arise as a result of a complex regimen, and/or from poor instructions from the health care provider. In the AIDS Clinical Trial Group, 25% of the participants failed to understand how their medications were to be taken (53). In another study, less adherent individuals reported significantly greater confusion than did adherent individuals over how many pills to take and how to take them (41).

The most commonly cited reason for nonadherence is forgetfulness (51,53,65); for example, Chesney and colleagues (53) reported that 66% of their respondents gave this as the main reason for nonadherence. Ostrop and colleagues (51) demonstrated that not only is forgetfulness the most common reason for nonadherence, but also that the middle dose in a three-times-a-day regimen is the most commonly forgotten. Although other studies have not confirmed this finding, doses are more commonly missed in three-times-daily regimens than in once-daily or twice-daily regimens.

Patient–provider relationship. A meaningful and supportive relationship between the patient and health care provider can help to overcome significant barriers to adherence (37,59,66), but few providers routinely ask about adherence or offer counselling (67). Factors that strengthen the relationship between patient and provider include perceptions of provider competence, quality and clarity of communication, compassion, involving the patient as an active participant in treatment decisions and convenience of the regimen (27). Conversely, patients become frustrated with health care providers when misunderstandings occur, treatment becomes complex, the patient is blamed for being a "bad patient" or side-effects go unmanaged. These frustrations may lead to poor adherence. Specific strategies for clinicians and health teams, as suggested in the NIH Antiretroviral Guidelines (62) are listed below:

- Establish trust.

- Serve as educator, source of information, continuous support and monitoring.

- Provide access between visits for questions or problems by giving the patient a pager number, and arranging for coverage during vacation periods and conferences.

- Monitor adherence; intensify management during periods of low adherence (e.g. by means of more frequent visits, recruitment of family and friends, deployment of other team members, referral for mental health or chemical-dependency services).

- Utilize health team for all patients, for difficult patients and for those with special needs (e.g. peer educators for adolescents or for intravenous drug users).

- Consider the impact of new diagnoses (e.g. depression, liver disease, wasting, recurrent chemical dependency), on adherence and include adherence intervention in their management.

- Enlist nurses, pharmacists, peer educators, volunteers, case managers, drug counsellors, physician's assistants, nurse practitioners and research nurses to reinforce the message of adherence.

- Provide training on antiretroviral therapy and adherence to the support team.

- Add adherence interventions to the job descriptions of HIV support-team members; add continuity-of-care role to improve patient access.

4. A framework for interventions to increase adherence

Experiences with HAART suggest that adherence is arguably the most important issue in successfully managing HIV/AIDs. A multifaceted approach to improve adherence is the most likely to be beneficial, particularly a combination of actively involving patients in their own health care decisions, provision of appropriate supports, multidimensional educational programmes that teach behavioural skills to the patient to enhance his or her adherence, and tailoring of the regimen to fit the patient *(13,27,68)* (see Table 6).

The provider must accurately assess both the patient's willingness to adhere in the context of possible side-effects, and his or her willingness to overcome potential barriers to taking the medications as prescribed. Furthermore, it is essential that the patient adequately understands the importance of adherence and the serious consequences of nonadherence (i.e. treatment failure, or in some cases, disease progression, drug-resistance or death).

Especially for a condition such as HIV, where poor adherence can cause resistance, it may prove wise to delay active treatment until the patient understands the demands of the regimen and feels truly committed to it. One way in which to gauge a person's readiness to adhere to a regimen, identify specific barriers to adherence, and to simultaneously strengthen the patient–provider relationship is to ask the patient an idea of a trial run of the regimen. This may be done using vitamin pills or jelly beans, with different tablets or different-coloured beans representing the various medications. Such a trial can give patients a perspective on how dosing schedules and other complexities, such as food restrictions or requirements will fit into their daily routine. A trial lasting a few weeks is usually sufficient for assessing a patient's ability to stick to the regimen and overcome the barriers. However, such a trial run is unable to mimic possible side-effects.

For children who rely on the support of caregivers to maintain their adherence, the caregivers must believe the rationale for the regimen and assume responsibility for maintaining it. Moreover, every attempt should be made to involve the children in the decision-making process to the extent of their capability. Although infants may have little influence on adherence, older children can have more influence on whether or not they take their medications as prescribed.

Whether developed or acquired, resistance complicates treatment decisions. As a variant becomes progressively resistant to current medications, the therapeutic options become limited. Then the only solution is to select medications from a new treatment class or prescribe medications from existing classes that have demonstrated efficacy against variants resistant to current medications. However, forced selection limits the ability to fit a regimen to patients' lifestyles and schedules.

Ideally, the health practitioner should work together with the patient to select a regimen that will fit with his or her lifestyle. If more than one regimen may be appropriate for a given patient, providers may want to discuss the regimen, the number of pills, the dosing schedule, instructions and potential side-effects with the patient. This discussion will foster a more collaborative and positive relationship between the practitioner and the patient, which is likely to enhance adherence *(68)*. Once the regimen is decided upon, practitioners must make certain that patients fully understand the dosing schedules and instructions.

Rather than associating doses of medication with times of the day, fitting the regimen to the patient's lifestyle calls for working with the patient to associate medication doses with routine activities performed at the times that the medication should be taken *(41)*. For example, morning doses can be associated with morning rituals (e.g. brushing teeth or reading the newspaper), and evening doses can be associated with evening routines (e.g. children's homework or watching television news programmes). In general it is likely that accomplishing this "fit" will be easier with regimens that require infrequent dosing (i.e. once or twice a day). However, the principle of associating medications with daily activities can also accommodate more frequent and complex regimens.

The most simple, effective and potent regimen will fail if patients experience side-effects that they perceive as problematic and terminate their medications. At the time that the regimen is prescribed, health professionals should be proactive and provide strategies to help patients manage any side-effects that may occur *(69)*. Given that experiencing side-effects is associated with nonadherence, providers and their team members should remain in close contact with the patient during early treatment with a new regimen to allow for the timely identification and management of all side-effects and toxicities. A further advantage of this approach is that it provides an opportunity for reinforcing adherence behaviour. A powerful reinforcer of adherence behaviour is positive feedback regarding medication efficacy *(70)*. Consequently, laboratory and other tests should be conducted soon after the initiation of treatment to show the extent to which it has been effective.

Health care providers and their teams should address the patient-related factors and psychosocial issues associated with nonadherence. While these may vary across conditions, screening for active substance abuse and depressed mood would be appropriate in many patient groups. Finally, enlisting the support of family members and "significant others", or employing "treatment buddies" to administer medications can greatly enhance adherence.

An example of a currently operational comprehensive approach to AIDS care, which includes access to free voluntary tests and counselling, the provision of zidovudine or nevirapine for the prevention of mother-to-child transmission, diagnosis and treatment of opportunistic infections, social assistance and directly observed provision of HAART (DOT-HAART) by trained community health workers to the most severely ill patients, has been implemented by Farmer et al. in a poor rural area in Haiti where HIV infection is endemic *(71,72)*.

Preliminary reports have suggested that adherence rates are almost 100%; 86% of patients have no detectable virus in peripheral blood. Clinical outcomes have been excellent in all patients receiving DOT-HAART, enabling up to 90% of them to resume normal daily activities within 3 months of initiation of treatment. Also, hospitalization rates have decreased by more than half since the start of the programme and a sharp decline in mortality has been observed *(73)*.

The implementation of demonstration projects of good HIV/AIDS care practice, using targeted research or evidence-based quality improvement processes, is urgently needed for effectively fighting against the disease. As Pablos-Mendez stated, "research need not hold back care, we should learn by doing" *(74)*.

Table 6 Factors affecting adherence to therapy for HIV/AIDS and interventions for improving it, listed by the five dimensions and the interventions used to improve adherence

HIV/AIDS	Factors affecting adherence	Interventions to improve adherence
Socioeconomic-related factors	(–) Women: stress of childcare *(36)*; low income *(49)*; African American men *(63)*; lack of social support *(6)* (+) Support of family and friends *(6)*; Caucasian men *(63)*	Family preparedness *(6)*; mobilization of community-based organizations; intensive education on use of medicines for patients with low levels of literacy; assessment of social needs
Health care team/health system-related factors	(–) Lack of clear instructions from health professionals; poor implementation of educational interventions *(61)* (+) Good relationship between patient and physician; support of nurses and pharmacists *(61)*	Good patient–physician relationship *(61,68)*; multidisciplinary care; training of health professionals on adherence; training of health professionals on adherence education; training in monitoring adherence; training caregivers; identification of the treatment goals and development of strategies to meet them *(68)*; management of disease and treatment in conjunction with the patients; uninterrupted ready availability of information; regular consultations with nurses/physicians; non-judgemental attitude and assistance; rational selection of medications *(62)*
Condition-related factors	(–) Asymptomatic patients *(32)* (+) Symptomatic patients *(32)*; understanding the relationship between adherence and viral load *(53)*	Education on use of medicines *(53,62)*; supportive medical consultation; screening for comorbidities; attention to mental illness, as well as abuse of alcohol and other drugs
Therapy-related factors	(–) Complex treatment regimens *(28)*; close monitoring; severe lifestyle alterations *(36)*; adverse events *(36)*; adverse effects of treatment *(27)*; lack of clear instructions about how to take the medications *(30,38,40–43,53)* (+) Less frequent dose *(6,33)*; fewer pills per day; fewer dietary restrictions *(36)*; fitting medication to individual's lifestyle *(35)*; belief that medication is effective *(35)*	Simplification of regimens; education on use of medicines; assessment and management of side-effects *(37,38)*; patient-tailored prescriptions *(41,68)*; medications for symptoms *(27)*; education on adherence *(68)*; continuous monitoring and reassessment of treatment *(70)*; management of side-effects *(69)*
Patient-related factors	(–) Forgetfulness *(53)*; life stress *(6,49)*; alcohol use; drug use *(53)*; depression *(6)*; hopelessness and negative feelings; beliefs that alcohol and drug use interfere with medications *(6,64)* (+) Positive beliefs regarding the efficacy of antiretroviral medications *(35)*	Monitoring drug and/or alcohol use; psychiatric consultation; behavioural and motivational intervention *(68)*; counselling/psychotherapy; telephone counselling; memory aids and reminders; self-management of disease and treatment *(68)*

(+) Factors having a positive effect on adherence; (–) factors having a negative effect on adherence.

5. Conclusions

The problems of adherence are ubiquitous across medicine. Because adherence is a complex process, attempts to improve it need to be multifaceted. Factors such as the complexity of the treatment regimen, patient-related factors and the relationship between the patient and the provider of care all affect adherence.

Health care providers should work to establish a collaborative treatment relationship with their patients. This can be fostered by involving the patients in selecting regimens with dosing schedules, pill burdens and side-effects that they believe are tolerable and will "fit" into their daily lives. Pharmaceutical companies are currently working diligently to develop once-daily and twice-daily regimens with fewer side-effects and higher tolerability that will better achieve this fit. Providers should openly discuss with patients their readiness to follow treatment, the potential barriers to adherence and possible solutions to problems. While the provider and his or her team can be a source of support, other possible sources (including family, friends and formal support services) should also be discussed with patients.

Clinicians should also be aware of the prevalence of mental health disorders and disorders related to psychoactive substance abuse in certain HIV-infected populations, as inadequate mental health treatment services may jeopardize the ability of affected individuals to adhere to their medical treatment. Appropriate attention to mental illness, as well as to abuse of alcohol and other drugs could greatly enhance adherence to medical treatment of HIV. Social and living conditions, fit of regimen to lifestyle, availability and nature of social support and treatment expectations can also affect adherence.

No patient should be excluded from consideration for antiretroviral therapy simply because he or she exhibits a behaviour, characteristic or risk factor that might be judged as predictive of nonadherence *(62)*. The health care team should make all possible efforts to ensure that patients adhere to therapies. Awareness of patients' risk factors for nonadherence can help to guide clinicians in tailoring regimens to maximize adherence.

Poor adherence to a regimen is only one of several possible reasons for its failure. Others that must be assessed include initial resistance to one or more of the therapeutic agents, altered absorption or metabolism, and multi-drug pharmacokinetics that adversely affect levels of therapeutic drugs. It is therefore important to assess patient adherence carefully before changing antiretroviral therapy. Case managers, social workers and other health care providers involved in the care of the patient may assist in this evaluation.

6. References

1. Bedell SE et al. Discrepancies in the use of medications: their extent and predictors in an outpatient practice. *Archives of Internal Medicine*, 2000, 160:2129–2134.

2. Lerner BH, Gulick RM, Dubler NN. Rethinking nonadherence: historical perspectives on triple-drug therapy for HIV disease. *Annals of Internal Medicine*, 1998, 129:573–578.

3. Stephenson BJ et al. Is this patient taking the treatment as prescribed? *Journal of the American Medical Association*, 1993, 269:2779–2781.

4. Bangsberg DR et al. Adherence to protease inhibitors, HIV-1 viral load, and development of drug resistance in an indigent population. *AIDS*, 2000, 14:357–366.

5. Montaner JSG et al. A randomized, double-blind trial comparing combinations of nevirapine, didanosine, and zidovudine for HIV-infected patients: the INCAS Trial. *Journal of the American Medical Association*, 1998, 279:930–937.

6. Paterson DL et al. Adherence to protease inhibitor therapy and outcomes in patients with HIV infection. *Annals of Internal Medicine*, 2000, 133:21–30.

7. Boden D et al. HIV-1 drug resistance in newly infected individuals. *Journal of the American Medical Association*, 1999, 282:1135–1141.

8. Hecht FM et al. Sexual transmission of an HIV-1 variant resistant to multiple reverse-transcriptase and protease inhibitors. *New England Journal of Medicine*, 1998, 339:307-311.

9. Little SJ et al. Reduced antiretroviral drug susceptibility among patients with primary HIV infection. *Journal of the American Medical Association*, 1999, 282:1142–1149.

10. Little SJ et al. Antiretroviral drug susceptibility and response to initial therapy among recently HIV-infected subjects in North America. In: *Program and Abstracts of the 8th Conference on Retroviruses and Opportunistic Infections*. Alexandria, VA, Foundation for Retrovirology and Human Health, 2001:273.

11. Hammer SM et al. A controlled trial of two nucleoside analogues plus indinavir in persons with human immunodeficiency virus infection and CD4 cell counts of 200 per cubic millimeter or less. *New England Journal of Medicine*, 1997, 337:725–733.

12. Palella FJJ et al. Declining morbidity and mortality among patients with advanced human immunodeficiency virus infection. *New England Journal of Medicine*, 1998, 338:853–860.

13. Chesney MA, Morin M, Sherr L. Adherence to HIV combination therapy. *Social Science & Medicine*, 2000, 50:1599–1605.

14. Ho DD et al. Rapid turnover of plasma virions and CD4 lymphocytes in HIV-1 infection. *Nature*, 1995, 373:123–126.

15. Perelson AS et al. HIV-1 dynamics in vivo: virion clearance rate, infected cell life-span, and viral generation time. *Science*, 1996, 271:1582–1586.

16. Finzi D et al. Identification of a reservoir for HIV-1 in patients on highly active antiretroviral therapy. *Science*, 1997, 278:1295–1300.

17. Zhang L et al. Quantifying residual HIV-1 replication in patients receiving combination antiretroviral therapy. *New England Journal of Medicine*, 1999, 340:1605–1613.

18. Voelker R. HIV drug resistance. *Journal of the American Medical Association*, 2000, 284:169.

19. Miller NH. Compliance with treatment regimens in chronic asymptomatic diseases. *American Journal of Medicine*, 1997, 102:43–49.

20. Gao X, Nau DP. Congruence of three self-report measures of medication adherence among HIV patients. *Annals of Pharmacotherapy*, 2000, 34:1117–1122.

21. Waterhouse DM et al. Adherence to oral tamoxifen: a comparison of patient self-report, pill counts, and microelectronic monitoring. *Journal of Clinical Oncology*, 1993, 11:1189–1197.

22. Rand CS et al. Metered-dose inhaler adherence in a clinical trial. *American Review of Respiratory Disease*, 1992, 146:1559–1564.

23. Haynes RB, McKibbon KA, Kanani R. Systematic review of randomised trials of interventions to assist patients to follow prescriptions for medications. *Lancet*, 1996, 348:383–386.

24. Wagner GJ, Rabkin JG. Measuring medication adherence: are missed doses reported more accurately then perfect adherence? *AIDS Care*, 2000, 12:405–408.

25. Du Pasquier-Fediaevsky L, Tubiana-Rufi N. Discordance between physician and adolescent assessments of adherence to treatment: influence of HbA1c level. *Diabetes Care*, 2002, 22:1445–1449.

26. Gilbert JR et al. Predicting compliance with a regimen of digoxin therapy in family practice. *Canadian Medical Association*, 1980, 123:119–122.

27. Chesney MA. Factors affecting adherence to antiretroviral therapy. *Clinical Infectious Diseases*, 2000, 30:S171–176.

28. Bartlett J, DeMasi R, Quinn J, Moxham C, Rousseau F. Correlation between antiretroviral pill burden and durability of virologic response: a systematic overview. *Program and abstracts of the XIII International AIDS Conference; 9–14 July, 2000*; Durban, South Africa. Abstract ThPeB4998.

29. Carr A. HIV protease inhibitor-related lipodystrophy syndrome. *Clinical Infectious Diseases*, 2000, 30:S135–S142.

30. D'Arminio A et al. Insights into the reasons for discontinuation of the first highly active antiretroviral therapy (HAART) regimen in a cohort of antiretroviral naïve patients. *AIDS*, 2000, 14:499–507.

31. Kaul DR et al. HIV protease inhibitors: advances in therapy and adverse reactions, including metabolic complications. *Pharmacotherapy*, 1999, 19:281–298.

32. Gao X et al. The relationship of disease severity, health beliefs and medication adherence among HIV patients. *AIDS Care*, 2000, 12:387–398.

33. Eldred LJ et al. Adherence to antiretroviral and pneumocystis prophylaxis in HIV disease. *Journal of Acquired Immune Deficiency Syndromes*, 1998, 18:117–125.

34. Greenberg RN. Overview of patient compliance with medication dosing: a literature review. *Clinical Therapeutics*, 1984, 6:592–599.

35. Wenger N et al. Patient characteristics and attitudes associated with antiretroviral (AR) adherence. Abstract No.98. *Presented at the VI Conference on retrovirus and opportunistic infections*. Washington DC, 1999.

36. Halkitis P et al. Characteristics of HIV antiretroviral treatments and adherence in an ethnically-diverse sample of men who have sex with men. *AIDS Care* (in press).

37. Stone VE et al. HIV/AIDS patients' perspectives on adhering to regimens containing protease inhibitors. *Journal of General Internal Medicine*, 1998, 13:586–593.

38. Stone V. Strategies for optimizing adherence to highly active antiretroviral therapy: Lessons from research and clinical practice. *Clinical Infectious Diseases*, 2001, 33:865–872.

39. Nieuwkerk PT, Gisolf EH, Wu AW. Quality of life in asymptomatic- and symptomatic HIV infected patients in a trial of ritonavir/saquinavir therapy. *AIDS*, 2000, 14:181–187.

40. Mocroft A et al. Reasons for modification and discontinuation of antiretrovirals: results from a single treatment centre. *AIDS*, 2001, 15:185–194.

41. Catz SL et al. Patterns, correlates, and barriers to medication adherence among persons prescribed new treatments for HIV disease. *Health Psychology*, 2000, 19:124–133.

42. Duran S et al. Self-reported symptoms after initiation of a protease inhibitor in HIV-infected patients and their impact on adherence to HAART. *HIV Clinical Trials*, 2001, 2:38–45.

43. Kasper TB, Arboleda CH, Halpern M. The impact of patient perceptions of body shape changes and metabolic abnormalities on antiretroviral therapy. *Program and abstracts of the XIII International AIDS Conference; July 9-14, 2000*; Durban, South Africa. Abstract WePpB1380.

44. Graham NM. Metabolic disorders among HIV-infected patients treated with protease inhibitors: a review. *Journal of Acquired Immune Deficiency Syndromes*, 2002, 25:S4–S11.

45. Mauss S. HIV-associated lipodystrophy syndrome. *AIDS*, 2000, 14:S197–S207.

46. Carr A et al. A syndrome of peripheral lipodystrophy, hyperlipidaemia and insulin resistance in patients receiving HIV protease inhibitors. *AIDS*, 1998, 12:F51–F58.

47. Gervasoni C, Ridolfo AL, Trifirò G. Redistribution of body fat in HIV-infected women undergoing combined antiretroviral therapy. *AIDS*, 1999, 13:465–471.

48. Mynarcik DC et al. Association of severe insulin resistance with both loss of limb fat and elevated serum tumor necrosis factor receptor levels in HIV lipodystrophy. *Journal of Acquired Immune Deficiency Syndromes*, 2000, 25:312–321.

49. Chesney MA. Adherence to drug regimens: a learned skill. *Improving the Management of HIV Disease*, 1997, 5:12.

50. Malow R et al. A Cognitive-behavioral intervention for HIV+ recovering drug abusers: The 2000-05 NIDA-funded AIDS Prevention Center study. *Psychology & AIDS Exchange*, 2001, 30:23–26.

51. Ostrop NJ, Hallett KA, Gill MJ. Long-term patient adherence to antiretroviral therapy. *Annals of Pharmacotherapy*, 2000, 34:703–709.

52. Mocroft A et al. A comparison of exposure groups in the EuroSIDA study: starting highly active antiretroviral therapy (HAART), response to HAART, and survival. *Journal of Acquired Immune Deficiency Syndromes*, 1999, 22:369–378.

53. Chesney MA et al. Self-reported adherence to antiretroviral medications among participants in HIV clinical trials: the AACTG adherence instruments. *AIDS Care*, 2000, 12:255–266.

54. Gordillo V et al. Sociodemographic and psychological variables influencing adherence to antiretroviral therapy. *AIDS*, 1999, 13:1763–1769.

55. Holzemer WL et al. Predictors of self-reported adherence in persons living with HIV disease. *AIDS Patient Care and STDs*, 1999, 13:185–197.

56. Murphy DA et al. Antiretroviral medication adherence among the REACH HIV-infected adolescent cohort in the USA. *AIDS Care,* 2001, 13:27–40.

57. Singh BN. Effects of food on clinical pharmacokinetics. *Clinical Pharmacokinetics,* 1999, 37:213–255.

58. Dunbar-Jacob J, Burke LE, Pyczynski S. Clinical assessment and management of adherence to medical regimens. In: Nicassio PM, Smith TW, eds. *Managing chronic illness: A biopsychosocial perspective.* Washington, DC, American Psychological Association, 1995:313–349.

59. Morse EV et al. Determinants of subject compliance within an experimental anti-HIV drug protocol. *Social Science & Medicine,* 1991, 32:1161–1167.

60. Stall R et al. Decisions to get HIV tested and to accept antiretroviral therapies among gay/bisexual men: Implications for secondary prevention efforts. *Journal of Acquired Immune Deficiency Syndromes and Human Retrovirology,* 1996, 11:151–160.

61. Chesney M et al. Adherence: A necessity for successful HIV combination therapy. *AIDS,* 1999, 13:S271–S278.

62. Panel on Clinical Practices for Treatment of HIV. Guidelines for the use of antiretroviral agents in HIV-infected adults and adolescents (NIH 2002). *Morbidity and Mortality Weekly Report.* Atlanta, GA, Centers for Diseases Control and Prevention, 2002, Vol. 51, No. RR07.

63. Siegel K, Karus D, Schrimshaw EW. Racial differences in attitudes toward protease inhibitors among older HIV-infected men. *AIDS Care,* 2000, 12:423–434.

64. Ng JJ et al. Adherence to highly active antiretroviral therapy in substance abusers with HIV/AIDS. *Journal of General Internal Medicine,* 2000, 15:165.

65. Samet JH et al. Compliance with zidovudine therapy in patients infected with human immunodeficiency virus, type 1: a cross-sectional study in a municipal hospital clinic. *American Journal of Medicine,* 1992, 92:495–502.

66. Sbarbaro JA. The patient–physician relationship: compliance revisited. *Annals of Allergy,* 1990, 64:321–331.

67. Hedge B, Petrak JA. Take as prescribed: a study of adherence behaviours in people taking anti-retroviral medications [abstract 32346]. Abstract Book. *Presented at the 12th World AIDS Conference; 28 June – 3 July,* 1998. Geneva, 1998: 590–591.

68. Caldwell JR. Drug regimens for long-term therapy of hypertension. *Geriatrics,* 1976, 31:115–119.

69. Fischl MA. Antiretroviral therapy in 1999 for antiretroviral-naive individuals with HIV infection. *AIDS,* 1999, 13:S49–S59.

70. Reiter GS et al. Elements of success in HIV clinical care: multiple interventions that promote adherence. *Topics in HIV Medicine,* 2002, 8: 21-30.

71. Farmer P et al. Community-based treatment of advanced HIV disease: introducing DOT-HAART (directly observed therapy with highly active antiretroviral therapy). *Bulletin of the World Health Organization,* 2001, 79:1145–1151.

72. Farmer P et al. Community-based approaches to HIV treatment in resource-poor settings. *Lancet,* 2001, 358:404-409.

73. Singler J, Farmer P. Treating HIV in resource-poor settings. *Journal of the American Medical Association,* 2002, 288:1652–1653.

74. Pablos-Mendez A. AIDS care is learnt by doing it. *Bulletin of the World Health Organization,* 2001, 79:1153–1154.

CHAPTER XIII

Hypertension

1. Prevalence of adherence to pharmacotherapy in patients with hypertension   108
2. Impact of adherence on blood pressure control and cardiovascular outcome   108
3. Adherence to non-pharmacological treatment   108
4. Factors contributing to adherence   109
5. Interventions for improving adherence   110
6. Conclusions   112
7. References   113

Clinical trials have demonstrated that the treatment of mild-to-moderate hypertension can reduce the risk of stroke by 30 to 43% *(1–4)* and of myocardial infarction by 15% *(5)*. Other costly consequences of untreated hypertension can also be prevented or minimized by effective treatment. Examples of the benefits of treatment include reduction in risk of cardiac failure, reduction in incidence of dementia *(6)*, preservation of renal function and prevention of blindness in diabetic patients with hypertension *(7–9)*.

Traditionally, the term compliance has been employed to mean the extent to which the patient, when taking a drug, complies with the clinician's advice and follows the regimen *(10)*. However, the new era of patient-oriented care has led to the use of this term being questioned, and alternative terms such as adherence, persistence and concordance have been suggested *(11–14)*.

In addition to the confusing terminology in the area of adherence, there has been controversy over the use of 80% as a cut-off point to distinguish adherence from nonadherence. In most studies, nonadherence has been considered to occur when patients do not take ≥ 80% of their prescribed antihypertensive drugs (15,16).

Whatever the definition, poor adherence to treatment is the most important cause of uncontrolled blood pressure *(13,14,17)* and only 20 to 80% of patients receiving treatment for hypertension in real-life situations are considered to be "good compliers" *(18)*.

1. Prevalence of adherence to pharmacotherapy in patients with hypertension

Despite the availability of effective treatment, over half of the patients being treated for hypertension drop out of care entirely within a year of diagnosis *(15)* and of those who remain under medical supervision only about 50% take at least 80% of their prescribed medications *(16)*. Consequently, because of poor adherence to antihypertensive treatment, approximately 75% of patients with a diagnosis of hypertension do not achieve optimum blood-pressure control *(13,18)*.

Estimates of the extent to which patients adhere to pharmacotherapy for hypertension vary between 50 and 70%. This variation relates to differences in study groups, duration of follow-up, methods of assessment of adherence and drug regimens used in different studies. For example, studies that defined adherence as an 80% ratio of days on which medication was dispensed to days in the study period, reported adherence rates ranging from 52 to 74% *(19,20)*. Other studies that have investigated discontinuation of antihypertensives have reported adherence rates of 43 to 88% *(21–24)*. Furthermore, it has been estimated that within the first year of treatment 16 to 50% of patients with hypertension discontinue their antihypertensive medications, and among those who continue their therapy in the long term, missed doses of medication are common *(25)*. These figures differ for newly-diagnosed patients and those with chronic, long-standing hypertension *(26)*.

Another source of variation that could explain the differences in rates of adherence is the method used to measure adherence. Examples of methods used include calculating the percentage of pills taken in a specific time period, the percentage of patients taking 80% of their pills, the improvement in number of pills taken, the dropouts from treatment and follow-up, and the missed appointments. There are also indirect proxy measures such as change in blood pressure and the achievement of target blood pressure *(27)*.

2. Impact of adherence on blood pressure control and cardiovascular outcome

Good adherence has been associated with improved blood pressure control *(17)* and reduced complications of hypertension *(28,29)*. For example, in one study, health education interventions for urban-poor patients with hypertension were introduced sequentially in a randomized factorial design to a cohort of 400 ambulatory outpatients with hypertension over a 5-year period. The interventions resulted in an improvement in adherence, which was associated with better blood pressure control and a significant reduction (53.2% less) in hypertension-related mortality rates *(28)*.

In another study, patients who did not adhere to beta-blocker therapy were found to be 4.5 times more likely to have complications of coronary heart disease than those who did *(23)*. However, whether this increased complication rate was directly related to poor adherence to antihypertensive medication is not certain.

3. Adherence to non-pharmacological treatment

The efficacy of non-pharmacological therapy, including reduction in dietary salt intake, weight reduction, moderation of alcohol intake and increased physical activity, in lowering blood pressure has been shown by several studies *(30,31)*. In general, among small, well-supervised and motivated groups of patients receiving counselling on moderate salt restriction, most of the patients followed the regimen *(30,32,33)*. There is limited information, however, on adherence to other lifestyle measures intended to lower blood pressure. Most of the problems related to adherence to non-pharmacological treatment are currently assumed to be similar to those related to adherence to antihypertensive drug therapy and this is an area that warrants further investigation.

4. Factors contributing to adherence

Many factors have been shown to contribute to adherence and these have been extensively reviewed *(34–36)*. Two of the most important factors contributing to poor adherence are undoubtedly the asymptomatic and lifelong nature of the disease. Other potential determinants of adherence may be related to:

– demographic factors such as age and education;

– the patient's understanding and perception of hypertension *(37)*;

– the health care provider's mode of delivering treatment;

– the relationships between patients and health care professionals;

– health systems influences; and

– complex antihypertensive drug regimens *(38)*.

Poor socioeconomic status, illiteracy and unemployment are important risk factors for poor adherence *(39,40)*. Other important patient-related factors may include understanding and acceptance of the disease, perception of the health risk related to the disease, awareness of the costs and benefits of treatment, active participation in monitoring *(41)* and decision-making in relation to management of the disease *(42)*.

The influence of factors related to the health care provider on adherence to therapy for hypertension has not been systematically studied. Some of the more important factors probably include lack of knowledge, inadequate time, lack of incentives and feedback on performance. Multifaceted educational strategies to enhance knowledge, audit with feedback on performance, and financial incentives are some of the interventions that should be tested for their effectiveness *(43–45)*.

The responsibility for adherence must be shared between the health care provider, the patient and the health care system. Good relationships between the patients and their health care providers are therefore imperative for good adherence. Empathetic and non-judgemental attitude and assistance, ready availability, good quality of communication and interaction are some of the important attributes of health care professionals that have been shown to be determinants of the adherence of patients *(46)*.

Health systems-related issues also play an important role in the promotion of adherence. In most low-income countries supplies of medications are limited and they often have to be bought out-of-pocket. Strategies for improving access to drugs such as sustainable financing, affordable prices and reliable supply systems have an important influence on patient adherence, particularly in poorer segments of the population *(47)*. Focusing on improving the efficiency of key health system functions such as delivery of care, financing and proper pharmaceutical management can make a substantial contribution to improving the adherence rates of patients with hypertension and patients with chronic illnesses in general.

Some of the better-recognized determinants of adherence to antihypertensive therapy are related to aspects of the drug treatment itself *(46,48–55)* and include drug tolerability, regimen complexity, drug costs and treatment duration.

Some investigators have speculated that poor adherence can be explained in part by properties of the medications such as tolerability. However, a discrepancy has been noted between data on adherence in relation to drug tolerability that are obtained from randomized controlled trials and those obtained from observational studies. For example pooled results from head-to-head randomized controlled trials that recorded discontinuation of medications due to adverse events have demonstrated that significantly fewer patients discontinued treatment with thiazide diuretics than discontinued treatment with beta-blockers and alpha-adrenergic blockers *(46,48)*. However a recent review based on observational studies has reported that initial treatment with newer classes of drug such as angiotensin II antagonists, angiotensin converting enzyme inhibitors and calcium channel blockers favoured adherence to treatment *(22)*.

It has been argued that information on adherence and the factors that contribute to it is better obtained from observational studies than from randomized clinical trials *(49)* because the stricter selection criteria and structured protocols used in randomized clinical trials may preclude generalization to patient behaviour in the real world. The role of drug tolerability in adherence to antihypertensive medication remains a topic for debate *(50–53)* and warrants further investigation.

The complexity of the regimen is another treatment-related factor that has been identified as a possible cause of poor adherence. Frequency of dosing, number of concurrent medications and changes in antihypertensive medications are some of the factors that contribute to the complexity of a regimen and these have been investigated in many observational studies *(46)*. Fewer daily doses of antihypertensives *(56,57)*, monotherapies and fewer changes in antihypertensive medications (less treatment turbulence) have all been associated with better adherence *(54,55)*.

5. Interventions for improving adherence

Adherence to treatment recommendations has a major impact on health outcomes and the costs of care for patients with hypertension. However, evidence to support any specific approach or intervention for improving patient adherence to antihypertensive drugs or prescribed lifestyle changes is lacking *(27)*.

Adherence to long-term medication regimens requires behavioural change, which involves learning, adopting and sustaining a medication-taking behaviour. Strategies such as providing rewards, reminders and family support to reinforce the new behaviour have been found to improve adherence in chronic illnesses *(58–60)* (see also table 7). Such behaviour-related interventions are likely to be key to improving adherence to antihypertensive medications and should be explored rigorously in clinical trials.

Until better insight into adherence is obtained, multifaceted measures to assist patients to follow treatment with antihypertensives have to be adopted. Health care providers need to be made aware of the low rates of adherence of patients with hypertension. They should receive training on how to counsel patients in a constructive and non-judgemental manner with the primary goal of helping the patient to adhere better to the treatment schedule.

Health care providers should also be trained to make a rational selection of antihypertensive drugs. The drug selected should be available, affordable, have a simple dosing regimen, and ideally, should not interfere with the quality of life of the patient.

Wherever feasible, patients should be taught to measure and monitor their own blood pressure and to assess their own adherence. Patients need to understand the importance of maintaining blood pressure control during the day and to use their drugs rationally. Furthermore, they need to learn how to deal with missed doses, how to identify adverse events and what to do when they occur.

Table 7 Factors affecting adherence to treatment for hypertension and interventions for improving it, listed by the five dimensions and the interventions used to improve adherence

Hypertension	Factors affecting adherence	Interventions to improve adherence
Socioeconomic-related factors	(–) Poor socioeconomic status; illiteracy; unemployment; limited drug supply; high cost of medication *(46,48–55)*	Family preparedness *(58–60)*; patient health insurance; uninterrupted supply of medicines; sustainable financing, affordable prices and reliable supply systems
Health care team/health system-related factors	(–) Lack of knowledge and training for health care providers on managing chronic diseases; inadequate relationship between health care provider and patient; lack of knowledge, inadequate time for consultations; lack of incentives and feedback on performance (+) Good relationship between patient and physician *(46)*	Training in education of patients on use of medicines; good patient–physician relationship; continuous monitoring and reassessment of treatment; monitoring adherence; non-judgemental attitude and assistance; uninterrupted ready availability of information; rational selection of medications; training in communication skills; delivery, financing and proper management of medicines; pharmaceuticals: developing drugs with better safety profile; pharmaceuticals: participation in patient education programmes and developing instruments to measure adherence for patients
Condition-related factors	(+) Understanding and perceptions about hypertension *(37)*	Education on use of medicines *(58)*
Therapy-related factors	(–) Complex treatment regimens *(38,46,48–55)*; duration of treatment; low drug tolerability, adverse effects of treatment *(46,48–55)* (+) Monotherapy with simple dosing schedules; less frequent dose *(56)*; fewer changes in antihypertensive medications *(54)*; newer classes of drugs: angiotensin II antagonists, angiotensin converting enzyme inhibitors, calcium channel blockers *(22)*	Simplification of regimens *(38,46)*
Patient-related factors	(–) Inadequate knowledge and skill in managing the disease symptoms and treatment; no awareness of the costs and benefits of treatment; non-acceptance of monitoring (+) Perception of the health risk related to the disease *(37)*; active participation in monitoring *(41)*; participation in management of disease *(42)*	Behavioural and motivational intervention *(58–60)*; good patient–physician relationship; self-management of disease and treatment *(58)*; self-management of side-effects; memory aids and reminders *(58–60)*

(+) Factors having a positive effect on adherence; (–) factors having a negative effect on adherence.

6. Conclusions

Patients need advice, support and information from health professionals in order to be able to understand the importance of maintaining blood pressure control during the day, to use their drugs rationally, to learn how to deal with missed doses and how to identify adverse events and what to do when they occur. Sharing this responsibility with health professionals is a must – the patient does not need to cope alone.

There is a direct need for research to fill gaps in knowledge on adherence. In general such research should aim at gaining a better understanding of the determinants of adherence discussed above so that effective interventions that address barriers can be developed.

In addition, research should focus on the following important areas:

– validation and standardization of various measures of adherence to prescribed drug therapy and non-pharmacological therapy for hypertension;

– development of valid and reliable questionnaires to obtain information on determinants of adherence;

– investigation of health-related quality-of-life indicators related to patients' adherence to antihypertensive therapy;

– identification of predictors of adherence to pharmacological and non-pharmacological therapy;

– determination of the factors related to behaviour that influence adherence to antihypertensive therapy, such as patient preferences and patient beliefs;

– identifying common risk factors for nonadherence in patients with hypertension, in both developing and developed countries, to study strategies for improving patient adherence;

– understanding of behaviour change principles and mechanisms that promote adherence;

– development of interventions to promote adherence to antihypertensive medication;

– development of materials to involve patients more in managing and regulating their adherence and therefore their hypertension; and

– determination of the reductions in costs and hypertension-related complications resulting from adherence to antihypertensive therapy – issues that are relevant to the needs of patients, managed care organizations and governments.

7. References

1. Hennekens CH, Braunwald E. Clinical trials in cardiovascular disease: A companion to Braunwald´s heart disease. Philadelphia, W.B. Saunders, 1999.
2. Singer RB. Stroke, in the elderly treated for systolic hypertension. *Journal of Insurance Medicine*, 1992, 24:28–31.
3. Medical Research Council Working Party. Medical Research Council Trial of treatment of hypertension in older adults. Principal results. *British Medical Journal*, 1992, 304:405–412.
4. Collins R, MacMahon S. Blood pressure, antihypertensive drug treatment and the risks of stroke and coronary heart disease. *British Medical Bulletin*, 1994, 50:272–298.
5. Collins R et al. Blood pressure, stroke and coronary heart diseases. Part II: Effects of short-term reduction in blood pressure – An overview of the uncounfounded randomised drug trials in an epidemiological context. *Lancet*, 1990, 335:827–838.
6. Peterson JC et al. For the Modification of Diet in Renal Disease Study Group. Blood pressure control, proteinuria, and the progression of renal diseases. *Annals of Internal Medicine*, 1995, 123:754–762.
7. Bergstrom J et al. Progression of renal failure in man is retarded with more frequent clinical follow-ups and better blood-pressure control. *Clinical Nephrology*, 1985, 25:1–6.
8. Holman R et al. Efficacy of atenolol and captopril in reducing the risk of macrovascular and microvascular complications in type 2 diabetes: UKPDS 39. *British Medical Journal*, 1998, 317:713–720.
9. Forette F et al. Systolic Hypertension in Europe Investigators. The prevention of dementia with antihypertensive treatment: new evidence from the Systolic Hypertension in Europe (Syst-Eur) study. *Archives of Internal Medicine*, 2002, 162:2046–2052.
10. Spence JD, Hurley TC, Spence JD. Actual practice in hypertension: implications for persistence with and effectiveness of therapy. *Current Hypertension Reports*, 2001, 3:481–487.
11. Sackett DL et al. Patient compliance with antihypertensive regimens. *Patient Counselling & Health Education*, 1978, 1:18–21.
12. Haynes RB et al. Improvement of medication compliance in uncontrolled hypertension. *Lancet*, 1976, 1:1265–1268.
13. Burt VL et al. Prevalence of hypertension in the US adult population. Results from the Third National Health and Nutrition Examination Survey, 1988–1991. *Hypertension*, 1995, 25:305–313.
14. Hershey JC et al. Patient compliance with antihypertensive medication. *American Journal of Public Health*, 1980, 70:1081–1089.
15. Mapes RE. Physicians' drug innovation and relinquishment. *Social Science & Medicine*, 1977, 11:619–624.
16. Sackett DL et al. Randomised clinical trial of strategies for improving medication compliance in primary hypertension. *Lancet*, 1975, 1:1205–1207.
17. Lucher TF et al. Compliance in hypertension: facts and concepts. *Hypertension*, 1985, 3:S3–S9.
18. Costa FV. Compliance with antihypertensive treatment. *Clinical & Experimental Hypertension*, 1996, 18:463–472.
19. Bittar N. Maintaining long-term control of blood pressure: the role of improved compliance. *Clinical Cardiology*, 1995, 18:312–316.
20. Okano GJ et al. Patterns of antihypertensive use among patients in the US Department of Defense database initially prescribed an angiotensin converting enzyme inhibitor or calcium channel blocker. *Clinical Therapeutics*, 1997, 19:1433–1435.
21. Christensen DB et al. Assessing compliance to hypertensive medications using computer-based pharmacy records. *Medical Care*, 1997, 35:1252–1262.
22. Caro JJ et al. Effect of initial drug choice on persistence with antihypertensive therapy: the importance of actual practice data. *Canadian Medical Association Journal*, 1999, 160:41–46.
23. Caro JJ, Payne K. Real-world effectiveness of antihypertensive drugs. *Canadian Medical Association Journal*, 2000, 162:190–191.
24. Psaty BM et al. Temporal patterns of antihypertensive medication use among elderly patients. The Cardiovascular Health Study. *Journal of the American Medical Association*, 1993, 270:1837–1841.
25. Flack JM, Novikov SV, Ferrario CM. Benefits of adherence to antihypertensive drug therapy. *European Heart Journal*, 1996, 17:16–20.
26. Caro JJ et al. Persistence with treatment for hypertension in actual practice. *Canadian Medical Association Journal*, 1999, 160:31–37.
27. Ebrahim S. Detection, adherence and control of hypertension for the prevention of stroke. *Health Technology Assessment*, 1998, 2:1–80.
28. Morisky DE, Levine DM, Green LW et al. Five year blood pressure control and mortality following health education for hypertensive patients. *American Journal of Public Health*, 1963, 73:153–162.
29. Psaty BM et al. The relative risk of incident coronary heart diseases associated with recently stopping the use of ß-blockers. *Journal of the American Medical Association*, 1990, 73:1653–1657.
30. Jeffery RW et al. Low-sodium, high-potassium diet: feasibility and acceptability in a normotensive population. *American Journal of Public Health*, 1984, 74:492–494.
31. Nugent CA et al. Salt restriction in hypertensive patients. Comparison of advice, education, and group management. *Archives of Internal Medicine*, 1984, 144:1415–1417.
32. Weinberger MH et al. Dietary sodium restriction as adjunctive treatment of hypertension. *Journal of the American Medical Association*, 1988, 259:2561–2565.
33. Feldman R et al. Adherence to pharmacologic management of hypertension. *Canadian Journal of Public Health*, 1998, 89:I16–I18.
34. Rudd P. Compliance with antihypertensive therapy: raising the bar of expectations. *American Journal of Managed Care*, 1998, 4:957–966.
35. Schneider M, Fallab Stubi C, Waeber B. The place of microelectronic system in measuring compliance. In: Metry J, Meyer U, eds. *Drug regimen compliance: issues in clinical trials and patient management*. Chichester, John Wiley and Sons, 1999:85–86.
36. Nessman DG, Carnahan JE, Nugent CA. Increasing compliance. Patient-operated hypertension groups. *Archives of Internal Medicine*, 1980, 140:1427–1430.
37. Conrad P. The meaning of medications: another look at compliance. *Social Science & Medicine*, 1985, 20:29–37.
38. Kjellgren KI, Ahlner J, Saljo R. Taking antihypertensive medication – controlling or co-operating with patients? *International Journal of Cardiology*, 1995, 47:257–268.
39. Saounatsou M et al. The influence of the hypertensive patient's education in compliance with their medication. *Public Health Nursing*, 2001, 18:436–442.
40. Bone LR et al. Community health survey in an urban African-American neighborhood: distribution and correlates of elevated blood pressure. *Ethnicity & Disease*, 2000, 10:87–95.
41. Johnson AL et al. Self-recording of blood pressure in the management of hypertension. *Canadian Medical Association Journal*, 1978, 119:1034–1039.
42. Fleiss JL. The statistical basis of meta-analysis. *Statistical Methods in Medical Research*, 1993, 2:121–145.
43. Davis DA et al. Evidence of the effectiveness of CME. A review of 50 randomized controlled trials. *Journal of the American Medical Association*, 1992, 268:1111–1117.
44. Davis DA et al. Changing physician performance. A systematic review of the effect of continuing medical education strategies. *Journal of the American Medical Association*, 1995, 274:700–705.
45. Oxaman AD. No magic bullets: a systematic review of 102 trials of interventions to improve professional practice. *Canadian Medical Association Journal*, 1995, 153:1423–1431.

46. Wright JM, Lee C, Chambers GK. Real-world effectiveness of antihypertensive drugs. *Canadian Medical Association Journal*, 2000, 162:190–191.

47. Schafheutle EI et al. Access to medicines: cost as an influence on the views and behaviour of patients. *Health & Social Care in the Community*, 2002, 10:187–195.

48. Wright JM. Choosing a first line drug in the management of elevated blood pressure. What is the evidence? I. Thiazide diuretics. *Canadian Medical Association Journal*, 2000, 163:57–60.

49. Revicki DL, Frank L. Pharmacoeconomic evaluations in the real world. Effectiveness versus efficacy studies. *Pharmacoeconomics*, 1999, 15:123–134.

50. Myers MG. Compliance in hypertension: why don't patients take their pills? *Canadian Medical Association Journal*, 1999, 160:64–65.

51. Materson BJ et al. Single drug therapy for hypertension in men. A comparison of six antihypertensive agents with placebo. The Department of Veterans Affair Cooperative Study group on Antihypertensive Agents. *New England Journal of Medicine*, 1993, 328:914–921.

52. Phillipp T et al. Randomised, double blind multicentre comparison of hydrochlorothiazide, atenolol, nitredipine, and enalapril in antihypertensive treatment: results of the HANE study. *British Medical Journal*, 1997, 315:154–159.

53. McInnes GT. Integrated approaches to management of hypertension: promoting treatment acceptance. *American Heart Journal*, 1999, 138:S252–S255.

54. Monane M et al. The effects of initial drug choice and comorbidity on antihypertensive therapy compliance. Results from a population-based study in the elderly. *American Journal of Hypertension*, 1997, 10: 697–704.

55. Bloom BS. Continuation of initial antihypertensive medication after 1 year of therapy. *Clinical Therapeutics*, 1998, 20:671–681.

56. Nuesch R et al. Relation between insufficient response to antihypertensive treatment and poor compliance with treatment: a prospective case-control study. *British Medical Journal*, 2001, 323:142–146.

57. Eisen SA et al. The effect of prescribed daily dose frequency on patient medication compliance. *Archives of Internal Medicine*, 1990, 150:1881–1884.

58. Cholesterol, diastolic blood pressure, and stroke: 13,000 strokes in 450,000 people in 45 prospective cohorts. Prospective studies collaboration. *Lancet*, 1995, 346:1647–1653.

59. White A, Nicolass G, Foster K. *Health Survey for England, 1991*. London, Her Majesty's Stationery Office, 1993.

60. Five-year findings of the hypertension detection and follow-up program. I. Reduction in mortality of persons with high blood pressure, including mild hypertension. Hypertension Detection and Follow-up Program Cooperative Group. *Journal of the American Medical Association*, 1979, 242:2562–2571.

CHAPTER XIV

Tobacco smoking

1. The burden of tobacco smoking   115

2. Clinical guidelines and therapies available for tobacco smoking cessation   116

3. Definitions   117

4. Epidemiology of adherence   118

5. Factors affecting adherence   119

6. Interventions for improving adherence   119

7. Cost, effectiveness and cost-effectiveness of adherence   120

8. Conclusions   121

9. References   121

1. The burden of tobacco smoking

The health risks of tobacco use, particularly cigarette smoking, are well-recognized. Tobacco smoke is the single most important factor contributing to poor health, and it is widely believed that a reduction in the prevalence of tobacco smoking would be the single most effective preventive health measure (1). An estimated 70–90% of lung cancer, 56–80% of chronic respiratory diseases and 22% of cardiovascular diseases are attributable to tobacco smoking (2).

Cigarette smoking remains the most important preventable cause of premature death and disability worldwide (3). Each year, tobacco use causes some 4.9 million premature deaths (2,4). Whereas until recently this epidemic of chronic disease affected the wealthy countries, it is now rapidly becoming a problem in the developing world (5). About 80% of the world's 1.1 billion smokers live in low-income and middle-income countries. By 2030, seven out of every 10 deaths from smoking will occur in low-income countries (6).

The available evidence suggests that free trade in tobacco products has led to increases in tobacco smoking and other types of tobacco use, but measures to reduce its supply are difficult to implement. However, interventions to reduce the demand for tobacco are likely to succeed. These include higher tobacco taxes, antismoking education, bans on tobacco advertising and promotion, policies designed to prevent smoking in public spaces or workplaces, and pharmacological therapies to help smokers to quit *(5,6)*.

Hundreds of controlled scientific studies have demonstrated that appropriate treatment can help tobacco users to achieve permanent abstinence. Millions of lives could therefore be saved with effective treatment for tobacco dependence.

2. Clinical guidelines and therapies available for tobacco smoking cessation

Effective smoking-cessation therapy can involve a variety of methods, such as a combination of behavioural treatment and pharmacotherapy *(4)*. A number of strategies have been developed to help smokers to quit. These include self-help manuals, individual or group counselling, aversive conditioning, hypnosis, clonidine, nicotine replacement therapy *(7)* and the use of antidepressant medications.

The most widely reported treatment is nicotine replacement therapy (NRT), which is available in the form of nicotine gum, nicotine patches and, more recently, as an oral inhaler. Nicotine replacement therapy is an established pharmacological aid to quitting smoking and it has consistently been shown to almost double the rate of quitting, irrespective of additional interventions *(8)*. Many studies have confirmed these findings *(1,7,9–18)*. A brief description of each of the NRTs is given below.

Nicotine gum delivers nicotine through transbuccal absorption. The gum should be discarded, not swallowed, after 30 minutes. The patient can chew another piece when there is an urge to smoke *(19)*. The total recommended dose is 10 to 12 pieces of gum daily for 1–3 months. After 3 months, a gradual withdrawal from gum use is recommended, with completion of treatment within 6 months *(20)*.

Transdermal administration of nicotine is available in three active forms (21, 14 and 7 mg), each steadily delivering an average of 0.7 mg nicotine per cm^2 per 24 h *(21)*. The strength of the patch is reduced gradually (by reducing the size of the patch) over the course of therapy, 8–12 weeks per 24 h treatment or 14–20 weeks per 16 h treatment (with patches that are worn only during the day) *(19)*. To reduce the likelihood of local skin irritation, the manufacturers recommend that the patch site be changed daily and that the same site is used not more than once every 7–10 days *(19,22,23)*.

The 1996 Smoking Cessation Clinical Guideline, which compared the use of NRT patches to nicotine gum, considered the patch easier to use and also more likely to enhance adherence *(24)*.

Oral nicotine inhalers consist of a disposable cartridge containing 10 mg nicotine and 1 mg menthol inserted in a plastic mouthpiece. Nicotine is delivered at a rate of 13 mg of nicotine/puff (80 puffs = 1 mg). The recommended dose is 6–12 cartridges over 24 h *(10)*. In one study, participants were encouraged to decrease use of the inhaler after 4 months, but were permitted to continue treatment for 18 of the 24 months *(10)*.

Behavioural therapies have been used in combination with NRTs, to enhance adherence to treatment and to help patients stop smoking. The therapies employed have included individual counselling, group therapy sessions and telephone hotline support, all of which provide encouragement, guidance, and strategies to combat urges and cravings to smoke. The intensity of the behavioural sessions varied between studies (e.g. weekly or daily, lasting between 15 minutes and 1 hour, and provided by a nurse, a physician or an MS/PhD therapist *(5,7,8,11,12,15,17–20,24–26)*. Pharmacists have also been proposed as potential providers of information and guidance concerning NRTs and tobacco in general *(27)*.

3. Definitions

Smoking cessation is generally defined as complete abstinence from the use of smoked tobacco. The duration of the studies varied from 12 weeks to 24 weeks, and used patient self-report questionnaires or interview data to assess quitting smoking. Almost all studies confirmed the self-reported data using one or more of the following biological measurements: expired carbon monoxide £ 10 ppm from the quitting day until the end of treatment and follow-up *(1,3,10–12,15,17,21,25,26,28–32)*, salivary cotinine levels ≤ 20 ng/ml *(3,11,13,16,24,28,31,33,34)* and urinary cotinine levels of 317 ng/ml or less *(21)*.

Adherence to smoking cessation therapy. The most widely used definition of adherence to treatment was "using the nicotine replacement therapy continuously at the recommended dose in the instructed manner for the entire 16-h *(17)* (or 24-h) time period" *(1,10,12,13,17,20,29,30,32,35,36)*.

Some studies assessed adherence by comparing the number of used and unused systems returned each week with the number of days that had elapsed between visits *(18,21,29)*. Others counted the total number of days on which patients did not use the systems during the treatment period, more than 5 days missed, or not wearing patches at night, were considered nonadherence *(7)*.

Others defined adherence as "perfect compliance with treatment protocol and/or not missing any scheduled follow-up visits" *(1,8,18)*. Bushnel et al. defined adherence as attending ≥ 75% of smoking cessation classes *(26)*.

Few reports provided detailed data on adherence such as number of prescribed doses taken during a monitored period, monitored days during which the correct number of doses were taken or whether or not the prescribed intervals between doses taken were respected.

Drop-out. Patients may drop out from treatment for several reasons. These include patient-related factors, physician decision and adverse effects of the drug. Regardless of the reason for dropping out, patients who do so are usually found to be smoking at follow-up *(25)*.

The way in which dropouts are handled can make it difficult to compare studies in this area. It is important to consider the reasons for dropping out to achieve accurate estimates of adherence. Those who drop out for reasons related to the treatment need to be distinguished from those who dropped out for reasons related to the study itself. Some patients drop out because they experience adverse events or withdrawal symptoms. As with studies in other therapeutic areas, these patients should be classified as nonadherent. Another important reason for dropout is the failure to stop or reduce smoking despite following the treatment. Many relapsed smokers stop using the prescribed NRT *(37)* when they fail to quit smoking despite having been adherent to NRT *(21,36)*. We consider that these patients should be counted as treatment failures for the purpose of calculating smoking cessation rates, but not for adherence rates. Side-effects were the main reason given for dropout in the studies reviewed *(1,9,11–13,16–18, 22,35–40)*. Other patient-related reasons for stopping therapy were failure to recall the receipt of a prescription *(20)*, unwillingness to continue in the study *(1,9,10,13–17)* lack of a self-perceived need for treatment and lack of a perceived effect of treatment *(1,9,13,16,36–40)*. Physicians reported discontinuation of therapy due to lack of efficacy or complete failure to stop or to reduce smoking after therapy had been started *(1,3,8–10,17,18,21,22,24,29,36–38,41–43)* and elevated carbon monoxide *(17)*.

4. Epidemiology of adherence

The prevalence of adherence to smoking cessation therapy varied widely between studies (5–96%) and also varied between countries as shown in Table 8.

Table 8 Rates of adherence to smoking cessation therapy reported by country

Country	No. of values reported	Mean	Standard deviation	Minimum	Maximum
Australia	8	0.57	0.25	0.19	0.83
Denmark	23	0.59	0.14	0.33	0.86
Italy	1	0.34	–	0.34	0.34
New Zealand	4	0.86	0.16	0.63	0.96
Switzerland	2	0.53	0.10	0.46	0.60
United Kingdom	11	0.62	0.17	0.40	0.91
United States	31	0.52	0.23	0.05	0.96

This variation can be explained by the use of different interventions, adjunctive support and populations studied.

Figure 4 includes only studies that reported time-series data. It suggests that adherence to smoking cessation therapies is a logarithmic function of number of weeks. The suggested trend line shows a rapid decrease in adherence rates during the first 6 weeks and a very slow decrease after 24 weeks. (Adherence rates after week 20 are related to adherence to follow-up visits rather than therapy.)

Many studies have found a positive linear correlation between adherence and cessation rates (3,7,12,14,15,20,24,25,31–33,36,37,39,44). Both adherence and smoking cessation rates increased significantly when NRT was combined with antidepressant pharmacotherapy (3).

Figure 4 Adherence rates over time

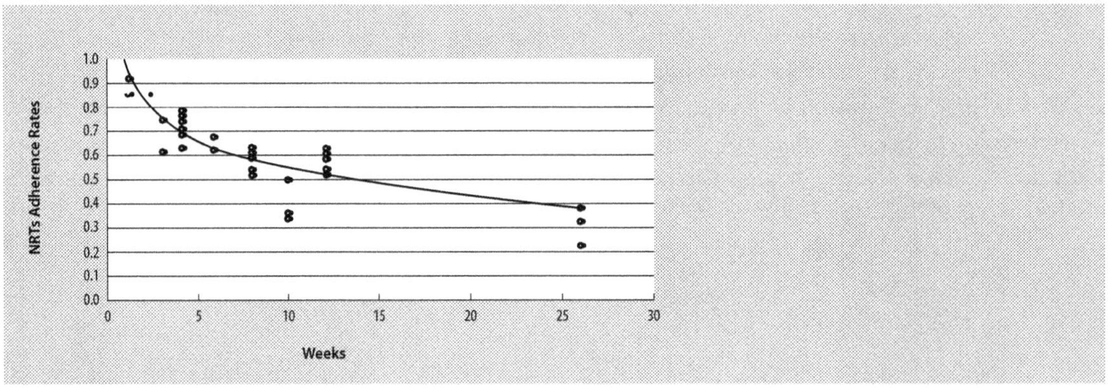

NRT, nicotine replacement therapy.

5. Factors affecting adherence

Some baseline variables apparently influence adherence to therapy. In one study, mean daily cigarette consumption, expired carbon monoxide, plasma nicotine and cotinine, and Fagerstrom Tolerance Questionnaire (FTQ) scores (44) were significantly higher in the dropout group than in the adherent group (1). Alterman et al. (25) concluded that greater dependence on tobacco was associated with less patch use, indicating that patients who smoked more cigarettes were less adherent to treatment with patches.

Depression is an important psychological factor associated with cessation of smoking. A higher prevalence of depressive symptoms would theoretically increase the risk of nonadherence to treatment (45). Differing results of studies of this association have been reported. Some studies showed that smokers with a history of major depression who were not depressed at the time of a 4-week treatment programme had a lower abstinence rate than did smokers without a history of depression. In another study, smokers with a history of major depression in an 8-week multicomponent cognitive behavioural group plus nicotine-gum programme, had a significantly higher abstinence rate than smokers with a history of depression who were treated with nicotine plus a standard programme of information (3,45). Ginsberg et al. suggested that cognitive–behavioural sessions emphasizing group cohesion and social support among smokers with a history of depression maintains adherence in this population (45). A satisfactory explanation of this link will require further research (3,24,31).

Other variables, such as gender, racial or ethnic background, history of psychiatric pathology (25), weight gain (29,30), craving and withdrawal symptoms are reported as being potential predictors of patch adherence. However, because there are no validated measures of these variables, the available data are insufficient to assess their effects on adherence.

During an NRT programme, investigators observed some factors that had a positive effect on adherence. These included motivation (25), attendance at cessation classes, access to free NRT, higher education levels, older age, advice from physicians (26), and more frequent contact with physicians and pharmacists (35). These factors were also reported as predictive of success in stopping smoking. The analysis of the studies showed that these factors have proven to be statistically significant in increasing abstinence rates, but there is no measure proving their association with adherence.

6. Interventions for improving adherence

The most frequently employed interventions for improving adherence reviewed were NRT, antidepressant therapy, pharmacist intervention, psychosocial/behavioural support and counselling, and diet counselling (low-calorie diet) (see also Table 9). Adjunctive psychosocial treatment or behavioural advice has been successfully used to support smoking cessation programmes (25).

Although Alterman et al. showed that patients receiving more intense adjunctive psychosocial or medical treatment were more adherent to treatment with patches (25), overall, the data reviewed suggested that minimal behavioural support also results in similar or higher adherence rates, at least for some types of smoker. Minimal behavioural support might offer a cost-effective way to implement first-line smoking cessation programmes at a population level. More controlled studies including cost-effectiveness analysis are needed to clarify this issue.

The monitoring of therapeutic drug levels, NRT and/or antidepressant may also be useful. This feedback might be used to identify poorly adherent patients for whom more intensive adherence-enhancing interventions would be helpful (46).

Intensive anti-smoking campaigns, such as the "Truth Denormalization Ads" might be extremely useful, especially among teenagers, as they change the social attitude towards tobacco smoking.

Table 9 Factors affecting adherence to smoking cessation therapy and interventions for improving it, listed by the five dimensions and the interventions used to improve adherence

Tobacco smoking	Factors affecting adherence	Interventions to improve adherence
Socioeconomic-related factors	(−) High treatment cost (41) (+) Higher education levels, older age (41)	Social assistance (25)
Health care team/health system-related factors	(−) Unavailability for follow up or lost to follow up (1,8,10,11,17,21); failure to recall the receipt of a prescription (20) (+) Access to free NRT; more frequent contact with physicians and pharmacists (35)	Pharmacist mobilization (41); access to free NRT; frequent follow-up interviews (35)
Condition-related factors	(−) Daily cigarette consumption; expired CO, plasma nicotine and cotinine levels; Fagerstrom Tolerance Questionnaire (FTQ) scores (44); greater tobacco dependence (25); psychiatric comorbidities; depression (3,25); failure to stop or reduce smoking during treatment (1,3,8–10,17,18,21,22,24,29,36–38,41–43)	Education on use of medications; supportive psychiatric consultation (3,25)
Therapy-related factors	(+) Attendance at behavioural intervention sessions (26); adverse events (1,9,16,37–40) or withdrawal symptoms (1,9,11,12,13,16–18,22,35–40)	NRT; antidepressant therapy; education on use of medications; adherence education; assistance with weight reduction (29); continuous monitoring and reassessment of treatment; monitoring adherence (46)
Patient-related factors	(−) Weight gain (29) (+) Motivation (25); good relationship between patient and physician (41)	Adjunctive psychosocial treatment; behavioural intervention (1,9–13,16–19,21–23,25,29,30, 32,38,39,47–52); assistance with weight reduction (29); good patient–physician relationship (41)

CO, Carbon monoxide; NRT, nicotine replacement therapy; (+) factors having a positive effect on adherence; (−) factors having a negative effect on adherence.

7. Cost, effectiveness and cost-effectiveness of adherence

There are few data available concerning the health economics of adherence to smoking cessation therapy. Westman et al. (7) reported that 4 weeks of high-dose and 2 weeks of low-dose nicotine treatment were cost-effective and sufficient to enhance cessation. This 6-week intervention achieved 6-month abstinence rates comparable with those of studies offering 12 or more weeks of treatment.

There is some debate as to whether it is necessary to have health professionals available in the clinic providing supportive counselling (7,53,54). However, the literature search suggested that providing minimal or moderate support resulted in higher adherence rates than providing no support. A separate discussion is required to decide which of the professionals in the health care team should be responsible for the provision of this support.

8. Conclusions

Adherence to NRTs and to other treatments for tobacco dependence is very low in the long term (< 40%), but it shows a strong positive correlation with better cessation outcomes. Unfortunately, these long-term cessation outcomes are still unsatisfactorily low (< 20%). The data presented in this chapter are based mainly on clinical trials and three population-based studies. Therefore the data on adherence and cessation rates presented here might be over-optimistic.

In order to improve the accuracy and comparability of measured adherence rates, further research is needed to establish explicit definitions of "adherence to treatment" and treatment dropout. A clearer understanding and distinction between the different factors that influence dropout is also needed.

The patterns of both adherence to therapy and cessation rates over time suggest that interventions for improving adherence would be more cost-effective the earlier they are introduced into the programme (i.e. during the first 3 weeks).

Surprisingly, lack of access to cheap NRTs has been reported as an important reason for smokers in developed countries failing to quit. This is unexpected because the cost of NRTs is usually equivalent to the cost of smoking. Substituting the demand at the same price should not be a reason not to adhere.

There are few data available for identifying effective adherence-promoting interventions, but the use of antidepressant drugs and psychosocial behavioural supports has shown good results. Studies to evaluate the cost-effectiveness of interventions for improving adherence are required.

9. References

1. Fornai E et al. Smoking reduction in smokers compliant to a smoking cessation trial with nicotine patch. *Monaldi Archives for Chest Disease*, 2001, 56:5–10.

2. *The World Health Report 2002: Reducing risks, promoting healthy life*. Geneva, World Health Organization, 2002.

3. Killen JD et al. Nicotine patch and paroxetine for smoking cessation. *Journal of Consulting & Clinical Psychology*, 2000, 68:883–889.

4. *WHO Tobacco Free Initiative Project*. Geneva, World Health Organization, 2001 (available on the Internet at http://tobacco.who.int/).

5. Jha P, Chaloupka FJ. *Curbing the epidemic: Governments and the economics of tobacco control*. Washington, DC, World Bank, 1999.

6. Jha P, Chaloupka FJ. The economics of global control. *British Medical Journal*, 2000, 321:358–361.

7. Westman EC, Levin ED, Rose JE. The nicotine patch in smoking cessation. A randomized trial with telephone counseling. *Archives of Internal Medicine*, 1993, 153:1917–1923.

8. Richmond RL, Harris K, de Almeida N. The transdermal nicotine patch: results of a randomised placebo-controlled trial. *Medical Journal of Australia*, 1994, 161:130–135.

9. Badgett RG, Tanaka DJ. Is screening for chronic obstructive pulmonary disease justified? *Preventive Medicine*, 1997, 26:466–472.

10. Bolliger CT et al. Smoking reduction with oral nicotine inhalers: double blind, randomised clinical trial of efficacy and safety. *British Medical Journal*, 2000, 321:329–333.

11. Effectiveness of a nicotine patch in helping people stop smoking: results of a randomised trial in general practice. Imperial Cancer Research Fund General Practice Research Group. *British Medical Journal*, 1993, 306:1304–1308.

12. Gourlay SG et al. Double blind trial of repeated treatment with transdermal nicotine for relapsed smokers. *British Medical Journal*, 1995, 311:363–366.

13. Kornitzer M et al. Combined use of nicotine patch and gum in smoking cessation: a placebo-controlled clinical trial. *Preventive Medicine*, 1995, 24:41–47.

14. Prochaska JO. *The transtheoretical approach: Crossing traditional boundaries of therapy*. Irwin, Homewood, IL, Dow Jones, 1984.

15. Russell MA et al. Targeting heavy smokers in general practice: randomised controlled trial of transdermal nicotine patches. *British Medical Journal*, 1993, 306:1308–1312.

16. Saizow RB. Physician-delivered smoking intervention. *Journal - Oklahoma State Medical Association*, 1992, 84:612–617.

17. Tonnesen P et al. Higher dosage nicotine patches increase one-year smoking cessation rates: results from the European CEASE trial. Collaborative European Anti-Smoking Evaluation. European Respiratory Society. *European Respiratory Journal*, 1999, 13:238–246.

18. Transdermal Nicotine Study Group. Transdermal nicotine for smoking cessation. Six-month results from two multicenter controlled clinical trials. *Journal of the American Medical Association*, 1991, 266:3133–3138.

19. Timmreck TC, Randolph JF. Smoking cessation: clinical steps to improve compliance. *Geriatrics*, 1993, 48:63–66.

20. Johnson RE et al. Nicotine chewing gum use in the outpatient care setting. *Journal of Family Practice*, 1992, 34:61–65.

21. Razavi D et al. Maintaining abstinence from cigarette smoking: effectiveness of group counselling and factors predicting outcome. *European Journal of Cancer*, 1999, 35:1238–1247.

22. Martin PD, Robinson GM. The safety, tolerability and efficacy of transdermal nicotine (Nicotinell TTS) in initially hospitalised patients. *New Zealand Medical Journal*, 1995, 108:6–8.

23. Rigotti NA et al. Smoking by patients in a smoke-free hospital: prevalence, predictors, and implications. *Preventive Medicine*, 2000, 31:159–166.

24. The Agency for Health Care Policy and Research Smoking Cessation Clinical Practice Guideline. *Journal of the American Medical Association*, 1996, 275:1270–1280.

25. Alterman AI et al. Nicodermal patch adherence and its correlates. *Drug & Alcohol Dependence*, 1999, 53:159–165.

26. Bushnell FK et al. Smoking cessation in military personnel. *Military Medicine*, 1997, 162:715–719.

27. Teräsalmi E et al. *Pharmacists against Smoking: Research Report 2001*. Copenhagen, World Health Organization, 2001.

28. Anthonisen NR et al. Effects of smoking intervention and the use of an inhaled anticholinergic bronchodilator on the rate of decline of FEV1. The Lung Health Study. *Journal of the American Medical Association*, 1994, 272:1497–1505.

29. Danielsson T, Rossner S, Westin A. Open randomised trial of intermittent very low energy diet together with nicotine gum for stopping smoking in women who gained weight in previous attempts to quit. *British Medical Journal*, 1999, 319:490–493.

30. Gourlay SG et al. Prospective study of factors predicting outcome of transdermal nicotine treatment in smoking cessation. *British Medical Journal*, 1994, 309:842–846.

31. Killen JD et al. Do heavy smokers benefit from higher dose nicotine patch therapy? *Experimental & Clinical Psychopharmacology*, 1999, 7:226–233.

32. Solomon LJ et al. Free nicotine patches plus proactive telephone peer support to help low-income women stop smoking. *Preventive Medicine*, 2000, 31:68–74.

33. Dornelas EA et al. A randomized controlled trial of smoking cessation counseling after myocardial infarction. *Preventive Medicine*, 2000, 30:261–268.

34. Kviz FJ, Crittenden KS, Warnecke RB. Factors associated with nonparticipation among registrants for a self-help, community-based smoking cessation intervention. *Addictive Behaviors*, 1992, 17:533–542.

35. Orleans CT et al. Use of transdermal nicotine in a state-level prescription plan for the elderly. A first look at 'real-world' patch users. *Journal of the American Medical Association*, 1994, 271:601–607.

36. Sonderskov J et al. Nicotine patches in smoking cessation: a randomized trial among over-the-counter customers in Denmark. *American Journal of Epidemiology*, 1997, 145:309–318.

37. Hatch CL, Canaan T, Anderson G. Pharmacology of the pulmonary diseases. *Dental Clinics of North America*, 1996, 40:521–541.

38. Meliska CJ et al. Immune function in cigarette smokers who quit smoking for 31 days. *Journal of Allergy & Clinical Immunology*, 1995, 95:901–910.

39. O'Hara P et al. Design and results of the initial intervention program for the Lung Health Study. The Lung Health Study Research Group. *Preventive Medicine*, 1993, 22:304–315.

40. Pierce JR, Jr. Stroke following application of a nicotine patch [Letter]. *Annals of Pharmacotherapy*, 1994, 28:402.

41. Millard RW, Waranch HR, McEntee M. Compliance to nicotine gum recommendations in a multicomponent group smoking cessation program: an exploratory study. *Addictive Behaviors*, 1992, 17:201–207.

42. Persico AM. Predictors of smoking cessation in a sample of Italian smokers. *International Journal of the Addictions*, 1992, 27:683–695.

43. Shiffman S et al. The efficacy of computer-tailored smoking cessation material as a supplement to nicotine patch therapy. *Drug & Alcohol Dependence*, 2001, 64:35–46.

44. Fagerstrom KO. Measuring degree of physical dependence to tobacco smoking with reference to individualization of treatment. *Addictive Behaviors*, 1978, 3:235–241.

45. Ginsberg JP et al. The relationship between a history of depression and adherence to a multicomponent smoking-cessation program. *Addictive Behaviors*, 1997, 22:783–787.

46. Killen JD et al. Nicotine patch and paroxetine for smoking cessation. *Journal of Consulting & Clinical Psychology*, 2000, 68:883–889.

47. Curry SJ. Self-help interventions for smoking cessation. *Journal of Consulting & Clinical Psychology*, 1993, 61:790–803.

48. Warnecke RB et al. The second Chicago televised smoking cessation program: a 24-month follow-up. *American Journal of Public Health*, 1992, 82:835–840.

49. Raw M. Smoking Cessation Guidelines for Health Professionals. *Thorax*, 1998, 53:S1–S19.

50. Torrecilla M et al. [The physician and the patient in the decision to quit smoking. Effect of the initiative on the result of the intervention.] [Spanish] *Archivos de Bronconeumologia*, 2001, 37:127–134.

51. Dresler CM et al. Smoking cessation and lung cancer resection. *Chest*, 1996, 110:1199–1202.

52. Smith TM, Winters FD. Smoking cessation: a clinical study of the transdermal nicotine patch. *Journal of the American Osteopathic Association*, 1996, 95:655–656.

53. Hajek P, Taylor TZ, Mills P. Brief intervention during hospital admission to help patients to give up smoking after myocardial infarction and bypass surgery: randomised controlled trial. *British Medical journal*, 324:1–6.

54. West R. Helping patients in hospital to quit smoking. *British Medical Journal*, 2002, 324:64.

CHAPTER XV

Tuberculosis

1. Definition of adherence   123

2. Factors that influence adherence to treatment   124

3. Prediction of adherence   125

4. Strategies to improve adherence to treatment   125

5. Questions for future research   128

6. References   129

The World Health Organization (WHO) declared tuberculosis (TB) a global public health emergency in 1993 and since then has intensified its efforts to control the disease worldwide *(1)*. Despite these efforts, there were an estimated 8.7 million new cases of TB worldwide during 2000 *(2)*. The rapidly increasing rates of HIV infection, combined with escalating poverty and the collapse of public health services in many settings have contributed to this serious situation *(3)*.

The therapeutic regimens recommended by WHO have been shown to be highly effective for both preventing and treating TB *(4)*, but poor adherence to anti-tuberculosis medication is a major barrier to its global control *(2,5,6)*. Tuberculosis is a communicable disease, thus poor adherence to a prescribed treatment increases the risks of morbidity, mortality and drug resistance at both the individual and community levels.

The purpose of this chapter is to describe the current insights into patients' treatment behaviour and the methods adopted by health providers to enhance adherence to anti-tuberculosis treatment. This has been done with the aim of contributing to the generation of knowledge leading to the production of guidelines for enhancing adherence to prescribed medication in patients receiving long-term care.

1. Definition of adherence

In terms of TB control, adherence to treatment may be defined as the extent to which the patient's history of therapeutic drug-taking coincides with the prescribed treatment *(7)*.

Adherence may be measured using either process-oriented or outcome-oriented definitions. Outcome-oriented definitions use the end-result of treatment, e.g. cure rate, as an indicator of success. Process-oriented indicators make use of intermediate variables such as appointment-keeping or pill counts to measure adherence *(7)*. The extent to which these intermediate outcomes correlate with the actual quantities of prescribed drugs taken is unknown *(8)*.

The point that separates "adherence" from "nonadherence" would be defined as that in the natural history of the disease making the desired therapeutic outcome likely (adherence) or unlikely (nonadherence) to be achieved. There is as yet no empirical rationale for a definition of nonadherence in the management of TB. Therefore, the definition of adherence to TB treatment needs to be translated into an empirical method of monitoring both the quantity and timing of the medication taken by the patient *(9)*. At the individual level this is desirable, but at the population level a more pragmatic approach is needed. Thus, the success of treatment, that is, the sum of the patients who are cured and those who have completed treatment under the directly observed therapy, short course (DOTS) strategy, is a pragmatic, albeit a proxy, indicator of treatment adherence.

2. Factors that influence adherence to treatment

Many factors have been associated with adherence to TB treatment including patient characteristics, the relationship between health care provider and patient, the treatment regimen and the health care setting *(10)*. One author has defined nonadherence as "an unavoidable by-product of collisions between the clinical world and the other competing worlds of work, play, friendships and family life" *(11)*. Factors that are barriers to adherence to TB drugs can be classified as shown below.

A. Economic and structural factors
TB usually affects people who are hard to reach such as the homeless, the unemployed and the poor. Lack of effective social support networks and unstable living circumstances are additional factors that create an unfavourable environment for ensuring adherence to treatment *(12)*.

B. Patient-related factors
Ethnicity, gender and age have been linked to adherence in various settings *(13–15)*. Knowledge about TB and a belief in the efficacy of the medication will influence whether or not a patient chooses to complete the treatment *(16)*. In addition, cultural belief systems may support the use of traditional healers in conflict with allopathic medicine *(10,17)*. In some TB patients, altered mental states caused by substance abuse, depression and psychological stress may also play a role in their adherence behaviour.

C. Regimen complexity
The number of tablets that need to be taken, as well as their toxicity and other side-effects associated with their use may act as a deterrent to continuing treatment *(18)*. The standard WHO regimen for the treatment of TB involves using four drugs for an initial "intensive phase" (2–3 months), and two or three drugs for a further "continuation" phase (6–8 months). Drugs may be taken daily or "intermittently" three times a week.

D. Supportive relationships between the health provider and the patient
Patient satisfaction with the "significant" provider of health care is considered to be an important determinant of adherence *(19)*, but empathic relationships are difficult to forge in situations where health providers are untrained, overworked, inadequately supervised or unsupported in their tasks, as commonly occurs in countries with a high TB burden *(20)*.

E. Pattern of health care delivery
The organization of clinical services, including availability of expertise, links with patient support systems and flexibility in the hours of operation, also affects adherence to treatment. Many of the ambulatory health care settings responsible for the control of TB are organized to provide care for patients with acute illnesses, and staff may therefore lack the skills required to develop long-term management plans with patients. Consequently, the patient's role in self-management is not facilitated and follow-up is sporadic.

3. Prediction of adherence

If the individuals at risk for poor adherence could be identified early in their management, health care providers should, in theory, be able to intervene by tailoring the provision of treatment to enable such patients to continue their therapy. Unfortunately, the available evidence indicates that health care providers are unable to predict accurately which patients are likely to be nonadherent (21–23).

The literature describes over 200 variables associated with patients who default on treatment. Many of the cited determinants of adherence are unalterable, and the demonstration of a consistent association between characteristics such as gender, age group or literacy and adherence does not lead to a logical approaching to remedy the situation. Furthermore, demographic, social and other patient characteristics often relate poorly to the patient's intention or motivation and do not explain why some TB patients adhere to treatment despite having several unfavourable characteristics. Patients with TB apparently fluctuate in the intensity of their motivation to complete their treatment and admit to considering defaulting many times during their long course of therapy (24).

Many epidemiological studies have explored correlates of adherence, often examining the issue from a biomedical perspective. Within this framework the TB patient has sometimes been seen as a recipient of a treatment regimen, who should obey the instructions of the health care worker. Nonadherent patients who do not conform to these expectations have sometimes been regarded as "deviant". This approach ignores the fact that treatment behaviour is complex and is influenced by a host of factors including the patients' sociocultural setting, health beliefs and subjective experience of the illness.

Numerous psychosocial constructs have been proposed that have attempted to provide a conceptual model for thinking about health behaviour (24–28). The information–motivation–behavioural (IMB) skills model (29) which integrates information, motivation and behavioural skills in explaining behaviour has, however, attracted some attention as a potentially useful guide to developing interventions for enhancing adherence to TB treatment. The IMB model demonstrates that information is a prerequisite for good adherence, but is not sufficient in itself to change behaviour. Motivation and the development of behavioural skills are also critical determinants of behavioural change.

4. Strategies to improve adherence to treatment

Concurrently with the efforts to improve our understanding of factors affecting adherence to TB treatment, numerous measures have been introduced in different settings in an attempt to improve it (30,31).

A. Classification of interventions

The interventions for improving adherence rates may be classified into the following categories:

- Staff motivation and supervision – includes training and management processes aimed at improving the way in which providers care for patients with tuberculosis.

- Defaulter action – the action to be taken when a patient fails to keep a pre-arranged appointment.

- Prompts – routine reminders for patients to keep pre-arranged appointments.

- Health education – provision of information about tuberculosis and the need to attend for treatment.

- Incentives and reimbursements – money or cash in kind to reimburse the expenses of attending the treatment centre, or to improve the attractiveness of visiting the treatment centre.

- Contracts – agreements (written or verbal) to return for an appointment or course of treatment.

- Peer assistance – people from the same social group helping someone with tuberculosis to return to the health centre by prompting or accompanying him or her.

- Directly observed therapy (DOT) – an identified, trained and supervised agent (health worker, community volunteer or family member) directly monitors patients swallowing their anti-TB drugs (see below).

B. Directly observed treatment as a component of the WHO DOTS strategy

The concept of "entirely supervised administration of medicines", first developed by Wallace Fox in the 1950s *(32)*, is now known as directly observed therapy (DOT). DOT was first adopted in TB drug trials in Madras (India) and Hong Kong as early as the 1960s *(33)* and is now widely recommended for the control of TB *(34–36)*. WHO recommends DOT as one of a range of measures to promote adherence to TB treatment *(37)*.

DOT has always meant much more than "supervised swallowing". Different projects in countries with a high prevalence of TB have shown that removing the socioeconomic barriers to DOT faced by patients increases adherence and cure rates *(38,39)*. In a country where the prevalence of TB is low, such as the United States, DOT programmes are complex and have several components including social support, housing, food tokens and legal measures and are highly cost-effective *(35,40)*.

Since 1991, WHO has promoted the strategy of "directly observed therapy, short course" (now known as the DOTS strategy) *(32)*. "DOTS" is the brand name for a comprehensive technical and management strategy consisting of the following five elements:

– political commitment;

– case detection using sputum microscopy among persons seeking care for prolonged cough;

– standardized short courses of chemotherapy under proper case-management conditions including DOT;

– regular drug supply; and

– a standardized recording and reporting system that allows assessment of individual patients as well as of overall programme performance (41).

C. Evidence for the effectiveness of interventions aimed at improving adherence

Unfortunately, there is a lack of rigorous experimental research on the effects of interventions to promote adherence to TB treatment. Quantitative research asks questions about efficacy and effectiveness. The choice of an appropriate experimental design methodology (whether individual or community randomization) depends on the nature of the intervention under evaluation. Quantitative research should be complemented by in-depth qualitative research to answer questions about why an intervention had an effect in a particular setting.

The extent to which DOT alone and various individual social support measures contribute to adherence is unknown. On the one hand, randomized controlled trials have shown no difference in adherence between TB patients randomly allocated to DOT alone or to self-administered treatment. Two recently published systematic reviews reported 16 randomized trials, of which only half were in countries with a high disease burden *(8,49)*. These reviews showed that DOT alone ("supervised swallowing") did not always promote adherence, and therefore the results do not support the use of this intervention in isolation from the other factors affecting adherence (e.g. good quality of communication between patient and health providers, transport costs and lay health beliefs about TB) (Table 10).

Table 10 Factors affecting adherence to treatment for tuberculosis and interventions for improving it, listed by the five dimensions and the interventions used to improve adherence

Tuberculosis	Factors affecting adherence	Interventions to improve adherence
Socioeconomic-related factors	(–) Lack of effective social support networks and unstable living circumstances (12); culture and lay beliefs about illness and treatment (10,17); ethnicity, gender and age (13); high cost of medication; high cost of transport; criminal justice involvement; involvement in drug dealing	Assessment of social needs, social support, housing, food tokens and legal measures (35,40,41); providing transport to treatment setting; peer assistance; mobilization of community-based organizations; optimizing the cooperation between services
Health care team/health system-related factors	(–) Poorly developed health services; inadequate relationship between health care provider and patient; health care providers who are untrained, overworked, inadequately supervised or unsupported in their tasks (20); inability to predict potentially nonadherent patients (21) (+) Good relationship between patient and physician (19); availability of expertise; links with patient support systems; flexibility in the hours of operation of treatment centers	Uninterrupted ready availability of information; flexibility in available treatment; training and management processes that aim to improve the way providers care for patients with tuberculosis; management of disease and treatment in conjunction with the patients; multidisciplinary care; intensive staff supervision (42); training in adherence monitoring; DOTS strategy (32)
Condition-related factors	(–) Asymptomatic patients; drug use; altered mental states caused by substance abuse; depression and psychological stress (+) Knowledge about TB (16)	Education on use of medications (43); provision of information about tuberculosis and the need to attend for treatment
Therapy-related factors	(–) Complex treatment regimen; adverse effects of treatment; toxicity (18)	Education on use of medications; adherence education; tailor treatment to needs of patients at risk of nonadherence; agreements (written or verbal) to return for an appointment or course of treatment; continuous monitoring and reassessment of treatment
Patient-related factors	(–) Forgetfulness; drug abuse, depression; psychological stress (+) Belief in the efficacy of treatment (16); motivation (24)	Therapeutic relationship; mutual goal-setting; memory aids and reminders; incentives and/or reinforcements (44,45); reminder letters (46), telephone reminders (47) or home visits (48) for patients who default on clinic attendance

DOT, Directly observed therapy; TB, tuberculosis; (+) factors having a positive effect on adherence; (–) factors having a negative effect on adherence.

On the other hand, programmatic studies of the effectiveness of the DOTS strategy have shown high rates of treatment success (2,50–52). In practice, the trial design necessary to properly evaluate the contribution of DOT alone to the effectiveness of the overall DOTS strategy requires assessment of the social aspects of patient support that surround DOT (as "supervised swallowing"). The outcomes of programmatic evaluations of the effectiveness of implementation of the DOTS strategy better reflect the social, behavioural and economic factors related to the patient, the health care services and characteristics of treatment.

Many other interventions have been found to significantly improve adherence. One study found that reminder letters sent to patients who failed to attend clinic, appeared to be of benefit even when patients were illiterate *(46)*. Another study reported that home visits by a health worker, though more labour-intensive, may be more effective than reminder letters for ensuring that defaulters complete their treatment *(48)*. Yet another study showed that prospective telephone reminders are useful for helping people to keep scheduled appointments *(47)*. Such studies are often location-specific and therefore often produce results that cannot be generalized. For example, studies demonstrating the benefit of telephone and mail reminders are of little relevance in many of the countries with a high prevalence of TB because most patients do not have telephones or mail boxes.

Although one trial found that assistance by a lay health worker increased adherence to a first appointment *(44)*, a subsequent study showed no impact on completion of preventive therapy at 6 months *(53)*. Studies in the USA have suggested that monetary incentives are an effective method for improving adherence. Appointment-keeping was significantly improved in homeless men *(44)* and in drug users *(45)* by offering US $5 in payment for returning to a clinic for TB evaluation, but the results of a study of offering monetary incentives to people recently discharged from prison were inconclusive, partly due to its small size *(54)*.

The evidence for an independent effect of health education on adherence of patients to treatment is weak. One trial did suggest some benefit *(55)* but the design of this study was flawed because individuals receiving health education were contacted or seen every 3 months, whereas those in the control group were seen only at the end of the study period. The relative contributions of health education and increased attention in this study are therefore hard to separate. A trial to examine the impact of intensive education and counselling on patients with active TB did, however, find a trend towards increased treatment completion rates for the patients who received intensive education and counselling compared with those who received routine care *(43)*. The study by Morisky and colleagues *(56)*, lent no support to the authors' claims for the benefit of health education as the results were confounded by the effects of a monetary incentive used in tandem with the educational intervention. In a more recent trial that has helped to disaggregate these effects *(45)* health education alone was found to be no better than routine case management for improving appointment-keeping and the impact of education combined with a monetary incentive was indistinguishable from that of the monetary incentive alone.

Finally, an intervention directed at clinic staff rather than patients was studied. Patients attending clinics in which staff were closely supervised were more likely to complete treatment than those attending clinics where there was only routine supervision of staff *(42)*.

5. Questions for future research

Useful research into human behaviour should take into account a wide range of approaches to enquiry, including qualitative and quantitative research methods. A review of the current literature on adherence to TB treatment has revealed a variety of research objectives, ranging from social and anthropological to clinical and programmatic studies. Further studies should be designed with the following aims:

- Define the theoretical models that underlie interventions to promote adherence to TB therapy.

- Describe the extent of various patterns of adherence (patients who take their medication sporadically, regularly take less than prescribed, and those who discontinue it completely).

- Explore the "active ingredients" of effective alliances between health providers and patients in a variety of sociocultural settings.

- Identify time-points in the case management at which different types of adherence strategy may have increased impact.

- Determine the efficacy and cost-effectiveness of specific interventions to improve adherence, as part of a complex health intervention necessary to achieve a high rate of treatment success.

- Priority should be given to studies in middle- and low-income countries to ensure the relevance of interventions to the settings in which most of the TB caseload occurs.

6. References

1. *TB – A Global Emergency.* Geneva, World Health Organization, 1994 (document WHO/TB/94.177).

2. *Global Tuberculosis Control: Surveillance, Planning, Financing.* Geneva, World Health Organization, 2002 (WHO/CDS/TB/2002.295).

3. Grange J. The global burden of disease. In: Porter J, Grange J, eds. *Tuberculosis: an international perspective.* London, Imperial College Press, 1999.

4. Fox W, Gordon A, Mitchison D. Studies on the treatment of tuberculosis undertaken by the British Medical Research Council Tuberculosis Units, 1946–1986, with relevant publications. *International Journal of Tuberculosis and Lung Diseases,* 1999, 3:S231–S270.

5. Fox W. The problem of self-administration of drugs: with particular reference to pulmonary tuberculosis. *Tubercle,* 1958, 39:269–274.

6. Addington W. Patient compliance: The most serious remaining problem in the control of tuberculosis in the United States. *Chest,* 1979, 76:741–743.

7. Urquhart J. Patient non-compliance with drug regimens: measurement, clinical correlates, economic impact. *European Heart Journal,* 1996, 17 (Suppl A):8–15.

8. Volmink J, Garner P. Interventions for promoting adherence to tuberculosis management. *Cochrane Database of Systematic Reviews,* 2000, (4):CD000010.

9. Urquhart J. Ascertaining how much compliance is enough with outpatient anti-biotic regimens. *Postgraduate Medical Journal,* 1992, 68:49–59.

10. Sumartojo E. When tuberculosis treatment fails. A social behavioral account of patient adherence. *American Review of Respiratory Disease,* 1993, 147:1311–1320.

11. Trostle JA. Medical compliance as an ideology. *Social Science & Medicine,* 1988, 27:1299–1308.

12. Liefooghe R et al. Perception and social consequences of tuberculosis: a focus group study of tuberculosis patients in Sialkot, Pakistan. *Social Science & Medicine,* 1995, 41:1685–1692.

13. Hudelson P. Gender differentials in tuberculosis: the role of socio-economic and cultural factors. *Tubercle & Lung Disease,* 1996, 77:391–400.

14. Farmer P. Social inequalities and emerging infectious diseases. *Emerging Infectious Diseases,* 1996, 2:259–269.

15. Diwan VK, Thorson A. Sex, gender, and tuberculosis. *Lancet,* 1999, 353:1000–1001.

16. Dick J, Lombard C. Shared vision – a health education project designed to enhance adherence to anti-tuberculosis treatment. *International Journal of Tuberculosis & Lung Disease,* 1997, 1:181–186.

17. Banerji D. A social science approach to strengthening India's national tuberculosis programme. *Indian Journal of Tuberculosis,* 2002, 40:61–82.

18. *Treatment of Tuberculosis: guidelines for National Programmes.* Geneva, World Health Organization, 1997 (document WHO/TB/94.177).

19. Lewin SA et al. Interventions for providers to promote a patient-centred approach in clinical consultations. *Cochrane Database Systematic Reviews,* 2001, CD003267.

20. Steyn M et al. Communication with TB patients; a neglected dimension of effective treatment? *Curationis,* 1997, 20:53–56.

21. Mushlin AI, Appel FA. Diagnosing potential noncompliance. Physicians' ability in a behavioral dimension of medical care. *Archives of Internal Medicine,* 1977, 137:318–321.

22. Caron HS, Roth HP. Patients' cooperation with a medical regimen. Difficulties in identifying the noncooperator. *Journal of the American Medical Association,* 1968, 203:922–926.

23. Davis MS. Predicting non-compliant behavior. *Journal of Health & Social Behavior,* 1967, 8:265–271.

24. Dick J et al. Development of a health education booklet to enhance adherence to tuberculosis treatment. *Tubercle & Lung Disease,* 1996, 77:173–177.

25. Bandura A. *Social learning theory.* Englewood Cliffs, NY, Prentice Hall, 1977.

26. Ajzen I, Fishbein M. *Understanding attitudes and predicting social behavior.* Englewood Cliffs, NY, Prentice Hall, 1980.

27. Green L, Krueter M. *Health promotion planning: an educational and environmental approach.* Mountainview, CA, Mayfield Publishing, 1991.

28. *Health behavior and health education: theory, research, and practice.* San Francisco, CA, Jossey-Bass, 1997.

29. Fisher JD, Fisher WA. Changing AIDS-risk behavior. *Psychological Bulletin,* 1992, 111:455–474.

30. From the Centers for Disease Control and Prevention. Approaches to improving adherence to antituberculosis therapy. *Journal of the American Medical Association,* 1998, 269:1096–1098.

31. Sbarbaro JA, Sbarbaro JB. Compliance and supervision of chemotherapy of tuberculosis. *Seminars in Respiratory Infections,* 1994, 9:120–127.

32. Raviglione M, Pio A. Evolution of WHO policies for tuberculosis control, 1948–2001. *Lancet,* 2002, 359:775–780.

33. Bayer R, Wilkinson D. Directly observed therapy for tuberculosis: history of an idea. *Lancet,* 1995, 345:1545–1548 [erratum published in *Lancet,* 1995, 346:322].

34. Bass JB, Jr. et al. Treatment of tuberculosis and tuberculosis infection in adults and children. American Thoracic Society and The Centers for Disease Control and Prevention. *American Journal of Respiratory & Critical Care Medicine,* 1994, 149:1359–1374.

35. Chaulk CP, Kazandjian VA. Directly observed therapy for treatment completion of pulmonary tuberculosis: Consensus Statement of the Public Health Tuberculosis Guidelines Panel. *Journal of the American Medical Association,* 1998, 279:943–948 [erratum published in *Journal of the American Medical Association,* 1998, 280:134].

36. Enarson D et al. *Management of tuberculosis: a guide for low income countries,* 5th ed. Paris, International Union Against Tuberculosis and Lung Disease, 2000.
37. Maher D et al. *Treatment of tuberculosis: guidelines for national programmes,* 2nd ed. Geneva, World Health Organization, 1997.
38. Farmer P et al. Tuberculosis, poverty, and "compliance": lessons from rural Haiti. *Seminars In Respiratory Infections,* 1991, 6:254–260.
39. Olle-Goig JE, Alvarez J. Treatment of tuberculosis in a rural area of Haiti: directly observed and non-observed regimens. The experience of Hôpital Albert Schweitzer. *International Journal of Tuberculosis & Lung Disease,* 2001, 5:137–141.
40. Burman WJ et al. A cost-effectiveness analysis of directly observed therapy vs self-administered therapy for treatment of tuberculosis. *Chest,* 1997, 112:63–70.
41. *An Expanded DOTS Framework for Effective Tuberculosis Control.* Geneva, World Health Organization, 2002 (document WHO/CDS/TB/2002.297).
42. Jin BW et al. The impact of intensified supervisory activities on tuberculosis treatment. *Tubercle & Lung Disease,* 1993, 74:267–272.
43. Liefooghe R et al. A randomised trial of the impact of counselling on treatment adherence of tuberculosis patients in Sialkot, Pakistan. *International Journal of Tuberculosis & Lung Disease,* 1999, 3:1073–1080.
44. Pilote L et al. Tuberculosis prophylaxis in the homeless. A trial to improve adherence to referral. *Archives of Internal Medicine,* 1996, 156:161–165.
45. Malotte CK, Rhodes F, Mais KE. Tuberculosis screening and compliance with return for skin test reading among active drug users. *American Journal of Public Health,* 1998, 88:792–796.
46. Paramasivan R, Parthasarathy R, Rajasekaran S. Short course chemotherapy: A controlled study of indirect defaulter retrieval method. *Indian Journal of Tuberculosis,* 1993, 40:185–190.
47. Tanke ED, Martinez CM, Leirer VO. Use of automated reminders for tuberculin skin test return. *American Journal of Preventive Medicine,* 1997, 13:189–192.
48. Krishnaswami KV et al. A randomised study of two policies for managing default in out-patients collecting supplies of drugs for pulmonary tuberculosis in a large city in South India. *Tubercle,* 1981, 62:103–112.
49. Volmink J, Garner P. Directly observed therapy for treating tuberculosis. *Cochrane Database of Systematic Reviews.* 2001 (4):CD003343.
50. Suarez PG et al. The dynamics of tuberculosis in response to 10 years of intensive control effort in Peru. *The Journal of Infectious Diseases,* 2001, 184:473–478.
51. Fujiwara PI, Larkin C, Frieden TR. Directly observed therapy in New York City. History, implementation, results, and challenges. *Clinics In Chest Medicine,* 1997, 18:135–148.
52. Results of directly observed short-course chemotherapy in 112,842 Chinese patients with smear-positive tuberculosis. China Tuberculosis Control Collaboration. *Lancet,* 1996, 347:358–362.
53. Tulsky JP et al. Adherence to isoniazid prophylaxis in the homeless: a randomized controlled trial. *Archives of Internal Medicine,* 2000, 160:697–702.
54. White MC et al. A clinical trial of a financial incentive to go to the tuberculosis clinic for isoniazid after release from jail. *International Journal of Tuberculosis & Lung Disease,* 1998, 2:506–512.
55. Salleras SL et al. Evaluation of the efficacy of health education on the compliance with antituberculosis chemoprophylaxis in school children. A randomized clinical trial. *Tubercle & Lung Disease,* 1993, 74:28–31 [erratum published in *Tubercle & Lung Disease,* 1993, 74:217].
56. Morisky DE et al. A patient education program to improve adherence rates with antituberculosis drug regimens. *Health Education Quarterly,* 1990, 17:253–267.

Annexes

Annex I

Behavioural mechanisms explaining adherence

What every health professional should know

1. Introduction   135
2. The nature of poor adherence   136
3. Determinants of adherence   137
4. Models   139
5. Interventions   143
6. Conclusions   145
7. References   147

1. Introduction

Optimal outcomes in population health require both efficacious treatments and adherence to those treatments. Whether the treatment involves taking medication properly, making and keeping health care appointments, or self-managing other behaviours that influence the onset, course or prognosis of an illness; all other things being equal, success is determined by adherence behaviour. Patients, health care providers, researchers, funders and policy-makers, all have an interest in ensuring that effective biomedical and behavioural therapies for chronic illnesses are "used as prescribed". However, empirical studies have consistently found that levels of compliance or adherence are often far from optimal *(1,2)*. Because the burden of illness in the population has shifted toward chronic diseases, the problem of poor adherence is of major concern to all stakeholders in the health care system. This is because the risk of poor adherence increases with the duration and complexity of treatment regimens and both long duration and complex treatment are inherent to chronic illnesses.

Across diseases, adherence is the single most important modifiable factor that compromises treatment outcome. The best treatment can be rendered ineffective by poor adherence. Our perspective is that an understanding of basic behavioural principles and models of behavioural change is relevant to adherence to treatment for all chronic medical conditions, and more helpful than a disease-specific approach to the issue.

Behavioural science offers useful theories, models and strategies that support best-practice approaches to delivering treatment. The effectiveness of adherence interventions based on behavioural principles has been demonstrated in many therapeutic areas. Examples include hypertension *(3)*, headache *(4)*, AIDS *(5)*, cancer *(6)*, heart transplantation *(7,8)*, chronic asthma *(9,10)*, diabetes *(11)*, high cholesterol *(12)*, obesity *(13)* and sun-protection behaviours *(14)* among others. Recent research has also evaluated interventions aimed at maintaining adherence to treatments targeting substance abuse in pregnancy *(15)*; alcohol abuse *(16)*; opioid addictions and methadone maintenance *(17,18)*; substance dependence *(19)*; cocaine abuse *(20)*, and tobacco smoking *(21)*.

Decades of behavioural research and practice have yielded proven strategies for changing people's behaviour. Such strategies can be used to help patients with diverse medical conditions *(22,23)*, and can also be effective in changing the behaviour of health care providers *(24)* and health care systems *(25)*.

Epidemiological research concerning the prevalence and correlates of poor adherence to treatment, and research on adherence to treatment for specific diseases is presented in the main text of this report. In this annex, the following are discussed from a behavioural perspective:

– the nature of poor adherence;

– a practical approach to conceptualizing and defining adherence;

– models to help explain determinants of adherence; and

– guidelines for assessment and intervention in clinical practice.

2. The nature of poor adherence

Treatment effectiveness is determined jointly by the efficacy of the treatment agent and the extent of adherence to the treatment. Despite the availability of efficacious interventions, nonadherence to treatment remains a problem across therapeutic areas.

Adherence is a complex behavioural process determined by several interacting factors. These include attributes of the patient, the patient's environment (which comprises social supports, characteristics of the health care system, functioning of the health care team, and the availability and accessibility of health care resources) and characteristics of the disease in question and its treatment.

There are many specific aspects of treatment to which a patient may not adhere, for example:

– health-seeking behaviours (such as appointment-keeping);

– obtaining inoculations;

– medication use (use of appropriate agents, correct dosing and timing, filling and refilling prescriptions, consistency of use, duration of use); and

– following protocols for changing behaviour (examples include modifying diet, increasing physical activity, quitting smoking, self-monitoring of symptoms, safe food handling, dental hygiene, safer sex behaviours and safer injection practices).

The most frequently cited conceptual definition of adherence is "the extent to which a person's behaviour – taking medication, following a diet, executing lifestyle changes – follows medical advice" *(26)*. Adherence has also been defined as "the extent to which patient behaviour corresponds with recommendations from a health care provider" *(27,28)*. It has also been suggested that a more practical approach is to define adherence as "following treatment at a level above which treatment goals are likely to be met". However, these broad definitions belie the complexity of the issue.

In research, adherence has been operationalized in many different ways: as the degree to which a regimen is followed expressed as a percentage or ratio, a categorical phenomenon (e.g. good versus poor adherence), or as an index score synthesizing multiple behaviours. However, for clinical purposes, these definitions lack specificity, and give no clear direction for assessment and intervention.

The treatments that patients are asked to follow vary according to the nature of the demands they impose. They range from requiring relatively simple and familiar behaviours, to more complex and novel ones. Some treatments involve one behaviour, while others carry multiple behavioural requirements. Protocols also vary in terms of the length of time for which they must be followed. This means that the nature and meaning of adherence change according to the specific treatment demands of a particular protocol. Assessment and intervention strategies will differ according to *the circumstances and/or intensity of the recommendations*. All treatments make demands of one type or another on patients. Patients differ in their ability to meet those demands, and the resources available and the environmental contexts outlined earlier also differ. Perhaps adherence might be better understood as reflecting the process of efforts, occurring over the course of an illness, to meet the treatment-related behavioural demands imposed by that illness. This behavioural conceptualization allows us to define adherence more explicitly according to the type of behaviour, an acceptable frequency, consistency, intensity and/or accuracy.

3. Determinants of adherence

A considerable amount of empirical, descriptive, research has identified correlates and predictors of adherence and nonadherence. These include aspects of the complexity and duration of treatment, characteristics of the illness, iatrogenic effects of treatment, costs of treatment, characteristics of health service provision, interaction between practitioner and patient, and sociodemographic variables. Many of these variables are static, and may not be amenable to intervention. They have been well described in the main text of this report and will not be discussed further here. While such findings help to identify risk factors, they tend to be discrete and atheoretical, and not very helpful in guiding a clinical approach to this problem.

This section describes several important variables that are behavioural in nature and are also dynamic, and therefore amenable to intervention. First we identify key behaviours of health care providers, health system factors and attributes of patients. Then we discuss promising behavioural science theories and models that help to explain behavioural change. These serve as helpful heuristics both for understanding nonadherence and for addressing it.

A. Provider behaviours

Variables related to how health care providers interact and communicate with their patients are key determinants of adherence and patient health outcomes *(4,6,17,29,30)*. The health care providers prescribe the medical regimen, interpret it, monitor clinical outcomes and provide feedback to patients *(31)*.

Correlational studies have revealed positive relationships between adherence of patients to their treatment and provider communication styles characterized by, providing information, "positive talk" and asking patients specific questions about adherence *(32)*. The clarity of diagnostic and treatment advice has been correlated with adherence to short-term but not to long-term regimens and chronic illnesses. Continuity of care (follow-up) is a positive correlate of adherence. Patients who view themselves as partners in the treatment process and who are actively engaged in the care process have better adherence behaviour and health outcomes *(33)*. Warmth and empathy of the clinician emerge time and again as being central factors *(34)*. Their patients of providers who share information, build partnerships, and provide emotional support have better outcomes than the patients of providers who do not interact in this manner *(35)*. Patients who are satisfied with their provider and medical regimen adhere more diligently to treatment recommendations *(36)*. Findings such as these can guide providers to create a treatment relationship that reflects a partnership with their patients and supports the discussion of therapeutic options, the negotiation of the regimen and clear discussion of adherence.

Health care providers often try to supply information to patients and to motivate them, and recognize the importance of behavioural skills in improving health. However, there is evidence that, in practice, they give limited information *(37)*, lack skills in motivational enhancement *(38)*, and lack knowledge and experience frustration in teaching patients behavioural skills *(39)*. More structured, thoughtful and sophisticated interactions between provider and patient are essential if improvements in adherence are to be realized.

B. Health system factors

The health care delivery system has great potential to influence the adherence behaviour of patients. The policies and procedures of the health system itself control access to, and quality of, care. System variables include the availability and accessibility of services, support for education of patients, data collection and information management, provision of feedback to patients and health care providers, community supports available to patients, and the training provided to health service providers. Systems direct providers' schedules, dictate appointment lengths, allocate resources, set fee structures and establish organizational priorities. The functioning of the health system influences patients' behaviour in many ways.

- *Systems direct appointment length and duration of treatment*, and providers often report that their schedules allow insufficient time to address adherence behaviour adequately *(40)*.

- *Health systems determine reimbursements and/or fee structures*, and many health systems lack financial coverage for patient counselling and education: this threatens or precludes many adherence-focused interventions.

- *Systems allocate resources* in ways that may result in heightened stress for, and increased demands upon, providers and that have, in turn, been associated with decreased patient adherence *(41)*.

- *Systems determine continuity of care* and patients demonstrate better adherence when they receive care from the same provider over time *(42)*.

- *Systems direct information sharing* – the ability of clinics and pharmacies to share information regarding patients' behaviour towards prescription refills has the potential to improve adherence.

- *Systems determine the level of communication with patients* – ongoing communication efforts (e.g. telephone contacts) that keep the patient engaged in health care may be the simplest and most cost-effective strategy for improving adherence *(43)*.

C. Patient attributes

Patient characteristics have been the focus of numerous investigations of adherence. However, age, sex, education, occupation, income, marital status, race, religion, ethnic background, and urban versus rural living have not been definitely associated with adherence *(26,44)*. Similarly, the search for the stable personality traits of a typical nonadherent patient has been futile – there is no one pattern of patient characteristics predictive of nonadherence *(34,42)*. With the exception of extreme disturbances of functioning and motivation, personality variables have not emerged as significant predictors. Recent studies of patients with mental health problems have provided evidence that depression and anxiety are predictive of adherence to medical recommendations *(45–48)*. Almost everyone has difficulty adhering to medical recommendations, especially when the advice entails self-administered care.

Illness-relevant cognitions, perceptions of disease factors, and beliefs about treatment have stronger relationships to adherence. In particular, factors such as perceived susceptibility to illness, perceived severity of illness, self-efficacy and perceived control over health behaviours appear to be correlates *(26,49)*. For adherence to occur, symptoms must be sufficiently severe to arouse the need for adherence, be perceived as being resolvable and acute, and remedial action must effect a rapid and noticeable reduction in symptoms *(50)*.

Knowledge about an illness is not a correlate of nonadherence, but specific knowledge about elements of a medication regimen is, although apparently only for short-term, acute illnesses *(51)*. Some of the above variables, and several others, form the basis of various theories and models of behaviour change and we now turn our attention to these.

4. Models

Leventhal and Cameron *(52)* provided a very useful overview of the history of adherence research. They outlined five general theoretical perspectives on adherence:

- biomedical perspective;
- behavioural perspective;
- communication perspective;
- cognitive perspective; and
- self-regulatory perspective.

The biomedical model of health and illness remains a dominant perspective in many health care settings and organizations. The biomedical approach to adherence assumes that patients are more-or-less passive followers of their doctor's orders, further to a diagnosis and prescribed therapy *(52,53)*. Nonadherence is understood in terms of characteristics of the patient (personality traits, sociodemographic background), and patient factors are seen as the targets of efforts to improve adherence. This approach has helped to elucidate the relationships between disease and treatment characteristics on the one hand, and adherence on the other. Technological innovations (e.g. assessing levels of adherence using biochemical measures, developing new devices to administer medications) have had this as their impetus. However, other important factors, such as patients' views about their symptoms or their medications have been largely ignored.

Behavioural (learning) theory emphasizes the importance of positive and negative reinforcement as a mechanism for influencing behaviour, and this has immediate relevance for adherence.

- The most basic, but powerful, principle is that of antecedents and consequences and their influence on behaviour (i.e. operant learning) (54,55).

- Antecedents, or preceding events, are internal (thoughts) or external (environmental cues) circumstances that elicit a behaviour.

- Consequences, or expected consequences, that can be conceptualized as rewards or punishments, also influence behaviour.

- The probability of a patient, provider, or health care system initiating or continuing a behaviour partially depends on what happens before and after the behaviour occurs.

- From a theoretical standpoint it would be possible to "control" the behaviour of patients, providers and health care systems if one could control the events preceding and following a specific behaviour. From a practical standpoint, behavioural principles can be used to design interventions that have the potential to incrementally shape behaviour at each level of influence (i.e. patient, provider and system) to address adherence problems.

Communication perspectives that emerged in the 1970s encouraged health care providers to try to improve their skills in communicating with their patients. This led to emphasis being placed on the importance of developing rapport, educating patients, employing good communication skills and stressing the desirability of a more equal relationship between patient and health professional. Although this approach has been shown to influence satisfaction with medical care, convincing data about its positive effects on compliance are scarce *(56)*. Adopting a warm and kind style of interaction with a patient is necessary, but is insufficient in itself to effect changes in the adherence behaviours of patients.

Various models emphasizing cognitive variables and processes have been applied to adherence behaviour *(53)*. Examples of these include the health belief model *(57)*, social–cognitive theory *(58)*, the theory of planned behaviour (and its precursor, the theory of reasoned action) *(59)*, and the protection–motivation theory *(60)*. Although these approaches have directed attention to the ways in which patients conceptualize health threats and appraise factors that may be barriers to, or facilitate, adherence they do not always address behavioural coping skills well.

Self-regulation perspectives attempt to integrate environmental variables and the cognitive responses of individuals to health threats into the self-regulatory model *(61,62)*. The essence of the model pertains to the central importance of the cognitive conceptualization of a patient (or a patient-to-be *(63)* of a health threat or an illness. Illness representations (the ideas patients have about the diseases they suffer) and coping are seen as mediating between the health threat and the action taken. Recent empirical studies seem to lend support to the importance of illness cognitions in predicting adherence *(64–66)*. Patients create personal representations of health threats and models of the illness and its treatment, and it is these that guide their decision-making and behaviour. Thus, adherence requires an appropriate model and the belief that one can manage one's own environment and behaviour, specific coping skills, and a belief that the issue requires one's attention and the modification of one's behaviour.

Although these theories and models provide a conceptual framework for organizing thoughts about adherence and other health behaviours, each has its advantages and disadvantages and no single approach may be readily translated into a comprehensive understanding of, and intervention for, adherence. More recent approaches that are more specific to health behaviours and the demands of following recommended health practices may provide more helpful frameworks.

Meichenbaum and Turk *(42)* suggested that four interdependent factors operate on adherence behaviour and that a deficit in any one contributes to risk of nonadherence.

- knowledge and skills: about the health problem and self-regulation behaviours required, their mechanisms of action, and the importance of adherence;

- beliefs: perceived severity and susceptibility (relevance), self-efficacy, outcome expectations, and response costs;

- motivation: value and reinforcement, internal attribution of success (positive outcomes are reinforcing, negative results seen not as failure, but rather as an indication to reflect on and modify behaviour);

- action: stimulated by relevant cues, driven by information recall, evaluation and selection of behavioural options and available resources.

The recently developed information–motivation–behavioural skills model (IMB model) *(67,68)*, borrowed elements from earlier work to construct a conceptually based, generalizable, and simple model to guide thinking about complex health behaviours. The IMB constructs, and how they pertain to patient adherence, are outlined below.

- Information is the basic knowledge about a medical condition that might include how the disease develops, its expected course and effective strategies for its management.

- Motivation encompasses personal attitudes towards the adherence behaviour, perceived social support for such behaviour, and the patients' subjective norm or perception of how others with this medical condition might behave.

- Behavioural skills include ensuring that the patient has the specific behavioural tools or strategies necessary to perform the adherence behaviour such as enlisting social support and other self-regulation strategies.

Note that information, motivation and behavioural skills must directly pertain to the desired behavioural outcome; they have to be specific.

Interventions based on this model have been effective in influencing behavioural change across a variety of clinical applications *(67–69)*. In both prospective and correlational studies, the information, motivation and behavioural skills constructs have accounted for an average of 33% of the variance in behaviour change *(68)*.

Figure 1 Information-motivation-behavioural skills model

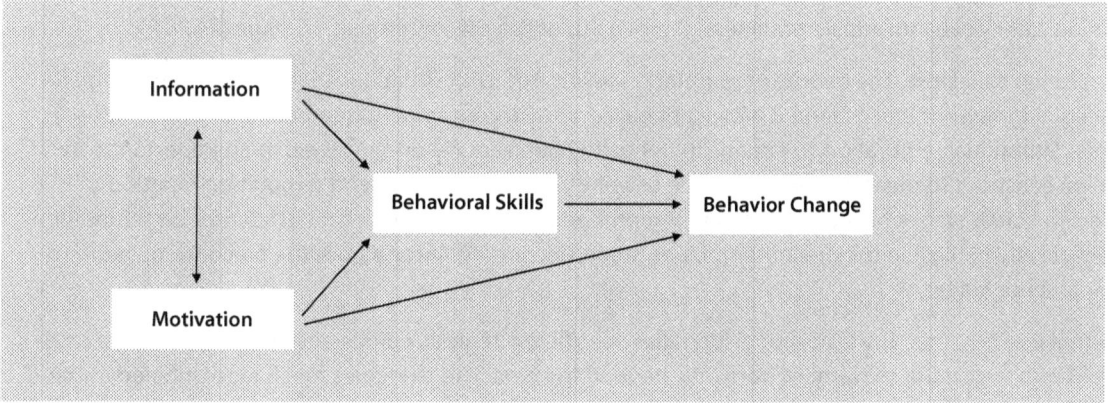

The IMB model demonstrates that information is a prerequisite for changing behaviour, but in itself is insufficient to achieve this change *(70)*. Motivation and behavioural skills are critical determinants and are independent of behaviour change *(67,68)*. Information and motivation work largely through behavioural skills to affect behaviour; however, when the behavioural skills are familiar or uncomplicated, information and motivation can have direct effects on behaviour (see diagram). In this case, a patient might fill a prescription (a simple, familiar behaviour) based on information given by the provider. The relationship between the information and motivation constructs is weak. In practical terms, a highly motivated person may have little information, or a highly informed person may have low motivation. However, in the IMB model, the presence of both information and motivation increase the likelihood of adherence.

The stages-of-change model (SOC – also referred to as the transtheoretical model) identifies five stages through which individuals progress as they change behaviours, and stage-matched strategies that predict progress to each subsequent stage of change *(71,72)*. The stages of change are: precontemplation (not considering changing behaviour in the next 6 months), contemplation (considering changing behaviour in the next 6 months), preparation (planning to change behaviour during the next 30 days), action (currently changing behaviour) and maintenance (successful behaviour change for at least 6 months). Stages of change describe an individual's motivational readiness to change.

The SOC model is useful for understanding and predicting intentional behaviour change. Most patients at one time or another make unintentional errors in taking their medication because of forgetfulness or misunderstanding of instructions. However, *intentional* non-adherence is a significant problem, particularly among patients with conditions requiring long-term therapy such as asthma, hypertension and diabetes.

Stage of change is an indicator of an individual's motivation to change, and is a powerful predictor of behaviour *(73–75)*, but variables that explain behavioural change are needed to develop actionable, effective strategies to help people change. The SOC model has proven useful in this regard because it utilizes key psychological constructs to characterize individuals at different levels of readiness for change. Some of these constructs are: decisional balance, temptation to relapse, and processes or strategies for change *(76)*. These constructs are briefly summarized below.

Decisional balance. Decisional balance consists of the pros and cons of behaviour change. Longitudinal research has established a characteristic relationship between stage of change and the pros and cons *(77,78)*. The pros of healthy behaviour are low in the early stages of change and increase as stage of change increases. Conversely, the cons of the healthy behaviour are high in the early stages of change and decrease as stage of change increases. The positive aspects of changing behaviour begin to outweigh the negative aspects of change late in the contemplation stage or early in the preparation stage. Scales measuring pros and cons are particularly useful when intervening with individuals in early stages of change (precontemplation, contemplation and preparation) because decisional balance is an excellent indicator of an individual's readiness to move out of the precontemplation stage *(74,78,79)*.

Temptation to relapse. The degree of temptation associated with situations that present a challenge for maintaining behavioural change is a concept based upon the coping models of relapse and maintenance. Situational temptation to engage in unhealthy behaviour is often viewed as an important companion construct to measures of confidence or self-efficacy. Confidence and temptation function inversely across stages of change *(80)*, and temptation predicts relapse better *(81)*. Scores on temptation are generally highest in the precontemplation stage, decreasing linearly from the precontemplation to maintenance stages *(81)*.

Strategies for change. The SOC model identifies specific strategies or processes of change that are associated with successful movement from one stage to the next. The strategies for change outlined in the SOC theory are based upon components of several theoretical models in behavioural science. Each of the strategies for change is categorized as either experiential or behavioural in nature *(82)*. Experiential strategies reflect cognitive, evaluative and affective planning for change whereas behavioural strategies reflect observable change strategies such as using reminders or rewards *(73)*.

Specific strategies for change are useful for intervening with individuals in particular stages of change; individuals who are thinking about change need different strategies from those who are actively involved in change.

Tailored interventions provide individualized information based upon a specific theoretical framework, demographic characteristics or a combination of variables. There is evidence that tailored communications are more effective for influencing health behaviours than non-tailored materials *(83)*, and comparisons of stage-tailored versus non-tailored interventions have shown that tailoring resulted in increased efficacy in influencing health behaviours *(84)*.

A recent review found that interventions to improve adherence to medication were more effective when they included multiple components such as more convenient care, information, counselling, reminders, self-monitoring, reinforcement or family therapy *(43)*. SOC tailoring may be a useful strategy for implementing complex, multi-component interventions in a cost-effective manner. Identification of stage of change can help determine the most relevant intervention components for each person, thus eliminating the need to deliver all intervention components to all patients. The availability of valid measures to assess stage of change provides a foundation for the development of stage-matched interventions for the promotion of adherence to medication. Stage-tailored communication has been shown to be an effective method for changing health behaviour, but has yet to be applied to the problem of nonadherence with medication.

5. Interventions

The "state-of-the-art" adherence interventions target the patient, the provider, and the health care system. Several programmes have demonstrated good results using multilevel team approaches *(85–87)*. Adequate evidence exists to support the utility of innovative, modified health care system teams in addressing the problem *(25,88)*.

However, research on interventions to promote adherence has focused largely on modifying patient behaviour. According to several published reviews on adherence, no single intervention targeting patient behaviour is effective, and the most promising methods of improving adherence behaviour use a combination of the strategies listed below *(89–91)*:

– patient education *(92)*;

– behavioural skills *(93,94)*;

– self-rewards *(95)*;

– social support *(96)*; and

– telephone follow-up *(97)*.

Various combinations of these techniques have been shown to increase adherence and improve treatment outcomes. However, even the most efficacious patient-focused interventions have no substantial effects on adherence behaviour over the long term *(43)* and few randomized controlled trials targeting patient adherence behaviour have been reported *(91)*.

A. Patient interventions

The most effective adherence-enhancing interventions directed at patients aim to enhance self-regulation or self-management capabilities. Self-management programmes offered to patients with chronic diseases can improve health status and reduce health care utilization and costs. Some data suggest a cost-to-savings ratio of 1:10 *(98)*. Such approaches are grounded in basic principles of learning *(99,100)*. This is critical in the management of patients with chronic illness, as over the long term patients must rely on unassisted effort and self-regulation to maintain their behaviour. Several strategies appear to be effective, at least in the short term. These include:

– self-monitoring;

– goal-setting;

– stimulus control;

– behavioural rehearsal;

– corrective feedback;

- behavioural contracting;

- commitment enhancement;

- creating social support;

- reinforcement; and

- relapse prevention.

Since the early 1980s there has been sufficient evidence to support the use of these strategies. These are most effective when used as components of multi-modal programmes and implemented in an individualized tailored manner, including creating social support, reorganization of the service-delivery environment, increasing accessibility of services, and a collaborative treatment relationship.

A meta-analysis of 28 studies revealed that the key intervention components were providing reinforcement for patients' efforts to change, providing feedback on progress, tailoring education to patients' needs and circumstances, teaching skills and providing access to resources, and continuity of care (proactive) *(101)*. An earlier review, Garrity & Garrity *(102)* identified four intervention themes associated with successful outcomes: active patient theme (promote self-care), social support theme (help in meeting illness-related demands), fear arousal theme (increase concern about the consequences of the disease), and patient instruction theme. The self-care (contingency contracting element) and social support themes were associated with the strongest effects on treatment outcome.

There has been little research on the most effective methods for improving adherence to recommended treatment in children. Education alone does not promote the desired patient outcomes and the format of the educational programme may be less important than the actual presentation and understanding of the information *(103)*. However, when behavioural strategies were used in conjunction with patient education, adherence to recommended treatment improved by an average of 25% *(104)*. Multi-component behavioural strategies that have been found to be successful in promoting adherence include self-monitoring, contingency contracting, reinforcing, tailoring and cueing. In addition, individual rather than group educational sessions can be better adapted to the specific needs of a child and his or her family, and are therefore anticipated to have a greater impact on outcomes *(105)*. There is a need for research to identify and test developmentally-appropriate interventions to remedy the problem of paediatric nonadherence and improve health care outcomes for children.

The need for research to further our understanding of the differences in adherence behaviour at different stages of development has been only partially met. While some progress has been made in understanding and modifying adherence among paediatric populations there remains much to be learned. The research to date has suffered from a lack of methodological rigour and attention to theoretically-based investigations, particularly the utilization of developmentally-based theory to guide adherence interventions. Children are not small adults; children and adolescents have specific needs that differ from those of their adult counterparts. Advances in the area of adherence will be dependent upon:

- designing and testing tools for objectively measuring adherence that are non-intrusive (e.g. electronic monitoring), and that children and adolescents are willing and able to use;

- addressing psychosocial and family factors that modify adherence in children and adolescents;

- designing and testing age- and disease-specific quality-of-life scales for children and adolescents; and

- designing and testing educational and behavioural strategies appropriate for children and adolescents.

The desired outcome is for practitioners to tailor scientifically-based adherence interventions to the developmental stage of the patient. As interdisciplinary expertise is brought to bear on developing scientifically-based policy for addressing the developmental aspects of adherence and managing care, the gaps in the understanding of nonadherence should begin to close.

B. Interventions directed to providers

Because providers have such a significant role in adherence, designing interventions to influence their behaviour seems a reasonable strategy. However, few investigations on this subject have been reported in the literature. Training providers in patient-centred methods of care may be effective, but the strongest effects of such training appear to be on patient satisfaction with treatment. Some recent studies suggest that adherence interventions based on behavioural principles can be successfully implemented by social workers and nurses *(106,107)*. Studies of physicians trained to use goal-setting, feedback and ongoing education reveal better patient outcomes, though such studies have seldom measured adherence as an outcome.

C. Health system

Interventions in the health system are higher order interventions affecting health policy; organization and financing of care and quality of care programmes. One example is the creation and adoption of chronic care models of service delivery, which, at least in patients with diabetes and asthma, have been shown to result in better patient outcomes. However the extent to which these models are related to adherence is not yet clear.

6. Conclusions

Nonadherence to treatment is a problem of increasing concern to all stakeholders in the health system. Since the early 1970s, the extent and consequences of poor adherence have been well documented in terms of impact on population health and health expenditure. Poor adherence limits the potential of efficacious treatments to improve patients' health and quality of life. This is a particular problem in the context of the chronic conditions that currently dominate the burden of illness in our society. Across health disciplines, providers experience considerable frustration over the high proportion of their patients who fail to follow treatment recommendations.

Adherence is a behavioural problem observed in patients, but with causes beyond the patient. It occurs in the context of treatment-related demands that the patient must attempt to cope with. These demands are characterized by the requirement to learn new behaviours, alter daily routines, tolerate discomforts and inconveniences, and persist in doing so while trying to function effectively in their various life-roles *(108–110)*. While there is no behavioural magic bullet, there is substantial evidence identifying effective strategies for changing behaviour.

Practitioners (and other health enablers) often assume that the patient is, or should be, motivated by his or her illness to follow a treatment protocol. However, recent research in the behavioural sciences reveals this assumption to be erroneous. In fact, the patient population can be segmented according to level-of-readiness to follow health recommendations. The lack of concordance between patient readiness and practitioner behaviour means that treatments are frequently offered to patients who are not ready to follow them. This reflects an understandable bias towards treating the biomedical problem and an under-emphasis on addressing the behavioural requirements of the treatment protocol.

Prochaska *(71)* argued that people move through stages of increasing readiness to follow recommendations as they develop the motivation and skills required to change their behaviour. The SOC model provides a sensible and clear framework upon which to tailor treatment to patients' needs, and organize the delivery of the range of cognitive and behavioural interventions that are supported by the evidence base. Miller and Rollnick *(111)* noted that motivation to adhere to treatment is influenced by the value that a person places on following the regimen (cost–benefit ratio) and their degree of confidence in being able to follow it. If either the perceived value of adhering, or confidence, is low the likelihood of adherence will also be low.

First-line interventions to optimize adherence can go beyond the provision of advice. Building on a patient's intrinsic motivation by increasing the perceived importance of adherence, and strengthening confidence by intervening at the level of self-management skills are behavioural treatment targets that must be addressed concurrently with biomedical ones if overall effectiveness of treatment is to be improved. This approach offers a way of increasing the sophistication of the adherence interventions offered to patients. Pharmacists, case managers, health educators and others involved in patient care should be made familiar with these basic concepts. Non-physician providers have an important role to play and an opportunity to dramatically improve health by specifically targeting issues of patient adherence.

In every situation in which patients are required to administer their own treatment, nonadherence is likely. Consequently, the risk for nonadherence for all patients should be assessed as part of the treatment-planning process and their adherence should be monitored as part of treatment follow-up. The traditional approach has been to wait to identify those patients who demonstrate nonadherence and then try to "fix" the problem. The risk for nonadherence is ever present. Interventions based on non-adherence risk-stratification should be offered from the start, as opposed to using a stepped-care approach.

Poor adherence persists largely because it is a complex problem and is resistant to generic approaches to dealing with it. Adherence-promoting interventions are not consistently implemented in practice; practitioners report lack of time, lack of knowledge, lack of incentives and lack of feedback on performance as barriers. Clearly, non-adherence is not simply a "patient" problem. At the points of initial contact and follow-up, providers can have a significant impact by assessing risk and delivering interventions to optimize adherence. To make this way of practice a reality, practitioners must have access to specific training in adherence management, and the systems in which they work must design and support delivery systems that respect this objective. Health care providers can learn to assess the potential for nonadherence, and to detect in their patients. They can then use this information to implement brief interventions to encourage and support progress towards adherence.

Interventions aimed at particular diseases need to target the most influential and core determinants among the various factors. Given available resources, these targets will invariably be the patient and provider, at least in the immediate term. Disease-specific protocols for patients can be tailored to their needs. Practitioner protocols can convey the key requirements for the creation of optimal treatment relationships and behaviour assessment and management skills. Beyond this, the system in which providers work must be organized in such a way as to enable a consistent and systematic focus on adherence. A major focus for future research should be the clarification of the best mode, or modes, of delivering adherence interventions. There are many points of contact with patients and times at which such interventions are required, and delivering them outside the traditional health system may enhance their overall effectiveness.

7. References

1. Bloom BS. Daily regimen and compliance with treatment. *British Medical Journal*, 2001, 323:647.

2. Myers LB, Midence K. *Adherence to treatment in medical conditions.* Amsterdam, Harwood Academic, 1998.

3. Burnier M, Brunner HR. Impact on clinical outcomes. Compliance in healthcare and research. Monograph series. Armonk, NY, Blackwell, 2001:299–309.

4. Scopp A. Clear communication skills with headache patients. *Headache Quarterly*, 2000, 11:269–274.

5. Rudman LA, Gonzales MH, Borgida E. Mishandling the gift of life: Noncompliance in renal transplant patients. *Journal of Applied Social Psychology*, 1999, 29:834–851.

6. Wright S. Patient satisfaction in the context of cancer care. *Irish Journal of Psychology*, 1998, 19:274–282.

7. Dew MA. Behavioral factors in heart transplantation: Quality of life and medical compliance. *Journal of Applied Biobehavioral Research*, 1994, 2:28–54.

8. Harper RG et al. Self-report evaluation of health behavior, stress vulnerability, and medical outcome of heart transplant recipients. *Psychosomatic Medicine*, 1998, 60:563–569.

9. Godding V, Kruth M, Jamart J. Joint consultation for high-risk asthmatic children and their families, with pediatrician and child psychiatrist as co-therapists: model and evaluation. *Family Process*, 1997, 36:265–280.

10. Wamboldt FS et al. Parental criticism and treatment outcome in adolescents hospitalized for severe, chronic asthma. *Journal of Psychosomatic Research*, 1995, 39:995–1005.

11. Romero MI, Portilla L, Martin E. El apoyo social y su papel en la Diabetes Mellitus: consideraciones teoricas y resultados. [Social support, its role in diabetes mellitus: Theoretical considerations and results.] *Avances en Psicologia Clinica Latinoamericana*, 1992, 10:81–86.

12. Wilson MG, Edmunson J. Characteristics of adherers of a worksite cholesterol intervention program. *Health Values*, 1993, 17:10–20.

13. Burnett KF, Taylor CB, Agras WS. Ambulatory computer-assisted behavior therapy for obesity: An empirical model for examining behavioral correlates of treatment outcome. *Computers in Human Behavior*, 1992, 8:2–3.

14. Cockburn J et al. Behavioural dynamics of a clinical trial of sunscreens for reducing solar keratoses in Victoria, Australia. *Journal of Epidemiology and Community Health*, 1997, 51:716–721.

15. Clark HW. Residential substance abuse treatment for pregnant and postpartum women and their children: treatment and policy implications. *Child Welfare*, 2001, 80:179–198.

16. Mattson ME et al. Compliance with treatment and follow-up protocols in project MATCH: predictors and relationship to outcome. *Alcoholism: Clinical and Experimental Research*, 1998, 22:1328–1339.

17. Abbott PJ et al. Retrospective analyses of additional services for methadone maintenance patients. *Journal of Substance Abuse Treatment*, 1999, 17:129–137.

18. Griffith JD et al. Implications of family and peer relations for treatment engagement and follow-up outcomes: An integrative model. *Psychology of Addictive Behaviors*, 1998, 12:113–126.

19. Grella CE et al. Patient histories, retention, and outcome models for younger and older adults in DATOS. *Drug and Alcohol Dependence*, 1999, 57:151–166.

20. Hoffman JA et al. Psychosocial treatments for cocaine abuse. 12-month treatment outcomes. *Journal of Substance Abuse Treatment*, 1996, 13:3–11.

21. Whitlock EP et al. Does gender affect response to a brief clinic-based smoking intervention? *American Journal of Preventive Medicine*, 1997, 13:159–166.

22. Dunbar-Jacob J, Burke LE, Pyczynski S. Clinical assessment and management of adherence to medical regiments. In: Nicassio PM, Smith TW, eds. *Managing chronic illness: A biopsychosocial perspective.* Washington, DC, American Psychological Association, 1995.

23. Nessman DG, Carnahan JE, Nugent CA. Increasing compliance. Patient-operated hypertension groups. *Archives of Internal Medicine*, 1980, 140:1427–1430.

24. Oxman AD et al. No magic bullets: a systematic review of 102 trials of interventions to improve professional practice. *CMAJ (Canadian Medical Association Journal)*, 1995, 153:1423–1431.

25. DeBusk RF et al. A case-management system for coronary risk factor modification after acute myocardial infarction. *Annals of Internal Medicine*, 1994, 120:721–729.

26. Haynes RB. *Determinants of compliance: The disease and the mechanics of treatment. Compliance in health care.* Baltimore, MD, Johns Hopkins University Press, 1979.

27. Rand CS. Measuring adherence with therapy for chronic diseases: implications for the treatment of heterozygous familial hypercholesterolemia. *American Journal of Cardiology*, 1993, 72:68D–74D.

28. Vitolins MZ et al. Measuring adherence to behavioral and medical interventions. *Controlled Clinical Trials*, 2000, 21:188S–194S.

29. Brown VJ. The association of concordance between physician and patient medical concepts and patient satisfaction, compliance and medical outcomes. *Humanities and Social Sciences*, 1994, 54:2632.

30. Horne R. Patients' beliefs about treatment: the hidden determinant of treatment outcome? *Journal of Psychosomatic Research*, 1999, 47:491–495.

31. *Interventions to improve adherence to medical regimens in the elderly.* Washington, DC, Center for the Advancement of Health, National Institute on Aging, 1999.

32. Hall JA, Roter DL, Katz NR. Meta-analysis of correlates of provider behavior in medical encounters. *Medical Care*, 1988, 26:657–675.

33. Schulman BA. Active patient orientation and outcomes in hypertensive treatment: application of a socio-organizational perspective. *Medical Care*, 1979, 17:267–280.

34. Dunbar J, Agras W. Compliance with medical instructions. In: Ferguson J, Taylor C, eds. *The comprehensive handbook of behavioural medicine.* New York, Springer, 1980:115–145.

35. Stewart MA. Effective physician–patient communication and health outcomes: A review. *Canadian Medical Association Journal*, 1996, 153:1423.

36. Whitcher-Alagna S. Receiving medical help: A psychosocial perspective on patient reactions. In: Nadler A, Fisher JD, DePaulo BM, eds. *New directions in helping.* New York, Academic Press, 2002.

37. Waitzkin H, Stoeckle JD. Information control and the micropolitics of health care. *Social Science and Medicine*, 1976, 10:263–276.

38. Botelho RJ, Skinner H. Motivating change in health behavior. Implications for health promotion and disease prevention. *Primary Care: Clinics In Office Practice*, 1995, 22:565–589.

39. Alto WA. Prevention in practice. *Primary Care: Clinics In Office Practice*, 1995, 22:543–554.

40. Ammerman AS et al. Physician-based diet counseling for cholesterol reduction: current practices, determinants, and strategies for improvement. *Preventive Medicine*, 1993, 22:96–109.

41. DiMatteo MR, DiNicola DD. *Achieving patient compliance.* New York, Pergamon, 1982.

42. Meichenbaum D, Turk DC. *Facilitating treatment adherence: A practitioner's guidebook*, New York, Plenum Press, 1987.

43. Haynes RB, McKibbon KA, Kanani R. Systematic review of randomised trials of interventions to assist patients to follow prescriptions for medications. *Lancet*, 1996, 348:383–386 [erratum published in Lancet, 1997, 349:1180].

44. Kaplan RM, Simon HJ. Compliance in medical care: Reconsideration of self-predictions. *Annals of Behavioral Medicine*, 1990, 12:66-71.

45. Chesney M, et al. Not what the doctor ordered: Challenges individuals face in adhering to medical advice/treatment. *Congressional Briefing*. Washington, DC, Consortium of Social Science Associations, 1999.

46. DiMatteo MR, Lepper HS, Croghan TW. Depression is a risk factor for noncompliance with medical treatment: meta-analysis of the effects of anxiety and depression on patient adherence. *Archives of Internal Medicine*, 2000, 160:2101–2107.

47. Lustman PJ et al. Effects of alprazolam on glucose regulation in diabetes. Results of double-blind, placebo-controlled trial. *Diabetes Care*, 1995, 18:1133–1139.

48. Ziegelstein RC et al. Patients with depression are less likely to follow recommendations to reduce cardiac risk during recovery from a myocardial infarction. *Archives of Internal Medicine*, 2000, 160:1818–1823.

49. Becker M, Rosenstock I. Compliance with medical advice. In: Steptoe A, Mathews A, eds. *Health care and human behaviour*. London, Academic Press, 1984:175–208.

50. Turk D, Salovey P, Litt M. Adherence: a cognitive behavioural perspective. In: Gerber K, Nehemkis A, eds. *Compliance: the dilemma of the chronically ill*. New York, Springer, 1986:44–72.

51. Kirscht J, Rosenstock I. Patient's problems in following recommendations of health experts. In: Stone C, eds. *Health Psychology*. San Francisco, Jossey-Bass, 1979:189–216.

52. Leventhal H, Cameron L. Behavioral theories and the problem of compliance. *Patient Education and Counseling*, 1987, 10:117–138.

53. Horne R, Weinman J. Predicting treatment adherence: an overview of theoretical models. In Myers LB, Midence K, eds. *Adherence to treatment in medical conditions*. UK, Harwood Academic, 1998.

54. Skinner BF. *The behavior of organisms*. New York, Appleton-Century-Crofts, 1938.

55. Skinner BF. *Science and human behavior*. New York, Free Press-Macmillan, 1953:23–42.

56. Ley P. *Communicating with patients*. Croom Helm, London, 1988.

57. Becker M, Maiman L. Patient perceptions and compliance; recent studies of the Health Belief Model. In: Haynes RB, Taylor DW, Sackett DL, eds. *Compliance in health care*. Baltimore, MD, Johns Hopkins University Press, 1979:78–112.

58. Bandura AJ, Simon KM. The role of proximal intentions in self-regulation of refractory behavior. *Cognitive Therapy and Research*, 1977, 1:177–184.

59. Ajzen I, Fishbein M. *Understanding attitudes and predicting social behavior*, Englewood Cliffs, NY, Prentice Hall, 1980.

60. Rogers R, Prentice-Dunn S. Protection Motivation Theory. In: Gochman G, eds. *Handbook of health behavior research: Vol. 1. Determinants of health behavior: Personal and social*. New York, NY, Plenum, 1997.

61. Leventhal H, Leventhal EA, Cameron L. Representations, procedures, and affect in illness self-regulation: A perceptual-cognitive model. In: Baum A, Singer JE, eds. *Handbook of health psychology*. Mahwah, NJ, Erlbaum, 2001:19–47.

62. Leventhal H, Leventhal EA, Contrada RJ. Self-regulation, health, and behavior: A perceptual-cognitive approach. *Psychology and Health*, 1998, 13:717–733.

63. Petrie KJ et al. Thoroughly modern worries: the relationship of worries about modernity to reported symptoms, health and medical care utilization. *Journal of Psychosomatic Research*, 2001, 51:395–401.

64. Kaptein AA, Scharloo M, Weinman JA. Assessing illness perceptions. In: Vingerhoets A, ed. *Assessment in behavioral medicine and health psychology*. London, Psychology Press, 2001:179–194.

65. Scharloo M et al. Illness perceptions, coping and functioning in patients with rheumatoid arthritis, chronic obstructive pulmonary disease and psoriasis. *Journal of Psychosomatic Research*, 1998, 44:573–585.

66. Schmaling KB, Blume AW, Afari N. A randomized controlled pilot study of motivational interviewing to change attitudes about adherence to medications for asthma. *Journal of Clinical Psychology in Medical Settings*, 2001, 8:167–172.

67. Fisher JD, Fisher WA. Changing AIDS-risk behavior. *Psychological Bulletin*, 1992, 111:455–474.

68. Fisher JD et al. Changing AIDS risk behavior: effects of an intervention emphasizing AIDS risk reduction information, motivation, and behavioral skills in a college student population. *Health Psychology*, 1996, 15:114–123.

69. Carey MP et al. Enhancing motivation to reduce the risk of HIV infection for economically disadvantaged urban women. *Journal of Consulting and Clinical Psychology*, 1997, 65:531–541.

70. Mazzuca SA. Does patient education in chronic disease have therapeutic value? *Journal of Chronic Diseases*, 1982, 35:521–529.

71. Prochaska JO, DiClemente CC, Norcross JC. In search of how people change. Applications to addictive behaviors. *American Psychologist*, 1992, 47:1102–1114.

72. Prochaska JO. Strong and weak principles for progressing from precontemplation to action. *Health Psychology*, 1992, 13:47–51.

73. Prochaska JO, Redding C, Evers K. The Transtheoretical Model. In: Glanz KLF, Rimer BK, eds. *Health behavior and health education: theory, research, and practice*. San Francisco, Jossey-Bass, 1997.

74. Redding, CA. Et al. Health behavior models. In: Hyner GC et al., eds. *SPM handbook of health assessment tools*. Pittsburgh, PA, Society of Prospective Medicine and Institute for Health and Productivity Management, 1999.

75. Velicer WF et al. Testing 40 predictions from the transtheoretical model. *Addictive Behaviors*, 1999, 24:455–469.

76. Willey C. Behavior-changing methods for improving adherence to medication. *Current Hypertension Reports*, 1999, 1:477–481.

77. Rakowski W, Fulton JP, Feldman JP. Women's decision making about mammography: a replication of the relationship between stages of adoption and decisional balance. *Health Psychology*, 1993, 12:209–214.

78. Prochaska JO. Strong and weak principles for progressing from precontemplation to action on the basis of twelve problem behaviors. *Health Psychology*, 1994, 13:47–51.

79. Prochaska JO et al. Stages of change and decisional balance for 12 problem behaviors. *Health Psychology*, 1994, 13:39–46.

80. Velicer WF et al. Relapse situations and self efficacy: an integrative model. *Addictive Behavior*, 1990, 15:271–283.

81. DiClemente CC et al. The process of smoking cessation: an analysis of precontemplation, contemplation, and preparation stages of change. *Journal of Consulting and Clinical Psychology*, 1991, 59:295–304.

82. Prochaska JO et al. Measuring processes of change: applications to the cessation of smoking. *Journal of Consulting and Clinical Psychology*, 1988, 56:520–528.

83. Skinner CS et al. How effective is tailored print communication? *Annals of Behavioral Medicine*, 1999, 21:290–298.

84. Campbell MK et al. Improving dietary behavior: the effectiveness of tailored messages in primary care settings. *American Journal of Public Health*, 1994, 84:783–787.

85. Multiple risk factor intervention trial. Risk factor changes and mortality results. Multiple Risk Factor Intervention Trial Research Group. *Journal of the American Medical Association*, 1982, 248:1465–1477.

86. Five-year findings of the hypertension detection and follow-up program. I. Reduction in mortality of persons with high blood pressure, including mild hypertension. Hypertension Detection and Follow-up Program Cooperative Group. *Journal of the American Medical Association*, 1979, 242:2562–2571.

87. Anonymous. Prevention of stroke by antihypertensive drug treatment in older persons with isolated systolic hypertension: final results of the Systolic Hypertension in the Elderly Program (SHEP). *Journal of the American Medical Association*, 1991, 265:3255–3264.

88. Peters AL, Davidson MB, Ossorio RC. Management of patients with diabetes by nurses with support of subspecialists. *HMO Practice*, 1995, 9:8–13.

89. Roter DL et al. Effectiveness of interventions to improve patient compliance: a meta-analysis. *Medical Care*, 1998, 36:1138–1161.

90. Miller NH et al. The multilevel compliance challenge: recommendations for a call to action. A statement for healthcare professionals. *Circulation*, 1997, 95:1085–1090.

91. Haynes RB et al. Interventions for helping patients follow prescriptions for medications. *Cochrane Systematic Reviews*, 2001.

92. Morisky DE et al. Five-year blood pressure control and mortality following health education for hypertensive patients. *American Journal of Public Health*, 1983, 73:153–162.

93. Oldridge NB, Jones NL. Improving patient compliance in cardiac rehabilitation: Effects of written agreement and self-monitoring. *Journal of Cardiopulmonary Rehabilitation*, 1983, 3:257–262.

94. Swain MS, Steckel SB. Influencing adherence among hypertensives. *Research Nursing and Health*, 1981, 4:213–222.

95. Mahoney MJ, Moura NG, Wade TC. Relative efficacy of self-reward, self-punishment, and self-monitoring techniques for weight loss. *Journal of Consulting and Clinical Psychology*, 1973, 40:404–407.

96. Daltroy LH, Godin G. The influence of spousal approval and patient perception of spousal approval on cardiac participation in exercise programs. *Journal of Cardiopulmonary Rehabilitation*, 1989, 9:363–367.

97. Taylor CB et al. Smoking cessation after acute myocardial infarction: effects of a nurse-managed intervention. *Annals of Internal Medicine*, 1990, 113:118–123.

98. Holman HR et al. Evidence that an education program for self-management of chronic disease can improve health status while reducing health care costs: a randomized trial. *Abstract Book/Association for Health Services Research*, 1997, 14:19–20.

99. Bandura A. *Social learning theory*. Englewood Cliffs, NY, Prentice Hall, 1977.

100. Matarazzo JD. Behavioral health and behavioral medicine: frontiers for a new health psychology. *American Psychologist*, 1980, 35:807–817.

101. Mullen PD, Mains DA, Velez R. A meta-analysis of controlled trials of cardiac patient education. *Patient Education and Counseling*, 1992, 19:143–162.

102. Garrity TF, Garrity AR. The nature and efficacy of intervention studies in the National High Blood Pressure Education Research Program. *Journal of Hypertension* 1985, (Suppl)3:S91–S95.

103. Holtzheimer LMHMI. Educating young children about asthma: Comparing the effectiveness of a developmentally appropriate education videotape and picture book. *Child Care, Health, and Development*, 1998, 24:85–99.

104. Burkhart P, Dunbar-Jacob J. Adherence research in the pediatric and adolescent populations: A decade in review. In: Hayman L, Mahom M, Turner R, eds. *Chronic illness in children: An evidence-based approach*. New York, Springer, 2002:199–229.

105. Bender BMH. Compliance with asthma therapy: A case for shared responsibility. *Journal of Asthma*, 1996, 33:199–202.

106. Rock BD, Cooper M. Social work in primary care: a demonstration student unit utilizing practice research. *Social Work in Health Care*, 2000, 31:1–17.

107. De los Rios JL, Sanchez-Sosa JJ. Well-being and medical recovery in the critical care unit: The role of the nurse-patient interaction. *Salud Mental*, 2002, 25:21–31.

108. Malahey B. The effects of instructions and labeling in the number of medication errors made by patients at home. *American Journal of Hospital Pharmacy*, 1966, 23:283–292.

109. Marlatt GA, George WH. Relapse prevention: introduction and overview of the model. *British Journal of Addiction*, 1984, 79:261–273.

110. Zola IK. Structural constraints on the doctor–patient relationship: The case of non-compliance. In: Eisenberg L, Kleinman A, eds. *The relevance of social science for medicine*. New York, D. Reidel, 1981.

111. Miller W, Rollnick S. *Motivational interviewing*. New York, Guilford Press, 1999.

ANNEX II

Statements by stakeholders

1. Family, community and patients' organizations   151
2. Behavioural medicine   153
3. General practitioners/family physicians   154
4. Industry   155
5. Nurses   158
6. Pharmacists   159
7. Psychologists   160

All statements expressed here are the sole responsibility of each individual or organization. None of these statements reflects the views of the World Health Organization on the topic discussed, or those of any other person or organization mentioned in this report.

The stakeholders are listed in alphabetical order, with the exception of patients, who should always come first.

1. Family, community and patients' organizations

Helping people with diabetes
By P. Lefebvre, President-Elect, The International Diabetes Federation (IDF)

Diabetes today represents an unprecedented epidemic. The number of people with diabetes worldwide is estimated to be more than 180 million, a figure likely to double in the next 20–25 years. Diabetes is currently a disease that can be treated, but unfortunately not cured.

The International Diabetes Federation (IDF) is the global advocate for people with diabetes. It comprises 182 patients' associations in more than 140 countries. The current mission of the IDF is to work with its member associations to enhance the lives of people with diabetes through awareness, education and improvement of health and well-being.

Several studies have shown that a gap presently exists between the goals recommended for diabetes care and the care that patients actually receive. Achieving the recommended targets for diabetes control requires informed patients who are motivated to work with their health care providers. The IDF stresses the importance of:

- helping people with diabetes, their families and communities to achieve better control of the condition; and

- helping to train health care professionals, people with diabetes and their families to improve management of the condition.

In this respect, the IDF fully endorses the recommendations of the WHO Adherence Report. The strategy of the IDF for helping to improve adherence includes the identification of core strategic messages and definition of communication objectives targeted at people with diabetes, their families and health care professionals. Specific programmes include the development of standardized and reliable measurement tools. Special emphasis is put on helping patients in developing countries and minority groups.

The IDF also stresses the need for making essential drugs, such as insulin, and monitoring material, such as home blood-glucose monitoring, available and affordable to all people with diabetes in all countries.

The Work of the South African Depression and Anxiety Support Group
By Linda Woods, General Manager, South African Depression and Anxiety Support Group (SADASG)

Seven years have given the SADASG a long time to work on the issues of depression and anxiety and to fulfil our goals, which have been:

Getting patients to treatment. By having a voice on the line, which is often that of someone who has been through the feelings and emotions the patient is currently experiencing, and by being independent and trustworthy listeners we are able to give the caller the confidence to take the next step which is to visit a professional psychiatrist or psychologist. Our referral list includes not only psychiatrists and psychologists, but also general practitioners with the special skills needed to help patients to find the right answers to becoming well again.

Screening. Through our counselling line which is operated from 8 a.m. to 7 p.m. on six days a week, we have been able to give callers advice on their symptoms, whether caused by depression, bipolar disorder, obsessive–compulsive disorder, social phobia, panic disorder, generalized anxiety disorder or post-traumatic stress disorder. Our counsellors have been trained to ask pertinent questions, to help the caller to understand that their symptoms could be those of a real illness and to tell them what it could possibly be.

Adherence. A voice with the time to listen to patients' concerns, their side-effects, their self-doubt, and that can reassure them – often from first-hand experience, for example, that the side-effects they are experiencing are transient, normal and non-threatening and will usually disappear in time. That even though they are feeling so much better after 3 months, we would encourage them to stay on their medication for 6 to 12 months, as recommended by WHO guidelines.

Destigmatization. Through a concerted and targeted effort we currently send out a press article *every single week*. These articles include statistics and quotes from local South African experts, and guidelines on how to get the help that patients may need. They emphasize that treatment is nothing to be ashamed of these days. They feature patients with names, jobs, business men, and women and media personalities who are not ashamed and who can confirm that mental illness is an illness just like diabetes, or heart disease, or asthma, and patients can be helped. Radio programmes, television shows and the screening of 30-second public service advertisements as well as magazine and newspaper articles help to get our message out. Through corporate education programmes that address a diversity of companies we are able to achieve a more caring and open atmosphere in which to tackle these disorders.

Our sponsors, local and national government, industry and certain foundations have helped us play a huge role in opening up this critical field for patients with depression and anxiety disorders throughout South Africa. We look forward to having the continued understanding and support of local government, with whom we could combine efforts to help patients at the community level.

Through our continued efforts, we can bring more people to treatment and improve levels of adherence. Thereby we can try to prevent some of the repercussions of depression becoming the number one illness causing death and disability in the world by 2020 as predicted by the World Bank and the World Health Organization.

2. Behavioural medicine

Health promotion, human behaviour and adherence to therapies
By Dr Aro Arja, Director, Education and Training Committee, International Society of Behavioural Medicine (ISBM)

Most long-term therapies combine medication with simultaneous instructions on health habits and lifestyle changes such as diet, physical activity and smoking cessation. Adherence to such lifestyle changes is often as important to optimal treatment outcome as adherence to medication. Furthermore, through lifestyle change, health promotion and disease prevention interventions can have a far-reaching impact in enhancing health beyond the specific condition being treated[1].

In comparison to the way in which adherence to medication has historically been addressed (in which the target behaviour is somewhat less multidimensional, but perhaps equally broadly determined), adherence to health-promoting or disease-preventing lifestyle changes now requires a different perspective. This perspective is quite broad in terms of the contexts or circumstances that directly influence these target behaviours; it requires a longer time horizon in which to evaluate benefits, consideration of a wider range of multi-level interventions, and a more varied theory-base.

The context extends beyond the person to the wider society, arrangement of working conditions and social processes. In practical terms it means that many factors outside the person, and perhaps beyond their volitional control must be considered. The *time horizon* means that the availability of data having a bearing on the effectiveness of programmes or procedures, in terms of recognizable health benefits, is often delayed by years or decades (as in the benefits of smoking cessation). This provides a challenge for motivation to adopt and maintain changes, especially in the absence of imminent threats to health.

The interventions needed are not only those that target the individual, but also those that act at the level of a society, community or group, and which are conveyed through a host of different channels of influence. For example using mass media, creating environmental changes, and regulations and laws such as smoking bans. Thus, multi-level approaches apply here too, but their range is wider than in compliance to medication.

---

[1] Tuomilehto J et al. Prevention of type 2 diabetes mellitus by changes in lifestyle among subjects with impaired glucose tolerance. New England Journal of Medicine, 2001, 344:1343–1350.

The theoretical basis for surveillance, monitoring and intervention also requires the adoption of a wider social and cultural framework (e.g. social marketing and communication theory) outside the individual, family and patient–clinician relationship[2]. Models explaining the inter-relations between different health-relevant behaviours, the factors that influence them, and the causal pathways of change in different contexts and over the life-course are needed.

Studying and enhancing adherence to preventive therapy and change towards a healthy lifestyle require building a bridge from the person-centred approaches to adherence to medical regimens with their traditional emphasis on individual volition and behavioural control, to the tools and concepts of health promotion which attempt to understand and intervene in a more systemic manner. This involves targeting causes at many levels of the processes that determine human behaviour, not just the behaviour of the individual.

3. General practitioners/family physicians

General practice/family medicine – our role in improving adherence
By Bjorn Gjelsvik, Hon. Secretary, World Organization of Family Doctors (Wonca), Europe Region

The general practitioner (GP) meets the patient in the first line. In many countries, the GP is the first point of contact with the health system.

One of the main goals of a GP is to follow the chronic ill "from birth to the grave", through his or her illnesses. This is in contrast with second-line or hospital medicine, where the patient is seen seldom and arbitrarily. "In hospitals patients come and go; the diseases persist. In general practice, the patients persist and diseases come and go."

Wonca is working very hard to improve quality of care. Every year, there are several Regional Conferences where thousands of GPs meet to discuss this issue. One of the items is, of course, adherence to therapy and the rational use of resources.

During the past 10 years, there has been a great wave of production of guidelines and treatment regimens for chronic diseases and risk conditions. These guidelines should be based on the best available evidence, but it is also necessary to assess their socioeconomic, ethical and political implications, and also what impact they will have on the corps of doctors working in the field.

Important principles to improve adherence are:

- maintaining and building good doctor–patient relationships;

- in consultations, emphasizing the concept of patient-centred method through education and research;

- strengthening the collaboration with home nurses and other services in the care of elderly patients; and

- developing better information technology and filing services for general practices to minimize the risk of failure.

Wonca is the most important international organization for General Practice/Family Medicine. There are member organizations in 66 countries and Wonca is divided into Regions, covering countries connected by geography, language and culture.

---

[2] Nutbeam D, Harris E. Theory in a nutshell. A guide to health promotion theory. Sydney, McGraw-Hill, 1999.

4. Industry

How better labels and package inserts could help people increase their adherence to therapies

By Jerome Reinstein, Director-General, World Self-Medication Industry (WSMI)

The literature on adherence to therapy has concentrated on specific therapies. There is at least one area, however, which is applicable to adherence to all therapies: improving the usability of medicine labels and package inserts. Along with all the specific interventions to improve adherence to therapy, the use of written information for the patient, which has been proven to result in appropriate behaviour with the medicine, is one that needs additional research and the application of what is already known about medicine information design.

WHO has stated on a number of occasions that about half of medicines are not used according to best practice. One of the reasons for this is that labels and leaflets are often not as useable as they should be. Currently, labelling regulations are content-based. That is to say, regulators in individual countries or the European Union decide on what should be on a label and what should be in a leaflet. Sometimes, the regulations even state that the information should be "in consumer-understandable language". However, no regulations currently require testing of labels and leaflets to determine their performance in real-life use. That is to say the labels and leaflets are not tested by members of the public to determine whether an acceptable standard of performance has been reached. One exception to this is in Australia where Consumer Medicines Information is performance-tested and where the contents of labels and leaflets are in the process of being regulated on a performance-test basis.

There are universal principles for producing usable medicines information, but in practice they are not followed by regulatory authorities. Information design principles can be used to produce labels that can be shown to be usable by people. The steps required are:

– *Scoping* – defining the problem to be solved.

– *Bench-marking* – setting performance requirements for the design.

– *Prototype development* – using the best writing and layout skills to develop a prototype.

– *Testing and refinement* – changing the prototype to meet performance requirements (this process may have to be repeated several times in iterative testing to reach the agreed standard).

– *Specification and production* – implementing the design for production and distribution.

– *Monitoring* – measuring the design's performance in use.

The application of these principles is not obvious and must be taught as a discipline. However, the principles can be learned in a short time and can then be applied and tested in any cultural environment, even in environments in which many people are illiterate, where communication agents such as children or village elders can be used to transmit the information on medicines.

How the pharmaceutical industry can help in enhancing adherence to long-term therapies

By H. Bale, Director-General, International Federation of Pharmaceutical Manufacturers Associations (IFPMA).

Medicines won't work if you don't take them. Even the best treatment plan will fail if it isn't followed. The most obvious consequence of nonadherence is that a person's illness may not be relieved or cured.

According to an estimate from the Office of the United States Inspector General, every year nonadherence to drug treatment results in 125 000 deaths from cardiovascular diseases such as heart attack and stroke. In addition, up to 23% of admissions to nursing homes, 10% of hospital admissions, many visits to doctors, many diagnostic tests and many unnecessary treatments could be avoided if people took their drugs as directed.

Unfortunately, people often don't take their medicines as prescribed. This nonadherence has serious and wide-reaching outcomes, ranging from the extra cost to whoever pays for the wasted medicines and additional treatment, to the cost to patients who will suffer avoidable illness and in serious cases, even death. For example, missed doses of a glaucoma drug can lead to damage to the optic nerve and blindness; missed doses of a heart drug may lead to an erratic heart rhythm and cardiac arrest; missed doses of a high blood-pressure drug can lead to stroke; and failure to take prescribed doses of an antibiotic can cause an infection to flare up again and can lead to the emergence of drug-resistant bacteria.

Studies of patient behaviour show that some 50% of medicines are not taken as prescribed. There are many reasons for this, and among the many reasons that patients give for not adhering to a treatment plan, forgetfulness is the most common. A key question is: why do people forget? The psychological mechanism of denial is often a reason, and sometimes something about the treatment may greatly concern the patient, resulting in a repression of the desire to follow the prescribed treatment. Illness in itself is a concern, and having to take medication is a constant reminder that you're ill. Other reasons for not adhering to a treatment plan include the cost of treatment, inconvenience and possible adverse effects.

Studies have shown that patients are more likely to be motivated to take their medicines correctly as prescribed when they:

- understand and accept the diagnosis;

- agree with the treatment proposed; and

- have been able to address and discuss seriously their concerns about the specific medicines.

Ways to improve adherence. Dr Joanne Shaw, director of the Medicines Partnership project (UK), points out that being part of the decision-making process involved in buying a home, household goods or a new car is obvious to most people, but this may not be as obvious when getting treatment for their illness. It has been shown that people normally adhere better to their prescribed treatment if they have a good relationship with their prescribing doctor. One reason for this is that when people participate in their health care planning, they also assume responsibility for it and are therefore more likely to stay with the plan. Getting clear explanations in a language they understand and understanding the rationale for the treatment also help to increase adherence.

A further important issue identified by the Medicines Partnership project, is that people are more likely to adhere if they believe that their doctor, nurse, physician assistant or pharmacist cares whether or not they stick with the plan. Studies show that people who receive explanations from a concerned doctor are more satisfied with the help they receive and like the doctor more; the more they like the doctor, the better they follow a treatment plan. Written instructions help people to avoid mistakes caused by poor recall of what the doctor said.

Creating a two-way relationship between patient and doctor can start with an information exchange. By asking questions, a patient can come to terms with the severity of his or her illness and intelligently weigh the advantages and disadvantages of a treatment plan. Misunderstandings can often be clarified simply by talking to an informed professional. Good communication also ensures that all caregivers can understand plans prescribed by other health care practitioners.

Patients who take responsibility for helping to monitor the good and bad effects of their treatment and discussing concerns with health care practitioners are likely have better results from a treatment plan. They should inform the doctor, pharmacist or nurse about unwanted or unexpected effects before adjusting or stopping the treatment on their own. A patient often has good reasons for not following a plan, and a doctor can make an appropriate adjustment after a frank discussion of the problem.

Patients may also form support groups for people suffering from similar conditions. Often the fact that there are other patients trying to cope with the same problems can be helpful, and the patient support groups can provide suggestions for coping with problems, building on the experiences of other patients.

Reasons for not adhering to a treatment plan. It is also important to try to understand the reasons for not adhering to a prescribed treatment. The patient could be misunderstanding or misinterpreting the instructions. Forgetting to take a medication is common, and experiencing adverse effects may be perceived as worse than the disease itself, especially if the disease is asymptomatic – the treatment of high blood pressure is a classic example of this. What may be represented as "misunderstanding or misinterpreting or forgetting", could be the expression of underlying beliefs and priorities about medicines in general, and the patient's regimen in particular. Denying the diagnosis and the illness, and not believing that the medicine will help are other factors. Patients may also fear adverse effects or becoming dependent on the drug (which may lead the patient to take a "medication holiday"). Sometimes patients may believe mistakenly – that the disease has been sufficiently treated, as is often the case when people take antibiotics for an infection, and the symptoms disappear before all the bacteria are eradicated. Other factors may be worries about the costs, or the patient experiences problems, for example, difficulty swallowing tablets, opening the medicine container, or following a cumbersome treatment plan.

For older people adherence may be a particular challenge, as they are often taking several drugs concurrently, making it harder for them to remember when to take each of them. It is also not unlikely that they could experience an adverse drug interaction. Doctors should take care to obtain information about all the drugs a person is taking, not only prescription medications, but also over-the-counter preparations.

A role for industry. The main role of the pharmaceutical industry is to develop safe and efficacious treatments. The development of drugs with few side-effects and easy or easier administration would promote adherence. Because medicines are for patients and their optimal use, the industry's role should go beyond the traditional one of bringing the medicines to the market. Industry also has a necessary role in helping to inform patients about their products. This should be in such a way that broader and increased knowledge and understanding can support the patient's relation to, and dialogue with, the prescribing doctor and the other health professionals involved, such as nurses and pharmacists, in following the prescribed treatment to achieve the best outcome for both the patient and the health care system.

5. Nurses

The role of the nurse in improving adherence
By Tesfamicael Ghebrehiwet, Nursing and Health Policy Consultant, International Council of Nurses (ICN)

Nonadherence to treatment regimens is a persistent challenge to nurses and other health professionals. It is estimated that the percentage of patients who fail to adhere to prescribed regimens ranges from 20 to 80%[1,2]. Nurses are aware of the consequences of nonadherence and its high cost to the patient, the community and the health care system. In addition, nurses are all too familiar with the frustrations about treatment failures, poor health outcomes and patient dissatisfaction that accompany poor adherence.

The International Council of Nurses (ICN) estimates that there are about 12 million nurses worldwide. And with a proper understanding of the dynamics of adherence, and techniques in assessing and monitoring the problems of nonadherence, these millions of nurses represent a formidable force in improving adherence and care outcomes. Their presence in all health care settings, their closeness to people and their large numbers combine to position nurses for sustained strategies to improve adherence.

Nursing interventions to scale up adherence need to be based on innovative approaches that involve nurse-prescribing, patient participation in self-care, and continuous assessment and monitoring of treatment regimens. Such approaches should foster therapeutic partnerships between patients and nurses that are respectful of the beliefs and choices of the patient in determining when and how treatment regimens are to be followed. Because much of the treatment for chronic conditions takes place in the home and community setting, nurses can provide a link and support through home visits, telephone and other reminders that facilitate adherence. Through sustained contact, nurses can form a therapeutic alliance with patients and their families and provide ongoing support for taking the recommended medications. Some techniques of monitoring adherence include directly observed therapy (DOT), pill counting, thoughtful and non-judgemental interviews, and reviewing medication cabinets[3].

Nursing strategies to improve adherence include:

- assessing the extent of adherence using non-threatening questions;

- asking about side-effects of medication and their effect on patient's quality of life;

- educating patients on their illness, the importance of adherence, how the treatment will help, possible side-effects and how deal with them;

- suggesting cues and reminders such as detailed schedules, integrating medication times with daily habits, using medication boxes and timers, alarms, beepers, etc;

- rewarding and reinforcing adherence behaviour, for example, through charts and graphics that show the impact of medication on clinical markers of disease: e.g. lower blood pressure, lower blood sugar, lower viral load, etc;

- encouraging the patient to cultivate therapeutic relationships with health professionals, and to talk with peer groups and family members.

Ensuring that treatment regimens are followed and administering medications and other treatments are some of the key roles in nursing. Nurses have diverse skills that must be tapped in improving adherence and care outcome. Continuing education programmes for nurses and other health professionals can improve their competence and awareness about the importance of adherence in health care.

[1,2] Cramer JA et al. How often is medication taken as prescribed? A novel assessment technique. Journal of the American Medical Association, 1989, 261:3273–3277 [erratum published in Journal of the American Medical Association, 1989, 262:1472]. Wright EC. Non-compliance – or how many aunts has Matilda? Lancet, 1993, 342:909–913.

[3] Williams AB. Adherence to HIV regimens: 10 vital lessons. American Journal of Nursing, 2001, 101:37–43.

6. Pharmacists

The role of the pharmacist in improving adherence
A.J.M. (Ton) Hoek, General Secretary, International Pharmaceutical Federation (FIP)

Medicines are an integral part of most courses of therapy, and their safe and appropriate use is an important aspect of optimizing health care outcomes. Medicines can be used effectively to prevent disease or the negative consequences of long-term chronic illness, but more needs to be done to improve the overall quality of their use. Pharmacists have a key role to play by providing assistance, information and advice to the public about medicines, as well as by monitoring treatment and identifying problems in close cooperation with other health care providers and the patients.

Pharmacists are well-positioned to play a primary role in improving adherence to long-term therapy because they are the most accessible health care professionals and they have extensive training in pharmaceuticals. Part of the professional responsibility of pharmacists is to provide sound, unbiased advice and a comprehensive pharmacy service that includes activities both to secure good health and quality of life, and to avoid ill-health.

Pharmaceutical care is a relatively new philosophy of practice, the goal of which is to optimize the patient's health-related quality of life and to achieve positive clinical outcomes.

Pharmaceutical care includes:
- educating the patient or the person caring for the patient about their medications and the conditions for which they are prescribed to ensure maximum therapeutic benefit and safety;
- reviewing the patient's medication history;
- continuous monitoring of the patient's therapy;
- screening for potential adverse effects; and
- monitoring the patient's ability to take his or her medications correctly and to adhere to the prescribed therapies.

Pharmacists, through the practice of pharmaceutical care, can prevent or stop interactions, monitor and prevent or minimize adverse drug reactions and monitor the cost and effectiveness of drug therapy as well as provide lifestyle counselling to optimize the therapeutic effects of a medication regimen. The concept of pharmaceutical care is particularly relevant to special groups of patients such as the elderly and chronically ill.

Intervention by the pharmacist and pharmaceutical care are effective approaches to improving adherence to long-term therapies. Adherence to immunosuppressive medications in renal transplant patients ranges from 50 to 95% and nonadherence can result in organ rejection[1]. Intervention by pharmacists has been demonstrated to improve average monthly compliance by more than 100% over a 12-month period[2]. Advice, information and referral by community pharmacists have been demonstrated to significantly improve adherence to antihypertensive medications and improve blood-pressure control[3]. Similar results have been demonstrated in patients with asthma[4,5].

---

[1] Greenstein S, Siegal B. Compliance and noncompliance in patients with a functioning renal transplant: a multicenter study. *Transplantation*, 1998, 66:1718–1726.

[2] Chisholm MA et al. Impact of clinical pharmacy services on renal transplant patients' compliance with immunosuppressive medications. *Clinical Transplantation*, 2001, 15:330–336.

[3] Blenkinsopp A et al. Extended adherence support by community pharmacists for patients with hypertension: A randomised controlled trial. *International Journal of Pharmacy Practice*, 2000, 8:165–175.

[4] Cordina M, McElnay JC, Hughes CM. Assessment of a community pharmacy-based program for patients with asthma. *Pharmacotherapy*, 2001, 21:1196–1203.

[5] Schulz M et al. Pharmaceutical care services for asthma patients: a controlled intervention study. *Journal of Clinical Pharmacology*, 2001, 41:668–676.

These are only examples of many indications where improved compliance and outcomes have been clearly demonstrated to result from pharmacists' interventions. Many studies on this subject have been published, especially during the last 10–15 years.

Pharmacists are an important resource for improving adherence to long-term therapy.

7. Psychologists

The role of psychologists in improving adherence to therapies
By Pierre L.-J. Ritchie. Secretary General. International Union of Psychological Sciences (IUPsyS)

Psychologists work as applied health researchers and practitioners in primary, secondary and tertiary care settings and as members of multidisciplinary teams of health service providers, as well as in independent practice. In these varied roles, the involvement of psychologists increases the effectiveness of programmes aimed at identifying and treating prevalent behaviourally-based health problems. Nonadherence is arguably the most widely distributed and prevalent of these problems.

The success of any treatment depends on both its efficacy and the manner in which a patient uses it. Adherence occurs in the process of adaptation to illness or to the threat of illness. While the past 50 years have witnessed considerable progress in developing powerful treatments for a wide variety of chronic and acute illnesses, patients' use of these treatments has been far from optimal. The global challenge now facing health systems is to become more effective in creating the conditions that enable people to derive maximum benefit from available treatments. Establishing the optimal conditions for adherence early in the treatment process sets the stage for long-term maintenance. Psychological science and practice concerning adherence focus on the systemic, biological, social, cognitive, behavioural and emotional contributing factors. Psychologists bring an understanding of both adaptive and maladaptive psychological, social and behavioural processes that are critical for understanding, preventing and treating nonadherence.

In every situation in which treatment involves an aspect of a patient's behaviour, adherence is a potential problem. This is the case for health-seeking behaviours, the self-administration of medication or making lifestyle changes. Adherence is a behavioural issue, and psychology is a behavioural discipline. It is therefore not surprising that psychologists have been very active in efforts to improve adherence since at least the 1950s. Furthermore, adherence to both medical and behavioural treatments has been a major subject of research and practice in health psychology and behavioural medicine since their emergence as specialty areas. Since the 1980s, many psychologists have embraced a population-health perspective, and have supported public health goals by putting psychological know-how to work at all levels of the health care system. Their work supports the development of effective health policy, surveillance of behavioural risk factors in the population, and the design, implementation and evaluation of interventions.

Psychologists have unique and specialized training. They are behavioural specialists, often trained as scientist–practitioners, who bring an evidence-based perspective to the problem of nonadherence. Through research and practice, psychologists have developed compelling, effective approaches to help patients to cope with the demands imposed by chronic illness that frequently contribute to nonadherence. Psychologists also possess expertise in interpersonal communication, and have contributed to knowledge concerning the importance of good communication between health providers and patients for promoting adherence. This has led to innovations in training in interpersonal skills for health service providers targeting this determinant. Recognition of the importance of psychological and behavioural skills in the training curricula of health disciplines has drawn further on the skills of psychologists as educators.

As a health discipline, psychology blends basic and applied scientific enquiry with clinical service delivery to increase knowledge about adherence behaviour and its determinants, and to improve people's health and well-being, and the quality and efficiency of health services. Psychology was founded in response to the need to understand, predict and influence such basic phenomena as human motivation, cognition and behaviour. Over time several sub-disciplines have emerged including, clinical, health, rehabilitation, community, experimental, organizational and social psychology. Each of these has made substantial contributions to the knowledge base on adherence.

As scientists, psychologists produce knowledge that helps to identify the causes of the nonadherence, develop and test theories that help to explain the mechanisms of causality and to design and evaluate interventions to increase adherence. In this regard, psychologists have contributed to adherence research and patient care in areas such as HIV/AIDS, diabetes, hypertension, obesity, ischaemic heart disease, stroke, chronic pain, asthma and chronic obstructive pulmonary disease, kidney disease, headache, addictions, seizure disorders, a range of mental illnesses and dental hygiene, as well as behavioural risk factors for illness such as poor diet, insufficient physical activity, smoking and risky sexual behaviours among others.

As health service providers and members of the health care team, psychologists bring unique skills in psychological assessment and behavioural measurement to help identify those patients at risk of nonadherence, and to identify the determinants of nonadherence where it has already become a problem. They bring sophisticated treatment skills to ameliorate these risk factors and determinants. These skills are applied to individuals, families, groups or communities in the service of illness prevention, acute and chronic care or rehabilitation. With regard to nonadherence, these skills are commonly used to address the cognitive, motivational, emotional and behavioural barriers to the self-management of illness, or the modification of health risk behaviours. In clinical service settings, psychologists function in varied roles; as providers of direct service, consultants to health care teams with respect to diagnosis and treatment planning, and patient advocacy.

In addition to the basic science, clinical and population health research described above, psychological practice in the area of adherence comprises:

– assessment of risk for nonadherence including the relative contributions of patient attributes, illness- and treatment-related factors, social context of illness, and health provider and system factors;

– assessment and treatment of mental health co-morbidities that confer additional risk for nonadherence;

– specific cognitive, motivational and behavioural interventions to enhance the ability of patients to manage their own illness or to reduce risk of illness;

– relapse prevention intervention to assist with the long-term maintenance of treatment;

– continuing education interventions for other health service providers that teach skills in communication, motivation enhancement, and behaviour modification; and

– systems interventions aimed at improving the availability, accessibility and acceptability of treatments.

Psychological service providers have an integral role in primary health care teams that aim to deliver optimal, cost-effective care. They contribute by monitoring the psychological and behavioural risks to patients' health, identifying and treating psychological and behavioural problems that threaten the effectiveness of treatment and they optimize treatment planning by helping to integrate behavioural science.

Annex III – Table of reported factors by condition and dimension

	Socioeconomic-related factors	Health care team/health system-related factors
Asthma	(–) Vulnerability of the adolescent to not taking medications; family conflict and a denial of severity of disease in adolescents; memory difficulties in older patients; polypharmacy in older patients; cultural and lay beliefs about illness and treatment; alternative medicine; fear of the health care system; poverty; inner-city living; lack of transport; family dysfunction	(–) Health care providers' lack of knowledge and training in treatment management and/or an inadequate understanding of the disease; short consultations; lack of training in changing behaviours of nonadherent patients
Cancer	(–) Long distance from treatment setting	(–) lack of knowledge of health professionals about pain management;' inadequate understanding of drug dependence by health professionals; health professionals' fears of investigation or sanction; poor delivery of care-education to the patient; poor delivery of care-education to family and caregivers; reluctance of health professionals to prescribe opioids for use at home (+) Good relationship between patient and physician
Depression	No information was found	(–) Poor health education of the patient (+) Multi-faceted intervention for primary care
Diabetes	(–) Cost of care; patients over 25 years (adherence to physical activity); older adolescents (insulin administration); older adolescents (SMBG); males (adherence to diet); females (adherence to physical activity); environmental high-risk situations (+) Patients aged less than 25 years (adherence to physical activity); younger adolescents (insulin administration); younger adolescents (SMBG); males (adherence to physical activity); females (adherence to diet); social support; family support	(–) Poor relationship between patient and physician
Epilepsy	(–) Long distance from treatment setting; under 60 years old; teenagers; poverty; illiteracy; unwillingness to pay the cost of medicines; high cost of medications; local beliefs or beliefs about the origin of illness (+) Elderly patients (over 60 years old); children from family reporting less parental education; non-English speaking in an English-speaking community; lower income; recent immigrants	(–) Inadequate or non-existent reimbursement by health insurance plans; irregular or poor drug supply; lack of supplies of free medicines; poorly developed health services; lack of education about AEDs (+) Good relationship between patient and physician

AEDs, Antiepileptic drugs; SMBG, self-monitoring of blood glucose; (+) factors having a positive effect on adherence;
(–) factors having a negative effect on adherence.

Condition-related factors	Therapy-related factors	Patient-related factors
(−) Inadequate understanding of the disease	(−) Complex treatment regimens; long duration of therapy; frequent doses; adverse effects of treatment	(−) Forgetfulness; misunderstanding of instructions about medications; poor parental understanding of children's asthma medications; patient's lack of perception of his or her own vulnerability to illness; patients' lack of information about the prescribed daily dosage/misconception about the disease and treatments; persistent misunderstandings about side-effects; drug abuse (+) Perceiving that they are vulnerable to illness
(−) Nature of the patient's illness; poor understanding of the disease and its symptoms	(−) Complex treatment regimens; taking too many tablets; frequency of dose; having no treatment instructions; misunderstanding instructions about how to take the drugs; bad tasting medication; adverse effects of treatment; inadequate treatment doses; perceived ineffectiveness; unnecessary duplicate prescribing (+) Monotherapy with simple dosing schedules	(−) Forgetfulness; misconceptions about pain; difficulty in taking the preparation as prescribed; fear of injections; anxieties about possible adverse events; no self-perceived need for treatment; not feeling it is important to take medications; undue anxiety about medication dependence; fear of addiction; psychological stress
(−) Psychiatric co-morbidity (+) Clear instructions on management of disease; nature of the patient's illness; poor understanding of the disease and its symptoms	(−) High frequency of dose; co-prescribing of benzodiazepines; inadequate doses of medication (+) Low frequency of dose; clear instructions on management of treatment	(−) Personality traits
(−) Depression; duration of disease	(−) Complexity of treatment (+) Less frequent doses; monotherapy with simple dosing schedules, frequency of the self-care behaviour	(−) Depression; stress and emotional problems; alcohol abuse (+) Self-esteem/self-efficacy
(−) Forgetfulness; memory deficits; duration and previous treatment failures; high frequency of seizures	(−) Complex treatment regimens; misunderstanding instructions about how to take the drugs; adverse effects of treatment (+) Monotherapy with simple dosing schedules	(−) Disbelief of the diagnosis; refusal to take medication, delusional thinking; inconvenience of treatment; denial of diagnosis; lifestyle and health beliefs; parental worry about a child's health; behavioural restrictions placed on the child to protect his/her health; fear of addiction; doubting the diagnosis; uncertainty about the necessity for drugs; anxiety over the complexity of the drug regimen; feeling stigmatized by the epilepsy; not feeling that it is important to take medications (+) Parents and child satisfied with medical care; not feeling stigmatized by epilepsy; feeling that it is important to take medications; high levels of stressful life events

Annex III – Table of reported factors by condition and dimension (cont)

	Socioeconomic-related factors	Health care team/health system-related factors
HIV/AIDS	(–) Women (stress of childcare); low income; African American men; lack of social support (+) Support of family and friends; Caucasian men	(–) Lack of clear instructions from health professionals; poor implementation of educational interventions (+) Good relationship between patient and physician; support from nurses and pharmacists
Hypertension	(–) Low socioeconomic status; illiteracy; unemployment; limited drug supply; high cost of medication	(–) Lack of knowledge and training for health care providers on managing chronic diseases; inadequate relationship between health care provider and patient; lack of knowledge; inadequate time for consultations; lack of incentives and feedback on performance (+) Good relationship between patient and physician
Tobacco smoking	(–) High cost of treatment (+) Higher levels of education, older age	(–) Unavailability for follow-up or lost to follow-up; failure to recall the receipt of a prescription (+) Access to free nicotine-replacement therapy; more frequent contact with physicians and pharmacists
Tuberculosis	(–) Lack of effective social support networks and unstable living conditions; cultural and lay beliefs about illness and treatment; ethnicity, gender and age; high cost of medication; high cost of transport; criminal justice involvement; involvement in drug dealing	(–) Poorly developed health services; inadequate relationship between health care provider and patient; health care providers who are untrained, overworked, inadequately supervised or unsupported in their tasks; inability to predict potentially non-adherent patients (+) Good relationship between patient and physician; availability of expertise; links with patient support systems; flexibility in the hours of operation
Common elements	(–) Long distance from treatment setting; low socioeconomic status; illiteracy; high cost of medication (+) Family support	(–) Lack of knowledge and training of health professionals about treatment management and/or an inadequate understanding of the disease; poor relationship between patient and physician; short consultations; poor implementation of educational interventions (+) Good relationship between patient and health professionals

CO, carbon monoxide; (+) factors having a positive effect on adherence; (–) factors having a negative effect on adherence.

Condition-related factors	Therapy-related factors	Patient-related factors
(–) Asymptomatic patients (+) Symptomatic patients; understanding the relationship between adherence and viral load	(–) Complex treatment regimens; close monitoring; severe lifestyle alterations; adverse effects of treatment; lack of clear instructions about how to take the medications (+) Less frequent dose; fewer pills per day; fewer dietary restrictions; fitting medication to individual's lifestyle; belief that medication is effective	(–) Forgetfulness; life stress; alcohol use; drug use; depression; hopelessness and negative feelings; beliefs that alcohol and drug use interfere with medications (+) Positive beliefs regarding the efficacy of antiretroviral medications
(+) Understanding and perceptions about hypertension	(–) Complex treatment regimens; duration of treatment; low drug tolerability, adverse effects of treatment (+) Monotherapy with simple dosing schedules; less frequent dose; fewer changes in antihypertensive medications; newer classes of drug: angiotensin II antagonists, angiotensin converting enzyme inhibitors, calcium channel blockers	(–) Inadequate knowledge and skill in managing the disease symptoms and treatment; no awareness of the costs and benefits of treatment, non-acceptance of monitoring (+) Perception of the health risk related to the disease; active participation in monitoring; participation in management of disease
(–) Daily cigarette consumption; expired CO; plasma nicotine and cotinine levels; Fagerstrom tolerance questionnaire (FTQ) scores; greater tobacco dependence; psychiatric co-morbidities; depression; failure to stop or reduce smoking during treatment	(–) Adverse events or withdrawal symptoms (+) Attendance at behavioural intervention sessions	(–) Weight gain, no self-perceived need for treatment; no perceived effect of treatment (+) Motivation; good relationship between patient and physician
(–) Asymptomatic patients; drug use; altered mental states caused by substance abuse; depression and psychological stress (+) Knowledge about tuberculosis	(–) Complex treatment regimen; adverse effects of treatment; toxicity	(–) Forgetfulness; drug abuse, depression; psychological stress (+) Belief in the efficacy of treatment; motivation
(–) Poor understanding of the disease and its "side-effects"; depressive illness; psychiatric co-morbidities; asymptomatic disease; long duration of the disease (+) Understanding and perception of the disease	(–) Complex treatment regimen; adverse effects of treatment; frequent doses; lack of clear instructions about how to take the medications (+) Monotherapy; less frequent doses; fewer pills per day; clear instructions on management of treatment	(–) Forgetfulness; misunderstanding instructions about how to take the medications; inadequate knowledge and skill in managing the disease symptoms and treatment; anxieties about possible adverse effects; lack of self-perceived need for treatment; psychosocial stress; depression; low motivation (+) Belief in the efficacy of treatment; motivation; perception of the health risk related to the disease

Annex IV Table of reported interventions by condition and dimension

	Socioeconomic-related interventions	Health care team-/ health care system-related interventions
Asthma	List-organized instructions; clear instructions about treatment for older patients	Education on use of medicines; management of disease and treatment in conjunction with patients; adherence education; multidisciplinary care; training in monitoring adherence; more intensive intervention by increasing number and duration of contacts
Cancer	Optimizing the cooperation between services; assessment of social needs; family preparedness; mobilization of community-based organizations	Training of health professionals on adherence; pain education component in training programmes; support to caregivers; multidisciplinary care; follow-up consultation by community nurses; supervision in home pain management; identification of the treatment goals and development of strategies to meet them
Depression	No information was found	Multidisciplinary care; training of health professionals on adherence; counselling provided by a primary care nurse; telephone consultation/counselling; improved assessment and monitoring of patients
Diabetes	Mobilization of community-based organizations; assessment of social needs; family preparedness	Multidisciplinary care; training for health professionals on adherence; identification of the treatment goals and development of strategies to meet them; continuing education; continuous monitoring and re-assessment of treatment; systems interventions: health insurance for nutrition therapy, telephone reminders to patients, chronic care models
Epilepsy	Assessment of social and career needs	A regular, uninterrupted supply of medicines in developing countries; good patient–physician relationship; instruction by nurses and physicians about methods of incorporating drug administration into patient's daily life; training health professionals on adherence; adherence education
HIV/AIDS	Family preparedness; mobilization of community-based organizations; intensive education on use of medicines for patients with low levels of literacy; assessment of social needs	Good patient–physician relationship; multidisciplinary care; training of health professionals on adherence; training for health professionals in adherence education; training in monitoring adherence; training caregivers; identification of the treatment goals and development of strategies to meet them; management of disease and treatment in conjunction with the patients; uninterrupted ready availability of information; regular consultations with nurses or physicians; non-judgemental attitude and assistance; rational selection of medications

Condition-related interventions	Therapy-related interventions	Patient-related interventions
Patient education beginning at the time of diagnosis and integrated into every step of asthma care	Simplification of regimens; education on use of medicines; adaptations of prescribed medications; continuous monitoring and re-assessment of treatment	Self-management programmes that include both educational and behavioural components; memory aids and reminders; incentives and/or reinforcements; self-monitoring
Education of the patient on adherence	Simplification of regimens; education on use of medications; giving clear instructions; clarifying misunderstandings about the recommendation of opioids; patient-tailored prescriptions; continuous monitoring and re-assessment of treatment; assessment and management of side-effects; coordination of prescribing	Interventions to redress misconceptions about pain treatment and to encourage dialogue about pain control between patient and oncologist; exploration of fears (e.g. about addiction); assessment of psychological needs; education on use of medications; behavioural and motivational intervention; self-management of disease and treatment; self-management of side-effects
Education of patients on use of medicines	Education on use of medicines; patient-tailored prescriptions; continuous monitoring and re-assessment of treatment	Counselling; relapse-prevention counselling; psychotherapy; family psychotherapy; frequent follow-up interviews; specific advice targeted at the needs and concerns of individual patients
Education on use of medicines	Patient self-management; simplification of regimens; education on use of medicines; weight reduction assistance; teaching prescribed physical activity	Behavioural and motivational interventions; assessment of psychological needs; telephone reminders to patients in order to reduce missed appointments
Education on use of medicines	Simplification of regimens; single antiepileptic therapy (monotherapy); education on use of medicines; patient-tailored prescriptions; clear instructions; use of educational materials; continuous monitoring and re-assessment of treatment	Self-management of disease and treatment; self-management of side-effects; behavioural and motivational intervention; education on adherence; providing the patients with control and choices; assessment of psychological needs; frequent follow-up interviews; memory aids and reminders
Education on use of medicines; supportive medical consultation; screening for co-morbidities; attention to mental illness, as well as abuse of alcohol and other drugs	Simplification of regimens; education of the patient on the use of medicines; assessment and management of side-effects; patient-tailored prescriptions; medications for symptoms; adherence education; continuous monitoring and re-assessment of treatment	Monitor drug and/or alcohol use; psychiatric consultation; behavioural and motivational intervention; counselling/psychotherapy; telephone counselling; memory aids and reminders; self-management of disease and treatment

Annex IV Table of reported interventions by condition and dimension (cont)

	Socioeconomic-related factors	Health care team/health system-related factors
Hypertension	Family preparedness; patient health insurance; uninterrupted supply of medicines; sustainable financing, affordable prices and reliable supply systems	Training in education of patients on use of medicines; good patient–physician relationship; continuous monitoring and re-assessment of treatment; monitoring adherence; non-judgemental attitude and assistance; uninterrupted ready availability of information; rational selection of medications; training in communication skills; delivery, financing and proper management of medicines; development of drugs with better safety profile by pharmaceutical industry; participation of pharmaceutical industry in patient education programmes and in developing instruments to measure adherence for patients
Tobacco smoking	Social assistance	Pharmacist mobilization; free access to nicotine-replacement therapy; frequent follow-up interviews
Tuberculosis	Assessment of social needs; social support, housing, food tokens and legal measures; providing transport to treatment setting; peer assistance; mobilization of community-based organizations; optimizing the cooperation between services	Uninterrupted ready availability of information; flexibility in available treatment; training and management processes that aim to improve the way providers care for patients with tuberculosis; management of disease and treatment in conjunction with the patients; multidisciplinary care; intensive staff supervision; training in monitoring adherence; DOTS strategy
Common elements	Assessment of social needs; social support; family support and preparedness; mobilization of community-based organizations; uninterrupted supply of medicines	Multidisciplinary care; training in educating patients about adherence; good patient–provider relationship; management of disease and treatment in conjunction with the patients; more intensive intervention in terms of number and duration of contacts; adherence education; training in monitoring adherence; uninterrupted ready availability of information

DOTS, Directly observed therapy, short course.

Condition-related factors	Therapy-related factors	Patient-related factors
Education on use of medicines	Simplification of regimens	Behavioural and motivational intervention; self-management of disease and treatment; self-management of side-effects; memory aids and reminders
Therapeutic patient education; supportive psychiatric consultation	Nicotine replacement therapy; antidepressant therapy; education on use of medications; adherence education; assistance with weight reduction; continuous monitoring and re-assessment of treatment; monitoring adherence	Adjunctive psychosocial treatment; behavioural intervention; assistance with weight reduction; good patient–physician relationship
Education on use of medicines; provision of information about tuberculosis and the need to attend for treatment	Education on use of medications; adherence education; tailor the treatment to the needs of patients at risk of nonadherence; agreements (written or verbal) to return for an appointment or course of treatment; continuous monitoring and re-assessment of treatment	Mutual goal-setting; memory aids and reminders; incentives and/or reinforcements; reminder letters, telephone reminders or home visits for patients who fail to attend clinic
Education on use of medicines	Simplification of regimens; adherence education; education on use of medicines; patient-tailored prescriptions; continuous monitoring and re-assessment of treatment; monitoring adherence	Mutual goal-setting; incentives and/or reinforcements; behavioural and motivational intervention; counselling/psychotherapy; assessment of psychological needs; self-management of the disease and treatment that includes both educational and behavioural components; memory aids and reminders

ANNEX V

Global Adherence Interdisciplinary Network (GAIN)

1. Scientists   171

2. Professional, industry and patient's organizations   173

3. Policy-makers   175

Scientists

Alvarez-Gordillo, Guadalupe • Senior Researcher • Colegio de la Frontera Sur (Chiapas) • Mexico

Arnsten, Julia • Assistant Professor of Medicine • Montefiore Medical Center • USA

Aro, Arja • Assistant Professor and Senior Researcher • National Public Health Institute • Finland

Ashida, Terunao • Senior Researcher • Institute for Adult Diseases, Asahi Life Foundation • Japan

Ayuso-Mateos, Jose Luis • Professor of Psychiatry • University Hospital "La Princesa", Autonomous University of Madrid • Spain

Bamberger, Josh • Medical Director • Housing and Urban Health • USA

Basile, Jan • Associate Professor of Medicine • Ralph H. Johnson VA Medical Center, Medical University of South Carolina • USA

Bender, Bruce • Head, Pediatric Behavioral Health • National Jewish Medical and Research Center • USA

Bernsten, Cecilia • Director • Medicines Unit, National Board of Health and Welfare • Sweden

Betancourt, Joseph • Senior Scientist • Institute for Health Policy • USA

Blake, Max • CORE Center for Prevention of Infectious Diseases • USA

Blank, Karen • Senior Research Psychiatrist • Hartford Hospital's Mental Health Network • USA

Bogart, Laura • Assistant Professor • Kent State University • USA

Borgdorff, Martien • Epidemiologist • Royal Netherlands Tuberculosis Association (KNCV) • Netherlands

Bosco de Oliveira, Helenice • Professor • Campina State University • Brazil

Botelho, Richard J. • Associate Professor of Family Medicine • Family Medicine Center • USA

Boulet, Louis-Philippe • Professor • Laval University Hospital • Canada

Bovet, Pascal • Epidemiologist Consultant • Unit for Prevention and Control of Cardiovascular Disease, Ministry of Health • Seychelles

Branco Ferreira, Manuel • Clinical Practitioner • Immuno-allergology Unit • Santa Maria Hospital • Portugal

Broers, Barbara • Researcher • Department of Community Health, University Hospital of Geneva • Switzerland

Burkhart, Patricia • Assistant Professor and Nurse Researcher • University of Kentucky • USA

Cameron, Tebbi • Medical Director • Tampa Children's Hospital • USA

Caplehorn, John • Clinical Epidemiology • University of Sydney • Australia

Chapman, Kenneth • Director • Asthma Center and Pulmonary Rehabilitation Program • Canada

Chaustre, Ismenia • Attending Physician and Professor • "JM de los Ríos" Children's Hospital • Venezuela

Chen, Junwen • Research Associate • School of Human Sciences, Waseda University • Japan

Chesney, Margaret A. • Professor of Medicine • University of California at San Francisco Prevention Sciences Group • USA

Choo, Peter • Researcher • Brigham and Women's Hospital • USA

Coker, Richard • Senior Lecturer, Public Health • London School of Hygiene and Tropical Medicine • England

Conway, Alison • Respiratory Nurse Specialist • Glenfield Hospital • England

Crystal, Stephen • Research Professor, Director AIDS Research Group and Associate Director for Health Services Research • Institute for Health, Health Care Policy, and Aging Research/ Rutgers University • USA

Dean, Linda • Director of Clinical Education • MCP Hahnemann University • USA

de Boer, Hanneke M. • Global Campaign Co-Chair • The International Bureau for Epilepsy/Stichting Epilepsie Instellingen Nederland • Netherlands

De Geest, Sabina • Professor of Nursing and Director • Institute of Nursing Science, University of Basel • Switzerland

Di Pollina, Laura • Chief, Clinical Geriatrics • University Hospital of Geneva • Switzerland

Dick, Judy • Senior Researcher • Medical Research Centre of South Africa • South Africa

Dilorio, Colleen • Professor • Center for Nursing Research, Emory University • USA

DiMatteo, Robin • Professor • Department of Psychology, University of California • USA

Erlen, Judith • Professor • University of Pittsburgh • USA

Esparis, Belen • Clinical Practitioner • University Hospital of Caracas • Venezuela

Farmer, Paul • Professor • Harvard Medical School • USA

Farmer, Paul • Director • Partners in health, Harvard University • USA

Fitzgerald, Mark • Director of Clinical Epidemiology and Evaluation • Vancouver General Hospital • Canada

Fodor, George • Head of Research • Heart Institute, University of Ottawa Heart Institute • Canada

Fox, Steven • Researcher • Agency for Healthcare Research and Quality • USA

Gabriel, Rafael • Director • Clinical Epidemiological Unit, Hospital "La Princesa" • Spain

Garfield, Frances • Researcher • Caro Research Institute • USA

Garnett, William • Professor of Pharmacy and Neurology • Virginia Commonwealth University • USA

George, Stephen • Deputy Director • The Regional Laboratory for Toxicology • England

Gerc, Vjekoslav • Medical Practitioner • Klinika za bolesti srca i reumatizam • Bosnia and Herzegovina

Glasgow, Russell • Senior Researcher • AMC Cancer Research Center • USA

Godding, Veronique • Medical Practitioner • University Clinic St-Luc • Belgium

Gomes, Marleide • Professor • Federal University of Rio de Janeiro • Brazil

Gourevitch, Marc • Associate Professor • Albert Einstein College of Medicine/Montefiore Medical Center • USA

Green, David • General Practitioner • South Africa

Haaga, David • Professor • Department of Psychology, American University • USA

Hanhoff, Nikola • Clinical Practitioner • Germany

Hays, Ron • Professor of Medicine • University of California at Los Angeles • USA

Henman, Martin • Centre for the Practice of Pharmacy, Trinity College • Ireland

Herborg, Hanne • Director, Research and Development • Pharmakon • Denmark

Hernan, Miguel • Associate Director • Program on Causal Inference, Harvard University • USA

Holland, Ross • Pharmacy Education Specialist • Independent Consultant • Australia

Horne, Rob • Director and Professor of Psychology in Health Care • Centre for Health Care Research, University of Brighton • England

Hotz, Stephen • University Research Fellow • University of Ottawa • Canada

Hyland, Michael • Professor • University of Plymouth • England

Jeffe, Donna • Assistant Professor of Medicine • Washington University School of Medicine • USA

Jordhoy, Marit • Clinical Practitioner • Norwegian University of Science and Technology • Norway

Joshi, Prashant • Director, Clinical Epidemiology Unit • Government Medical College • India

Kaptein, Ad A. • Head • Psychology Unit, Leiden University Medical Center (LUMC) • Netherlands

Karkashian, Christine • Dean • School of Psychology, Universidad latina • USA

Kennedy, Stephen • Project Manager • Helix Group • USA

Khan, Muhammad Amir • Chairman • Association for Social Development • Pakistan

Kidorf, Michael • Associate Professor • Johns Hopkins University School of Medicine • USA

Kihlstrom, Lucy • Institute for the Study of Healthcare Organizations and Transactions • USA

Kim, Jim Yong • Program Director • Program on Infectious Diseases and Social Change • Harvard Medical School • USA

Kjellgren, Karin • Assistant Professor • Institute of Nursing • Göteborg University • Sweden

Klesges, Robert • Executive Director • University of Memphis for Community Health • USA

Knobel, Hernando • Professor • Universidad Autonoma de Barcelona • Spain

Kos, Mitja • Chair, Social Pharmacy • Faculty of Pharmacy, University of Ljubljana • Slovenia

Lam, Tai Hing • Professor, Head of Department of Community Medicine and Behavioural Sciences • The University of Hong Kong • China

Lannon, Susan • Epilepsy Nurse Clinician • University of North Carolina at Chapel Hill • USA

Leandre, Fernet • Director • Zanmi Lazante Health Care • Haiti

Lebovits, Allen • Associate Professor • New York University Pain Management Center • USA

Leickly, Frederick • Clinical Professor of Pediatrics • James Whitcomb Riley Hospital for Children • USA

Leppik, Ilo • Director • MINCEP Epilepsy Care • USA

Leroyer, Christophe • Clinical Practitioner • Department of Chest Medicine • Hôpital de la Cavale Blanche • France

Linden, Michael • Professor • BfA-Rehabilitation Centre • Germany

Lindner, Helen • Associate Professor • School of Psychological Science, La Trobe University • Australia

Lorvick, Jennifer • University of California • USA

Malow, Robert • Professor and Director • AIDS Prevention Program, Florida International University • USA

Marquez Contreras, Emilio • Coordinator of the Compliance Group • Spanish Society of Hypertension • Spain

Mazumdar, Sati • Researcher • University of Pittsburgh • USA

Mazur, Lynnette • Professor • University of Texas • USA

McGann, Elizabeth • Chair • Department of Nursing, Quinnipiac University • USA

Meinardi, Harry • Prof. Emeritus • Department of Physiology, Leids University Medical Centre • Netherlands

Mitchell, Wendy • Professor, Neurology and Pediatrics • Keck School of Medicine, University of Southern California • USA

Morisky, Donald E. • Professor and Vice-Chair • Department of Community Health Sciences, University of California at Los Angeles School of Public Health • USA

Niggemann, Bodo • Professor • Pediatric Clinic, Humboldt University Children's Hospital • Germany

Nimmo, Christine • Director, Educational Resources • American Society of Health System Pharmacists • USA

Nuño, Roberto • Health Economist • Independent Consultant • Spain

Osman, Liesl • Senior Research Fellow • Chest Clinic Aberdeen Royal Infirmary • Scotland

Otero, Soraya • Mental Health Program Coordinator • Child and Adolescent Mental Health Centre • Spain

Penedo, Frank • Assistant Professor • Department of Psychology, Miami University • USA

Peveler, Robert • Head • Mental Health Group, Community Clinical Sciences Division, School of Medicine, University of Southampton • England

Pfaffenbach, Grace • Researcher • Campinas (UNICAMP) State University • Brazil

Polo, Friz • Professor • National University of Cordoba • Argentina

Preston, Kenzie • Acting Chief • Department of Health and Human Services • USA

Price, John • Professor • King's College Hospital • England

Pruitt, Sheri • Director of Behavioral Medicine • The Permanente Medical Group • USA

Rand, Cynthia • Associated Professor • Johns Hopkins University • USA

Reddy, K. Srinath • Professor of Cardiology • All India Institute of Medical Sciences • India

Reynolds, Nancy • Associate Professor • Ohio State University • USA

Roca, Bernardino • Medical Practitioner • Castellon General Hospital • Spain

Salas, Maribel • Senior Researcher • Caro Research Institute • USA

Salvador Carulla, Luis • Professor of Psychiatry and Psychological Medicine • University of Cadiz • Spain

Sanchez Gomez, Luis Maria • Senior Researcher • Clinical Epidemiology Unit • University Hospital "La Princesa" • Spain

Sanchez Sosa, Juan José • Professor • National University of Mexico • Mexico

Sayer, Quentin • Senior Clinical Nurse Specialist • Respiratory Medicine, Eastbourne Hospitals NHS Trust • England

Sbarbaro, John • Researcher and Clinical Practitioner • Department of Medicine, University of Colorado • USA

Schlundt, David • Associate Professor of Psychology • Vanderbilt University • USA

Schneiderman, Neil • Professor and Program Chair • Department of Psychology, Miami University • USA

Schroeder, Knut • MRC Training Fellow • Division of Primary Health Care, University of Bristol • England

Sclar, David • Director, Pharmacoeconomics and Pharmacoepidemiology Research Unit, Washington State University • USA

Shope, Jean • Senior Research Scientist • University of Michigan • USA

Singh, Meenu • Professor • Institute of Medical Education and Research • India

Skaer, Tracy • Assistant Dean and Associate Director, Pharmacoeconomics and Pharmacoepidemiology Research Unit, Washington State University • USA

Smirnoff, Margaret • Nurse Practitioner • Mount Sinai Center • USA

Sommaruga, Marinella • Clinical Psychologist • Salvatore Maugeri Foundation, Care and Research Institute • Italy

Sorensen, Jim • Adjunct Professor • Instruction and Research Department, San Francisco General Hospital • USA

Starace, Fabrizio • Director • Consultation Psychiatry and Behavioural Epidemiology Service, Cotugno Hospital • Italy

Starr, Mike • Clinical Practitioner and Researcher • Department of Microbiology, British Columbia Children's Hospital • Canada

Stephen, Crystal • Research Professor and Director • AIDS Research Group, Rutgers University • USA

Stewart, Simon • Ralph Reader Fellow • University of Adelaide • Australia

Stone, Valerie • Associate Chief • General Medicine Unit, Massachusetts General Hospital • USA

Sumartojo, Esther • Leader • Community Intervention Research Team, Centers for Diseases Control • USA

Svensson, Staffan • Researcher and Clinical Practitioner • Department of Clinical Pharmacology, Sahlgrenska University Hospital • Sweden

Tai-Seale, Ming • Professor • Department of Health Policy and Management, Texas AandM School of Rural Public Health • USA

Tazeen, Jafar • Assistant Professor • Aga Khan University • Pakistan

Tomaszewski, Maciej • Researcher • Blood Pressure Group • University of Glasgow • Scotland and in the Department of Internal Medicine, Diabetology and Nephrology of Zabrze • Poland

Tseng, Alice • Clinical Pharmacist • Immunodeficiency Clinic, Toronto General Hospital • Canada

Turner, Barbara • Professor of Medicine • University of Pennsylvania • USA

Urquhart, John • Professor • Department of Pharmacoepidemiology, Maastricht University • Netherlands

Vázquez-Barquero, José Luiz • Professor of Psychiatry and Director • Psychiatric Research Unit, University Hospital "Marqués de Valdecillas", Cantabria University • Spain

Volmink, Jimmy • Director of Research and Analysis • Global Health Council • USA

Wagner, Ed • Director • MacColl Institute for Healthcare Innovation • USA

Wagner, Glenn • Behavioral Scientist • RAND • USA

Wahl, Lindi • Professor • University of Western Ontario • Canada

Weingarten, Micky • Professor • Tel Aviv University • Israel

Weinstein, Andrew • Researcher and Clinical Practitioner • Christiana Medical Center • USA

Whitehouse, William • Researcher and Clinical Practitioner • Queen's Medical Centre • England

Willey, Cynthia • Professor of Pharmacoepidemiology • University of Rhode Island • USA

Williams, Ann • Nurse Researcher and Clinical Practitioner • Yale School of Nursing • USA

Williams, Mark • Associate Professor of Behavioral Sciences • The University of Texas • USA

Williams, Rhys • Professor of Clinical Epidemiology • University of Wales Swansea • Wales

Windsor, Richard • Professor and Chairman • The George Washington University Medical Center • USA

Zeppetella, John • Deputy Medical Director • St Joseph's Hospice • England

Zwarenstein, Merrick • Senior Researcher • Medical Research Council, Health Systems Division • South Africa

Professional, industry and patients' organizations

Acanfora, Miguel Angel • Board Member • Argentine Society of Gerontology and Geriatrics • Argentina

Alberti, George • President, International Diabetes Federation • Belgium

Ambler, Sue • Head of Practice Research • The Royal Pharmaceutical Society of Great Britain • London

Aung, May • Cardiac Society of Myanmar Medical Association • Myanmar

Avanzini, Giuliano • President • International League against Epilepsy • Italy

Bassand, Jean-Pierre • President • European Society of Cardiology • France

Bernard, Owen • Executive Director • Diabetes Association of Jamaica • Jamaica

Blennerhassett, Mitzi • Secretary • Cancer Action Now • England

Bunde-Birouste, Anne • Scientific and Technical Director/Director of Programmes International Union of Health Promotion and Education • France

Burell, Gunilla • President • International Society of Behavioural Medicine • Sweden

Callahan, James • Executive Vice-President and Chief Executive Officer • American Society of Addiction Medicine • USA

Camp, Rob • Executive Director • European AIDS Treatment Group • Netherlands

Cavalheiro, Esper • Secretary-General • International Bureau for Epilepsy • Brazil

Chan, Bill Piu • Director • Beijing Institute of Geriatrics • China

Chan, Juliana • Society for the Study of Endocrinology, Metabolism Diabetes Division, The Chinese University of Hong Kong • China

Charles, Renév • Haitian Foundation for Diabetes and Cardiovascular diseases (FHADIMAC) • Haïti

Chavez, Rafael • Mexican Society of Cardiology • Mexico

Chung, Wai-Sau • Honorary Secretary • Hong Kong College of Psychiatrists • China

Costa e Forti, Adriana • President • Brazilian Diabetes Society • Brazil

Covanis, Athanasios • Vice-President • International Bureau for Epilepsy • Greece

De Backer, Guy • Appointed Representative • Belgian Society of Cardiology • Belgium

de Boer, Hanneke M. • Global Campaign Co-Chair • The International Bureau for Epilepsy • The Netherlands

Delefosse, Santiago Marie • Vice-President • French Psychology Society • France

Diaz Alvarez, Ernesto • President • Dominican Society of Cardiology • Dominican Republic

Du Melle, Fran • Consultant on International Health • American Thoracic Society • USA

El-Guebaly, Nady • President • International Society of Addiction Medicine • Canada

Engel, Jerome Jr • Global Campaign Co-Chair • International League Against Epilepsy and Director of the University of California at Los Angeles (UCLA) Seizure Disorder Centre, UCLA School of Medicine • USA

Erkka, Susanna • President • European Federation of Asthma and Allergy Association (EFA) • Finland

Fejerman, Natalio • Secretary-General • International League Against Epilepsy • Argentina

Frew, Anthony • Secretary-General • European Academy of Allergology and Clinical Immunology • Belgium

Gaffney, Terri • Executive Director • American Academy of Nursing • USA

Ghebrehiwet, Tesfamicael • Consultant on Nursing and Health Policy • International Council of Nurses • Switzerland

Gjelsvik, Bjorn • Honorary Secretary • World Organization of Family Doctors (WONCA) (Europe) • Norway

Gradisek, Anton • Member and Past President • National Board of General Practitioners • Slovenia

Hackshaw, Joycelyn • Chief Executive Officer • Trinidad and Tobago Registered Nurses Association • Trinidad

Harumi, Kenichi • Vice-Chairman • Japan Heart Foundation • Japan

Harvey, Bale, Jr. • Director-General • International Federation of Pharmaceutical Manufacturers Associations (IFPMA) • Switzerland

Hayes, Angela • Chief Executive • International Alliance of Patients' Organizations (IAPO) • England

Heikki, Huikuri • Professor of Cardiology • Finnish Cardiac Society • Finland

Henne, Genie • Program Manager • Asthma Society of Ireland • Ireland

Hirst, Jenny • Co-Chairman • Insulin Dependent Diabetes Trust (IDDT) • England

Hoek, A.J.M. (Ton) • General Secretary • International Pharmaceutical Federation (FIP) • Netherlands

Horne, Rob • Director and Professor of Psychology in Health Care • Centre for Health Care Research, University of Brighton, and Boardman, Concordance Committee, Royal Pharmaceutical Society of Great Britain • England

Ilves, Pille • Chair • Estonian Patients Advocacy Association • Estonia

Kane-Williams, Edna • Vice-President, Programs and Research • Epilepsy Foundation of America • USA

Kielgast J. Peter • President • International Pharmaceutical Federation • The Netherlands

Kurashvili, Ramaz B. • President • Georgian Diabetes Federation • Diabetes Centre of Georgia • Georgia

Kwok, Ching-Fai • Secretary- General • Chinese Taipei Diabetes Association • China

Lahti, Pirkko • Executive Director • World Federation of Mental Health • Finland

Lee, Warren • Secretary • Diabetic Society of Singapore • Republic of Singapore

Lee, Philip • President • International Bureau for Epilepsy • Ireland

Lefebvre, Pierre • Elected President • International Diabetes Federation • Belgium

Maksoud, Mahmoud Abdel • President • Emro Pharm Forum and General Secretary • Syndicate of Pharmacists of Egypt • Egypt

Maekawa, Yutaka • Secretary • Japanese Circulation Society • Japan

Maheshwari, M.C. • Honorary Secretary • Neurological Society of India • India

Manickan, Sam • Founder and Honorary Director • Centre for Applied Psychological Studies • India

Mannign, Chris • Chair • Depression Alliance • England

McMahon, Stephen • Chairman • Irish Patients' Association • Ireland

Mendelson, Daniel • Program Director • Depression and Bipolar Support Alliance • USA

Migliori, Giovanni • Director • WHO Collaborating Centre for Control of Tuberculosis and Lung Diseases in Europe • Italy

Muggeo, Michele • Societa Italiana di Diabetologia • (Italian Diabetology Society) • Italy

Ng, Richard • President • Singapore Cardiac Society • Singapore

Nielson, Faamanatu • President • Samoa Nursing Association • Samoa

Ogola, N • Professor • Kenya Cardiac Society • Kenya

O'Sullivan, Tony • Founder • Patient Focus • Ireland

Paoletti, Rodolfo • President • Italian Heart Foundation • Italy

Pollard, Russell • Executive Officer • Epilepsy Australia • Australia

Poppa, Anna • Chief Editor • British HIV Association and Medical Society for Study of Venereal Disease Antiretroviral Adherence Guidelines 2002/3 • England

Ramaiya, Kaushik • General Secretary • Tanzania Diabetes Association • Tanzania

Reinstein, Jerome • Director- General • World Self-Medication Industry • England

Rodger, Ginette • Canadian Nurses Association • Canada

Rodolfo Paoletti • President • Italian Heart Foundation • Italy

Salas Sanchez, Rodrigo • President • Pharmaceutical Forum of the Americas • Costa Rica

Samad, Abdus • Secretary • Pakistan Cardiac Society • Pakistan

Santoso, Karo Karo • President • Indonesian Heart Association • Indonesia

Schulz, Martin • Head • Centre for Drug Information and Pharmacy Practice, Federal Union of German Associations of Pharmacists • Germany

Senten, Marina • Head, Department of Patient Care • Netherlands Heart Foundation • Netherlands

Shields, Chuck • Executive Director • Canadian Cardiovascular Society • Canada

Silvado, Carlos • President • Brazilian Academy of Neurology • Brazil

Snoj, Joze • Chief Editor • Slovenian Diabetes Association (SLODA) • Slovenia

Spicak, Vaclav • Director • Czech Initiative for Asthma • Czech Republic

Stauder, Adrienne • Coordinator • Institute of Behavioural Sciences, Semmelweis University • Hungary

Tainio, Satu • Project Coordinator • International Pharmaceutical Federation (FIP) • Netherlands

Temel, Yilmaz M • President • Turkish Diabetes Foundation • Turkey

Torongo, Mabel • Secretary-General • Pharmaceutical Society of Zimbabwe • Zimbabwe

Ulrich, Susan • Executive Director • American College of Clinical Pharmacology • USA

Webber, D.E. • Director-General (elected) • World Self-Medication Industry • France

Williams, Simon • Director of Policy • The Patients Association • England

Wilson, Elinor • President • Heart and Stroke Foundation of Canada • Canada

Woodend, Kirsten • Director of Research • The Canadian Pharmacists Association • Canada

Woods, Lynda • General Director • South African Depression and Anxiety Support Group • South Africa

Yiangou • Chairman • Cyprus Diabetic Association • Cyprus

Yilmaz M, Temel • President •Turkish Diabetes Foundation • Turkey

Zhang, Wen Fan • Professor and President • Gerontological Society of China • China

Policy-makers

Ala Din Abdul Sahib, Alwan • WHO Country Representative • Jordan

Asiama, Divine • Programme Manager • Ghana National Drugs Programme, Ministry of Health • Ghana

Beaglehole, Bonita Ruth • Director • Surveillance • WHO-HQ

Bengoa, Rafael • Director Management of Noncommunicable Diseases • WHO-HQ

Bertolote, Jose Manoel • Coordinator • Mental and Behavioural Disorders • WHO-HQ

Bloem, Paul • Technical Officer • Child and Adolescent Health and Development • WHO-HQ

Canny, Judith • Technical Officer • Health Care for Chronic Conditions • WHO-HQ

Casey, Kathleen • Scientist • HIV Care • WHO-HQ

Corte, Georgina • Medical Officer • Ageing and Life Course • WHO-HQ

Da Costa E Silva, Vera • Director • Tobacco Free Initiative • WHO-HQ

De Castro, Silvana • Technical Officer • Adherence Project • WHO-HQ

Edejer-Tan Torres, Tessa • Coordinator • Choosing Interventions: Effectiveness, Quality and Costs • WHO-HQ

Epping-Jordan, JoAnne • Coordinator • Health Care for Chronic Conditions • WHO-HQ

Fahey, Michael • Adviser • Department of Drug Control • Ministry of Health • United Arab Emirates

Francesca, Celletti • Medical Officer • Cardiovascular Diseases • WHO-HQ

Gatti, Anna • Medical Officer • Ageing and Life Course • WHO-HQ

Gojka, Roglic • Technical Officer • Diabetes • WHO-HQ

Gustafsen, Ida • Manager • EuroPharmForum • Netherlands

Herrera, Natasha • Scientist • Tobacco Free Initiative • Venezuela

Jaramillo, Ernesto • Medical Officer • Stop TB • WHO-HQ

Jones, Jack • Technical Officer • Health Promotion and Prevention • WHO-HQ

Kalache, Alexandre • Coordinator • Ageing and Life Course • WHO-HQ

Kawar, Rania • Technical Officer • Management of Noncommunicable Conditions • WHO-HQ

Khaltaev, Nikolai • Team Leader • Chronic Respiratory Diseases • WHO-HQ

King, Hillary • Team Leader • Diabetes • WHO-HQ

Leonardi, Matilde • Medical Officer • Classification, Assessment, Surveys and Terminology • WHO-HQ

Lopez Acuña, Daniel • Coordinator • Health Systems • WHO-PAHO

McGill, Scott • Technical Officer • HIV Care • WHO-HQ

Macklai, Nejma • Scientist • Tobacco Free Initiative • WHO-HQ

Maher, Dermot • Medical Officer • Stop TB • WHO-HQ

Maringo, Charles • Regional Adviser Noncommunicable Diseases • WHO-AFRO

Meiners, Micheline Marie • Technical Officer • Pharmaceutical Forum of The Americas • USA

Mendis, Shanthi • Coordinator • Cardiovascular Diseases • WHO-HQ

Mesquita, Fabio • Director of the STD/AIDS Program • The City of São Paulo Public Health Department • Brazil

Monteiro, Maristela G. Coordinator • Management of Substance Dependence • WHO-HQ

O'Dell, Virginia • Medical Officer • HIV care • WHO-HQ

Peruga, Armando • Regional Adviser on Tobacco, Alcohol and Drugs • WHO-PAHO

Prilipko, Leonid L. • Coordinator • Epilepsy • WHO-HQ

Puska, Pekka • Director • Health Promotion and Prevention • WHO-HQ

Rai, Kumara • Acting Director • Department of Health Systems and Community Health • WHO-SEARO

Ramaboot, Sawat • Acting Regional Adviser on Noncommunicable Diseases • WHO-SEARO

Robles, Sylvia • Coordinator • Noncommunicable Diseases • WHO-PAHO

Ron, A. • Director • Health Systems Development • WHO-WPRO

Rovira, Joan • Senior Economist • World Bank, Health, Population and Nutrition Division/ Pharmaceutical Unit • Washington, DC

Ottmani, Salah • Medical Officer • Stop TB • WHO-HQ

Sabaté, Eduardo • Medical Officer • Adherence Project • WHO-HQ

Saraceno, Benedetto • Director • Mental Health and Substance Dependence • WHO-HQ

Saxena, Shekhar • Coordinator • Mental Health: Evidence and Research • WHO-HQ

Sepulveda, Cecilia • Coordinator • Cancer Control Programme • WHO-HQ

Shatchkute, Aushra • Regional Adviser Chronic Disease Prevention • WHO-Europe

Uplekar, Mukund • Stop TB • WHO-HQ

Vareldzis, Basil • Medical Officer HIV Care • WHO-HQ

Yach, Derek • Executive Director • Noncommunicable Diseases and Mental Health • WHO-HQ

Access to...

Where to find a copy of this book

DEPOSITARIES

Officially designated depository libraries for WHO publications

ALBANIA (the Republic of) • Biblioteka Kombetare (Bibliotheque Nationale) • Tirana

ALGERIA (The People's Democratic Republic of) • Bibliothèque Nationale d'Algérie • Hamma, El Annassers. Alger, BP 127

ANGOLA (the Republic of) • Biblioteca da Faculdade de Medicina, Universidade de Angola (the Republic of) • Luanda

ARGENTINA • Centro de Documentacion Internacional, Ministerio de Cultura y Educacion, Direccion General de Cooperacion Internacional • Aguero 2.502, 3a Piso. Buenos Aires CF, 1425

AUSTRIA (the Republic of) • Zentralbibliothek für Medizin in Wien Zeitschriftenabteilung • Währinger Gürtel 18-20. Wien A-1097

BAHAMAS (the Commonwealth of the) • Hilda Bowen Library, The College of the Bahamas (the Commonwealth of the) • Grosvenor Close Campus, P.O. BOX N4912. Nassau

BAHRAIN (the State of) • Ahmed Al-Farsi Library • Ministry of Health, PO Box 12. Manama

BANGLADESH • Library, Bangabandhu Sheikh Mujib Medical University • Shahbag, 1000. Dhaka

BELGIUM (the Kingdom of) • Bibliothèque Royale de Belgique, Section Collections Officielles • Boulevard de l'Empereur 4, B-1000. Bruxelles

BELIZE • WHO Programme Coordination, PAHO/WHO Documentation Center • P.O. Box 430, 93 Freetown Road. Belize City

BENIN (the Republic of) • Bibliotheque D'administration Generale, Direction de la Fonction Publique • Porto-Novo

BUTHAN (the Kingdom of) • Library Royal Institute of Health Sciences • PO Box 298. Thimphu

BOTSWANA (the Republic of) • Botswana (the Republic of) National Library Service, Ministry Of Labour And Home Affairs • Private Bag 0036 • Gaborone

MARIANA ISLANDS • Commonwealth Health Centre, Department Of Public Health and Environmental Services • Po Box 409 Ck. Saipan, 96950

BRAZIL (the Federative Republic of) • Biblioteca Nacional, Setor de Intercambio • Avenida Rio Branco 219/39. Rio de Janeiro RJ, 20.040-008

BRUNEI DARUSSALAM • Medical Library, Ripas Hospital, Ministry of Health • Bandar Seri Begawan Negara 2062. Darussalam

BURKINA FASO • Bibliothèque, Ecole Nationale de Santé Publique (ENSP) • 03 BP 7047. Ouagadougou, 03

CANADA • Official Publications Section, The Library of Parliament • Ottawa (Ontario), K1A 0A9

CENTRAL AFRICAN REP • Bibliotheque Faculte des Sciences de la Sante • B. P. 1383. Bangui

CHILE (the Republic of) • Seccion Organismos Internacionales, Biblioteca Nacional de Chile • Clasifirador. Santiago 1400

CHINA (the People's Republic of) • National Library of China, Section of publications of international organizations and foreign governments • 39 Baishiqiao Road. Beijing 100081

COLOMBIA (the Republic of) • Grupo de Selección y Adquisiciones, Servicio de Canje, Biblioteca Nacional de Colombia • Calle 24 5-60, Apartado Aereo 27600. Santafé de Bogota DC

CONGO (the Republic of) • Institut Superieur des Sciences de la Sante • Universite Marien Ngouabi • B.P. 2672. Brazzaville

COOK ISLANDS • Library, Department of Health • P.O. Box 109. Rarotonga

COTE D'IVOIRE • Bibliothèque, Faculté de Médecine, Université d'Abidjan • BP V-166. Abidjan

CROATIA (the Republic of) • Biblioteka, Skola Narodnog Zdravlja Andrija Stampar, University of Zagreb • Rockefellerova 4,Post. Pret. 770. Zagreb, 10000

CUBA (the Republic of) • Biblioteca Nacional Jose Marti • Plaza de la Revolucion. Ave Independ. E/ Aranguren Y, 20 Mayo. Habana, 10600

CYPRUS (the Republic of) • Cyprus Library • Eleftherias Square. Nicosia, 1011

CZECH REPUBLIC • Library, Statni Zdravotni Ustav • Srobarova 48. Praha 10, 10042

DEMOCRATIC PEOPLE'S REPUBLIC OF KOREA • Library, The Grand People's Study House of DPRK • PO Box 200. Central Pyongyang

DEMOCRATIC REPUBLIC OF CONGO • Bibliotheque Nationale De Kinshasa • B.P. 3090, Ave Colonel Tsatsi No 10, Kinshasa 1, Gombe. Kinshasa

DENMARK (the Kingdom of) • Statsbiblioteket Tidsskriftafdelingen (The State and University Library) • Universitetsparken, DK-8000. Aarhus C

EGYPT (the Arab Republic of) • Egyptian National Library, UN Depository Library • Corniche el Nil. Ramlet Boulak. Cairo

EL SALVADOR (the Republic of) • Biblioteca Nacional • San Salvador

ESTONIA (the Republic of) • National Library of Estonia • Tonismagi 2. Tallinn, EE-0100

FIJI (the Republic of) • Central Medical Research Library, Fiji (the Republic of) School of Medicine • Suva

FRANCE (the French Republic) • Bibliothèque nationale de France, GCA Périodiques Magasin • Quai François Mauriac. Paris F-75706 Cedex 13

FRENCH GUIANA • Bibliothèque hospitalo-universitaire, Centre hospitalier général de Cayenne • Rue des Flamboyants, BP 6006. Cayenne, 97306

GERMANY (the Federal Republic of) • Staatsbibliothek zu Berlin, Preussischer Kulturbesitz, Abteilung Amtsdruckschriften und Internationaler • Amtlicher Schriftentausch • Potsdamer Str. 33. Berlin, D-10785

GERMANY (the Federal Republic of) • UN Depository Library, DL-202, Max-Planck-Institut für Auslaendisches, Offentliches Recht und Voelkerrecht • Im Neuenheimer Feld 535. Heidelberg, D-69120

GHANA (the Republic of) • Ghana Medical School, University of Ghana • PO Box 4236. Accra

GREECE (the Hellenic Republic of) • National Library of Greece • 32 Panepistimiou St., 106 79 Athinai

GUADELOUPE • Bibliothèque hospitalo-universitaire, Centre hospitalier universitaire de Pointe à Pitre • Route de Chauvel. Pointe à Pitre Cedex, 97159

GUAM • Robert F. Kennedy Memorial Library, University of Guam • 303 University Drive, UOG Station. Mangilao, GU 96923

GUATEMALA (the Republic of) • Biblioteca Nacional de Guatemala. Guatemala

GUYANA • Library, University of Guyana, Turkey en Campus • Box 10-1110. Georgetown

HAITI (the Republic of) • Bibliothèque nationale • 193 Rue du Centre. Port-au-Prince

HONDURAS (the Republic of) • Biblioteca Nacional • Tegucigalpa

HONG KONG • Yu Chun Keung Medical Library, University of Hong Kong • 21 Sassoon Road, Pokfulam. Hong Kong

ICELAND (the Republic of) • Landsbokasafn Islands, Haskolabokasafn (The National and University Library of Iceland) • Arngrimsgotu 3. Reykjavik, Is-107

INDIA (the Republic of) • National Science Library • Indian National Scientific Documentation Centre • 14 Satsang Vihar Marg. New Delhi,110067

INDONESIA (the Republic of) • Perpustakaan Nasional Republik Indonesia • Jalan Salemba Raya 28 A . Jakarta, 3624

IRAN (the Islamic Republic of) • Library • Medical Sciences University of Teheran • Inghelab Ave. Teheran

IRELAND • National Library Of Ireland • Kildare Street. Dublin

ISRAEL (the State of) • Jewish National and University Library • PO Box 503. Jerusalem, 91999

ITALY (The Italian Republic) • Biblioteca Nazionale Centrale Vittorio Emanuele • Via de Castro Pretorio 105. Roma, I-00185

JAMAICA • Medical Library, University of the West Indies • PO Box 107. Kingston 7

JAPAN • International Documentation Center, General Library, The University of Tokyo • Hongo 7-3-1, Bunkyo-Ku. Tokyo, 113-0033

JORDAN (the Hashemite Kingdom of) • Library, Serials Department, The University of Jordan • Amman

KENYA (the Republic of) • Medical Library, University of Nairobi • PO Box 30197. Nairobi

KIRIBATI • The National Library, Kiribati • Bairiki. Tarawa

LAO PEOPLE'S DEMOCRATIC REPUBLIC • Bibliothèque, Université des Sciences Médicales • Vientiane, BP 131

LIBERIA (the Republic of) • Library, A.M. Dogliotti College of Medicine, University of Liberia • PO Box 9020. Monrovia

LITHUANIA (the Republic of) • Lithuanian Library of Medicine, Lietuvos Medicinos Biblioteka • Kastonu 7. Vilnius, 2600

LUXEMBOURG (the Grand Duchy of) • Bibliothèque Nationale de Luxembourg • 37 Boulevard F.-D. Roosevelt. Luxembourg, L-2450

MALAYSIA • Library, Public Health Institute (Institut Kesihatan Umum) • Jalan Bangsar. Kuala Lumpur, 50590

MALDIVES (the Republic of) • The Library, Institute of Health Sciences. Malé

MALTA (the Republic of) • Bibliothèque, Institut National de Recherche en Santé Publique • Bamako, BP 1771

MALI (the Republic of) • The Library, School of Medicine • Guardamangia

MARIANA ISLANDS • Commonwealth Health Centre, Department of Public Health and Environmental Services • Po Box 409 Ck . Saipan, 96950

MARTINIQUE • Bibliothèque hospitalo-universitaire, Centre hospitalier de Fort de France • BP 632/La Meynard. Fort de France Cedex, 97271

MAURITANIA (the Islamic Republic of) • Bibliothèque des Sciences de la Santé, Institut National des Spécialités Médicales • Nouakchott, BP 309

MAURITIUS (the Republic of) • Library, Mauritius Institute of Health • Powder Mill. Pamplemousses

MEXICO (The United Mexican States) • Hemeroteca Nacional, Centro Cultural Ciudad Universitaria • Delegacion Coyoacan. Mexico DF, 04510

MONGOLIA • Central Medical Research Library, Ministry of Health and Social Welfare • Enkhtaiwan St. • Post Office 48, Box 1. Ulaanbaatar

MOROCCO (the Kingdom of) • Centre de Documentation en Santé (CDS), Institut national d'Administration sanitaire (INAS), Rabat-Instituts • Rabat, BP 6329

MOZAMBIQUE (the Republic of) • Centro de Documentacao, Instituto Nacional de Saude Ministerio da Saude • Maputo, CP 264

NAURU (the Republic of) • Nauru General Hospital • Nauru

NETHERLANDS (the Kingdom of) • UB Randwijck, Verwerking • Universiteit Bibliotheek, Rijksuniversiteit Limburg • PO Box 616. Maastricht, NL-6200 MD

NEW CALEDONIA • Bibliothèque, Direction territoriale des Affaires sanitaires et sociales • BP 3278. Noumea Cedex, 98846

NEW ZEALAND • Parliamentary Librarian • Parliament Buildings, Wellington 1

NICARAGUA (the Republic of) • Biblioteca Nacional Ruben Dario • Apartado Postal 101. Managua

NIGERIA (the Federal Republic of) • National Library of Nigeria • P.M.B. 12626, 4, Wesley Street . Lagos State

NIUE (the Republic of) • Department for Community Affairs • Community Affairs • Alofi

NORWAY (the Kingdom of) • Norwegian Directorate for Health and Social Welfare (NDHS), WHO Documentation Centre • PO Box 8054 Dep. Oslo, N-0031

OMAN (The Sultanate of) • The Medical Library, Sultan Qaboos University • PO Box 35. Al-Khod, 123

PANAMA (the Republic of) • Biblioteca Nacional de Panama • Parque Recreativo y Cultural Omar, Via Porras, San Francisco, Apartado Postal 7906. Panama, Zona 9

PAPUA NEW GUINEA (the Republic of) • Medical Library, University of Papua New Guinea • PO Box 5623. Boroko

PERU (the Republic of) • Departamento de Publicaciones Oficiales, Biblioteca Nacional • Apartado 2335. Lima

POLAND (the Republic of) • Bibliothèque, Panstwowy Zaklad Higieny • Ul. Chocimska 24 • PL-00-791. Warszawa

PORTUGAL (The Portuguese Tepublic) • Biblioteca Nacional, Servico Portugues De Trocas Internacionais • Campo Grande 83. Lisboa, P-1751

PUERTO RICO • Library Medical Sciences Campus, University of Puerto Rico • GPO Box 365067. San Juan, 00936-5067

QATAR (the State of) • Medical Library, Hamad General Hospital • PO Box 3050. Doha

REPUBLIC OF KOREA • Medical Library, College of Medicine, Seoul National University • 28 Yeon Keun Dong, Chongro Ku. Seoul

ROMANIA • Computer, Sanitary Statistics and Medical Documentation Center • Str. Pitar Mos 7-15. Bucuresti 1, R-70151

RWANDA (THE RWANDESE REPULIC) • Bibliothèque, Faculté de Medecine, Université Nationale du Rwanda (the Rwandese Repulic) • Butare, BP 30

SAMOA (the Independate State of) • Library Health Department • Moto'Otua. Apia

SAUDI ARABIA (the Kingdom of) • Library, Ministry of Planning • PO Box 358. Riyad, 11182

SENEGAL (the Republic of) • Bibliothèque Centrale, Section Médecine et Pharmacie, Université Cheikh Anta Diop • Dakar Fann, BP 2006

SEYCHELLES (the Republic of) • Medical Library, Ministry of Health • Botanical Gardens, PO Box 52. Victoria

SIERRA LEONE (the Republic of) • Fourah Bay College Library, University of Sierra Leone • Freetown

SLOVAKIA (The Slovak Republic) • Slovak Medical Library • Lazaretska 26. Bratislava, 814 42

SLOVENIA (the Republic of) • Dokumentacijski Center SZO, Instiut za Varovanje Zdravja RS • Trubarjeva 2. Ljubljana, 61000

SOLOMON ISLANDS • Library, Solomon Islands Health Training and Research Centre • c/o Ministry of Health and Medical Services. PO Box 349. Honiara

SOUTH AFRICA • National Library of South Africa, Foreign Official Publication Section • PO Box 397. Pretoria, 0001

SRI LANKA (The Democratic Socialist Republic of) • Medical Library, Faculty of Medicine, University of Colombo • Kynsey Road. PO Box 271. Colombo 08

SUDAN (the Republic of THE) • The Library, Faculty of Medicine, University of Khartoum • PO Box 102. Khartoum

SWAZILAND (the Kingdom of) • Swaziland National Library Service • c/o WHO Representative. PO Box 903. Mbabane

SWEDEN (the Kingdom of) • Library, Karolinska Institutet University • Nobels Väg 8. Solna

SYRIAN ARAB REPUBLIC • Bibliothèque Médicale, Université Syrienne • Damascus

TOGO (the Togolese Republic) • National Library • Samsen Road. Bangkok 11000 •

THAILAND (the Kingdom of) • Institut Togolais Des Sciences, Humaines et de La Bibliotheque Nationale • Boite Postale 1002. Lome

Trinidad and Tobago (the Republic of) • Medical Library, General Hospital • Port-of-Spain

TURKEY (the Republic of) • Kütüphane ve Dokumentasyon Dairesi, Ankara Üniversitesi • Ankara Tandogan. Ankara, TR-06100

UGANDA (the Republic of) • Albert Cook Library, Medical School, Makerere University • PO Box 7072. Kampala

UKRAINE • Vernadsky National Library of Ukraine • Prospekt 40-richja Zhovtnja, 3. Kiev, 03039

UNITED ARAB EMIRATES • Dubai Public Library • PO Box 67. Dubai

UNITED REP. TANZANIA (The United republic of) • College Library, Muhimbili University College of Health Sciences • PO Box 65012. Dar es Salaam

UNITED STATES of AMERICA • The Library of Congress, European and Latin American Acquisitions Division, Northern European Acquisitions Section • Attn: Exchange. 101 Independence Ave SE. Washington, DC 20540-4183

UZBEKISTAN (the Republic of) • State Scientific Medical Library, Ministry of Health • Akhunbabaeva 30. M/Box 4820. Tashkent, 700015

VENEZUELA (The Bolivarian Republic of) • Biblioteca Nacional, Division de Canje y Donaciones • Final Avda. Panteon, Foro Libertador, San Jose. Caracas, 1010

VIET NAM (the Socialist republic of) • National Library, International Exchange Service • 31, Trang Thi. Ha Noi, 10000

YUGOSLAVIA • Narodna Biblioteka • Skerliceva I. Beograd, YU-11000

LIBRARIES

Reference libraries for WHO publications

These libraries figure among the regular recipients of a comprehensive collection of WHO books, series and/or periodicals. They have agreed to offer unrestricted access to their premises to all readers interested in WHO publications.

ALBANIA (the Republic of) • Library, University of TIran (the Islamic Republic of)a (Univ.Shteteror), Faculty of Medicine (Fakulteti I Mjekesise). Tirana

ALGERIA (the People's Democratic Republic of) • Bibliothèque, Institut National d'Enseignement Supérieur en Sciences Médicales, Université d'Alger • 18 Av. Pasteur , BP 542 ALGER GARE. Alger

ALGERIA (the People's Democratic Republic of) • Bibliothèque, Institut National de Santé Publique Al-Madania • 4, Chemin El-Bakr-El-Biar. Alger

ALGERIA (the People's Democratic Republic of) Bibliothèque • Institut National d'Enseignement Supérieur en Sciences Médicales • BP 205. Annaba, 23000

ALGERIA (the People's Democratic Republic of) • Bibliothèque, Unité de Recherches en Sciences Médicales, Institut des Sciences Médicales, Faculté de Médecine • BP 125. Constantine, 25000

ALGERIA (the People's Democratic Republic of) • Bibliothèque, Institut National d'Enseignement Supérieur en Biologie • Route Bel-Hacel, BP 114. Mostaganem, 27000

ALGERIA (the People's Democratic Republic of) • Bibliothèque, Institut National d'Enseignement Supérieur en Sciences Médicales • El Menaouer, BP 1510. Oran, 31000

ALGERIA (the People's Democratic Republic of) • Bibliothèque, Institut Supérieur en Sciences Médicales, Université de Setif • Setif

ANTIGUA BARBUDA • Library, Antigua School of Medicine, University of Health Sciences • Po Box 510 . St John's

ARGENTINA • Biblioteca Central, Facultad de Medicina. Universidad de Buenos Aires • Paraguay 2155, Piso 4, 1121 Buenos Aires CF

ARGENTINA • Biblioteca, Facultad de Medicina, Universidad de El Salvador • Tucuman 1845, 2 Piso. 1050 Buenos Aires CF

ARGENTINA • Biblioteca, Instituto Nacional de Enfermedades Parasitarias "Dr Mario Fatala Chabén" • Paseo Colon 568, 6to Piso. Buenos Aires CF, 1063

ARGENTINA • Biblioteca, Facultad de Ciencias Medicas, Universidad Nacional de Cordoba (Ciudad Universitaria) • Agencia Postal No 4, Cordoba CBA, 5000

ARGENTINA Biblioteca, Facultad de Medicina, Universidad Nacional del Nordeste • Moreno 1240. Corrientes CTS, 3400

ARGENTINA • Biblioteca Islas Maluinas, Facultad de Ciencias Medicas, Universidad Nacional de la Plata • Calle 60 Y 120. La Plata BA, 1900

ARGENTINA • Biblioteca Nacional Felicinda Barrionuevo, Facultad de Ciencias Médicas, Universidad Nacional de Cuyo • Parque General San Martin, CC 33. 5500 Mendoza

ARGENTINA -Centro de Informacion Biomedica del Chaco (CIBCHACO), Ministerio de Salud Publica • Marcelo T. De Alvear 20, 2 Piso. Resistencia CHO, 3500

ARGENTINA • Biblioteca, Universidad Nacional de Rio Cuarto • Enlace Rutas 8 y 36, Km 603. Rio Cuarto CBA, 5800

ARGENTINA • Biblioteca, Facultad de Ciencias Medicas, Universidad Nacional de Rosario • Cordoba 3160. Rosario SF, 2000

ARGENTINA • Centro de Informacion y Documentacion Cientifica (CIDOC), Universidad Nacional de Rosario • Moreno 750. Rosario SF, 2000

ARGENTINA • Biblioteca, Facultad de Medicina, Universidad Nacional de Tucuman • Lamadrid 875 • C.C. 159. 4000 San Miguel De Tucuman

AUSTRALIA • United Nations Information Center • 46-48 York Street, 5th Floor, GPO Box 4045. Sydney NSW, 2001

AUSTRIA (the Republic of) • Bibliothek and Dokumentation, Osterreichisches Bundesinstitut Fuer, Gesundheitswesen • Stubenring 6. Wien, A-1010

BANGLADESH • The Library, Chittagong Medical College • K.B. Fazlul Kader Road. Chittagong 4000

BANGLADESH • National Medical Library and Documentation Centre, Institute of Public Health Premises Mohakhali • Dhaka 12

BANGLADESH • The Library, Sir Salimullah Medical College • Dhaka, Mitford Road. Dhaka, 1100

BANGLADESH • Library, People's Health Centre (Gonoshasthaya Kendra) • Nayarhat Head Office. Dhaka, 1344

BANGLADESH • The Library, Mymensingh Medical College • Mymensingh, 2200

BANGLADESH • The Library, Rangpur Medical College • Rangpur, 5400

BARBADOS • Library, Faculty of Health Sciences, University of the West Indies, Queen Elizabeth Hospital • Martindales Road. St Michael

BELARUS (the Republic of) • Medical Library, Minsk Medical Institute • 83 Dzerzinksky Prospect. Minsk, 220116

BENIN (the Republic of) • Centre de Documentation, Faculté des Sciences de la Santé, Université nationale du Bénin • Cotonou, BP 188

BOLIVIA (the Republic of) • Biblioteca, Facultad de Ciencias de la Salud, Universidad Mayor de San Andrés • Avenida Saavedra 2246, Casilla 12148. La Paz

BOLIVIA (the Republic of) • Biblioteca, Universidad Nur • Av. Cristo Redentor Nro. 100, Casilla 3273. Santa Cruz de la Sierra

BRAZIL (the Federative Republic of) • Biblioteca Central "Prof. Jose Aloiso de Campos", Universidade Federal de Sergipe Cidade Universitaria • Caixa Postal 353. Aracaju SE, 49100

BRAZIL (the Federative Republic of) • Biblioteca "José Bonifácio Lafayette de Andrada", Faculdade de Medicina de Barbacena da Fundaçao • Praca Antonio Carlos No.8, Caixa Postal 45. Barbacena MG, 36200-970

BRAZIL (the Federative Republic of) • Biblioteca, Faculdade de Medicina, Universidade Federal de Minas Gerais • Avenida Alfredo Balena 190. Belo Horizonte MG, 30130-100

BRAZIL (the Federative Republic of) • Biblioteca, Faculdade de Ciencias Medicas, Universidade Sao Francisco (Campus de Braganca Paulista) • Av. Sao Francisco de Assis, 218. Braganca Paulista SP, 12.916-00

BRAZIL (the Federative Republic of) • Nucleo de Medicina Tropical, Faculdade de Ciências da Saude, Universidade de Brasilia • 70910 Brasilia DF

BRAZIL (the Federative Republic of) • Biblioteca, Faculdade de Ciencias Medicas, Univ. Estadual de Campinas • Hospital de Clinicas-Bloco F2-Sal.15, Cidade Univ., Caixa Postal 6111. Campinas SP, 13081

BRAZIL (the Federative Republic of) • Biblioteca Central, Universidad Federal de Mato Grosso do Sul • Cidade Universitaria , Caixa Postal 649. Campo Grande MT, 79070-900

BRAZIL (the Federative Republic of) • Biblioteca, Faculdade de Medicina de Campos, Fundacao Benedito Pereira Nunes • Rua Alberto Torres 217. Campos RJ, 28100

BRAZIL (the Federative Republic of) • Biblioteca, Faculdade de Medicina, Universidade de Caxias do sul Bairro Petropolis • Rua F.G. Vargas 1130, C.P. 1352. Caxias Do Sul RS, 95001

BRAZIL (the Federative Republic of) • Biblioteca Central, Divisao de Documentacao / Intercambio, Hospital Universitario Julio Muller, Universidade Federal de Mato Grosso • Rua L, s/n, Bairro Jardim Alvorada. Cuiaba MT, 78048-790

BRAZIL (the Federative Republic of) • Biblioteca, Faculdade Evangelica de Medicina do Parana • Alameda Princesa Isabel 1580. Curitiba PR, 80000

BRAZIL (the Federative Republic of) • Biblioteca Central, Centro de Ciencias Biologicas e da Saude Pontificia, Universidade Catolica do Parana • Rua Imaculada Conceicao 1155, Prado Velho, Caixa Postal 16.210. Curitiba PR, 80215-901

BRAZIL (the Federative Republic of) • Biblioteca Universitaria, Setor de Intercambio, Universidade Federal de Santa Catarina • Caixa Postal 476. Florianopolis SC, 88010-970

BRAZIL (the Federative Republic of) • Biblioteca Setorial de Ciencias de Saude, Universidade Federal do Ceara Porangabucu • Rua Alex. Barauna 1019, C. P. 688. Fortaleza CE, 60430-160

BRAZIL (the Federative Republic of) • Biblioteca, Faculdade de Medicina, Universidade Federal de Juiz de Fora • Rua Catulo Breviglieri s/n. Juiz De Fora MG, 36035

BRAZIL (the Federative Republic of) • Biblioteca, Faculdade de Medicina de Jundiai • Rua Francisco Telles 250, C.P. 1295. Jundiai SP, 13200

BRAZIL (the Federative Republic of) • Biblioteca Central/DFDC/Seçao de Doaçao, Universidade Estadual de Londrina, Campus Universitario • Caixa Postal 6001. Londrina PR, 86051-990

BRAZIL (the Federative Republic of) • Biblioteca, Escola de Ciencias Medicas de Alagoas, Fundacao Governador Lamenha Fil'Ho • Av. Siqueira Campos 2095. Maceio AL, 57000

BRAZIL (the Federative Republic of) • Biblioteca Setorial, Faculdade de Ciencias da Saude, Fundacao Universidade do Amazonas • Av. W. Pedrosa s/n Esq.Com. Apurina. Manaus AM, 69025

BRAZIL (the Federative Republic of) • Biblioteca, Faculdade de Medicina de Marilia • Av. Monte Carmelo, 800 • CP 2003. Marilia SP, 17519-030

BRAZIL (the Federative Republic of) • Biblioteca Central, Universidade de Mogidas Cruzes • C.X. de Almeida Souza, 200, APDO 411. Mogi Das Cruzes SP, 08700

BRAZIL (the Federative Republic of) • Biblioteca Hermes de Paula, Faculdade de Medicina, Universidade Estadual de Montes Claros (Unimontes) • Av. Dr Ruy Braga s/n, APDO 19 . Montes Claros MG, 39400

BRAZIL (the Federative Republic of) • Nucleo de Documentacao, Seçao de Aquisicao de Periodicos, Universidade Federal Fluminense • Ag.Sao Francisco, CP 107.001. Niteroi RJ, 24250

BRAZIL (the Federative Republic of) • Biblioteca, Faculdade de Ciencias Medicas de Nova Iguacu, Soc.de Ensino Sup. de Nova Iguacu • Av. Abilio Augusto Tavora 2134. Nova Iguacu RJ, 26000

BRAZIL (the Federative Republic of) • Biblioteca de Ciencias Biomedicas, Faculdade de Medicina, Universidade de Passo Fundo • Campus, Bairro Jose. Passo Fundo RS, 99050

BRAZIL (the Federative Republic of) • Biblioteca, Centro de Ciencias da Saude e Biologicas Universidade, Catolica de Pelotas • Rua Goncalves Chaves 373. Pelotas RS 96100

BRAZIL (the Federative Republic of) • Biblioteca Charles Alfred Esberard, Faculdade de Medicina de Petropolis, Fundaçao Octacílo Gualberto • Rua Machado Fagundes 326, Cascatinha. Petropolis RJ, 25716-970

BRAZIL (the Federative Republic of) • Biblioteca, Escola de Saude Publica • Avenida Ipiranga 6311, Partenon Porto Alegre RS. 90610-001

BRAZIL (the Federative Republic of) • Biblioteca Setorial, Instituto de Biociencias, Universidade Federal do Rio Grande do Sul • Sarmento Leite, s/no. Porto Alegre RS, 90049

BRAZIL (the Federative Republic of) • Biblioteca da Faculdade de Medecina, Universidad Federal do Rio Grande do Sul • Rua Ramiro Barcelos 2400, 3° andar. Porto Alegre RS, 90035-003

BRAZIL (the Federative Republic of) • Biblioteca, Faculdade de Medicina Pontificia, Universidade Catolica do Rio Grande so Sul • Avenida Ipiranga 6690. C.P. 1429. Porto Alegre RS, 90000

BRAZIL (the Federative Republic of) • Biblioteca "Dr Jose Antonio Garcia Coutinho", Faculdade de Ciencias Medicas. Fundacao de Ens.Sup. Vale de Sapucai • Av. Alfredo Custodio de Paula 320. Pouso Alegre MG, 37550-000

BRAZIL (the Federative Republic of) • Bibioteca, Faculdade de Ciencias Medicas de Pernambuco, Hospital Oswaldo Cruz • Rua Arnobio Marques 310. Recife PE, 50000

BRAZIL (the Federative Republic of) • Biblioteca, Faculdade de Medicina de Ribeirao Preto, Universidade de Sao Paulo • Avenida Bandeirantes s/n. Ribeirao Preto SP, 14049

BRAZIL (the Federative Republic of) • Biblioteca Setorial, Instituto de Medicina Social, UERJ Univ. de Estado do Rio de Janeiro • 7 Andar, Bloco E, Maracana, Rua Sao Fco Xavier, 524. Rio De Janeiro RJ, 20550

BRAZIL (the Federative Republic of) • Biblioteca Centro Biomedico, Faculdade de Ciencias Medicas, Universidade Estado Rio de Janeiro • Rua Teodoro da Silva 48-2 Piso. Rio De Janeiro RJ, 20560

BRAZIL (the Federative Republic of) • Biblioteca • Escola de Medicina • Fundacao Tecnico-Educacional Souza Marques • Rua do Catete 6, Gloria. Rio De Janeiro RJ, 22220

BRAZIL (the Federative Republic of) • Biblioteca Central, Centro de Ciencias da Saude, Universidade Federal do Rio de Janeiro (Cidado Universitaria) • Ilha do Fundao, CP 68032. Rio de Janeiro RJ, 21949-900

BRAZIL (the Federative Republic of) • Divisao de Biblioteca e Documentaçao, Universidade Estadual Paulista (UNESP) • Campus de Botucatu, Caixa Postal 502. Rubiao Jr SP, 18618.000

BRAZIL (the Federative Republic of) • Biblioteca Faculdade de Medicina, Universidade Federal Da Bahia • Av. Reitor Miguel Calmon S/n. 40000 Salvador BA

BRAZIL (the Federative Republic of) • Biblioteca, Escola de Medicina e Saude Publica, Fundacao Bahiana para o Desenvolvimento da Medicina • Rua Frei Henrique No.8, Nazare. Salvador BA, 40050

BRAZIL (the Federative Republic of) • Biblioteca do Hospital Universitario, Biblioteca Central, Universidade Federal de Santa Maria • Cidade Universitaria, Camobi. Santa Maria RS, 97100

BRAZIL (the Federative Republic of) • Biblioteca, Faculdade Ciencias Medicas de Santos. Fundacao Lusiada Boqueirao • Rua Oswaldo Cruz 179, C.P. 459. Santos SP, 11100

BRAZIL (the Federative Republic of) • Faculdade de Medicina de Sao Jose do Rio Preto • Avenida Brigadeiro Faria Lima 5416. Sao José do Rio Preto SP, 15090-000

BRAZIL (the Federative Republic of) • Biblioteca, Instituto Butantan • Av. Vital Brasil 1500. Sao Paulo SP, 05503-900

BRAZIL (the Federative Republic of) • Biblioteca/CIR, Faculdade de Saúde Pública, Universidad de Sao Paulo • Av Dr Arnaldo 715. Sao Paulo SP, 01246-904

BRAZIL (the Federative Republic of) • Servico de Biblioteca/documentacao, Faculdade de Medicina, Universidade de Sao Paulo • Av. Dr Arnaldo 445, CP 54.199. Sao Paulo SP, 01296

BRAZIL (the Federative Republic of) • Biblioteca, Centro de Ciencias Medicas e Biologicas de Sorocaba • Praca Dr Jose Ermirio de Moraes 290, Caixa Postal 1570. Sorocaba SP, 18030-230

BRAZIL (the Federative Republic of) • Biblioteca, Centro de Ciências Biológicas e da Saúde, Universidade de Taubaté • Av. Tiradentes 500, Centro. Taubaté SP, 12030-180

BRAZIL (the Federative Republic of) • Biblioteca, Centro de Ciencias da Saude, Fundacao Universidade Federal do Piaui • Avenida Frei Serafim 2280. Teresina PI 64000

BRAZIL (the Federative Republic of) • Biblioteca Frei Eugenio Faculdade de Medicina Do • Triangulo Mineiro, Rua Frei Paulino 80. Uberaba MG, 38025

BRAZIL (the Federative Republic of) • Administracao Central das Bibliotecas, Fundacao Educacion "Dom A. Arcoverde", Faculdade de Medicina de Valenca Bairro de Fatima • Rua Sargento Vitor Hugo 161. Valenca RJ, 27600

BRAZIL (the Federative Republic of) • Biblioteca Central, Faculdade de Medicina de Vassouras, Universidade Severino Sombra • Av. Expedicionario o. de Almeida, 280. Vassouras RJ, 27700.000

BRAZIL (the Federative Republic of) • Biblioteca, Escola de Medicina da Santa Casa de Misericordia de Vitoria • Av.Nossa Senhora da Penha • CP 36. Vitoria ES, 29000

BRITISH VIRGIN ISLANDS • Health Department Library, BVI Health Department, Ministry of Health, Education and Welfare, Govt of the British Virgin Islands • Road Town. Tortola

BULGARIA • Bibliothèque, Institut Supérieur de Médecine • 63 Rue K. Zlatarev. Pleven, 5800

BULGARIA • Library and Information Center, Exchange Department, Medical University • Plovdiv, 15A V. Aprilov Street. Plovdiv, 4002

BULGARIA • Bibliotheque, Centre National de Maladies Infectieuses et Parasitaires • Boulevard Yanko Sakuzov 26. Sofia, 1504

BULGARIA • Library, Medical University • Ul. armeiska 11. Stara Zagora, 6000

BULGARIA • Bibliothèque, Institut Supérieur de Médecine • Ul. Marin Drinov 55. Varna, 9002

BURKINA FASO • Centre de Documentation, Organisation Ouest Africaine de la Santé, WAHO/OOAS • 01 BP 153. Bobodioulasso 01

CAMEROON (the Republic of) • Institut panafricain pour le Développement, Afrique Centrale Francophone • BP 4078. Douala

CANADA • Ministère de la Santé et des Services Sociaux, Service Documentation Périodiques • 1075 Chemin Ste-Foy, 5ème étage. Québec (Québec), G1S 2M1

CHILE (the Republic of) • Biblioteca (SERBYMAV), Canje y Donacion, Universidad de Antofagasta • Casilla 170. Antofagasta

CHILE (the Republic of) • Biblioteca Medica, Facultade de Medicina, Universidad de Concepcion • Casilla 160-C. Concepcion

CHILE (the Republic of) • Biblioteca Biomédica, Pontificia Universidad Católica de Chile, Campus Casa Cebtral • Av. Libertador Bernardo O'Higgins 340, Casilla 114-D. Santiago

CHILE (the Republic of) • Biblioteca Central, Facultad de Medicina, Universidad de Chile • Avenida Independencia 1027, Casilla 7000, Correo 7. Santiago

CHILE (the Republic of) • Biblioteca Central • Universidad de la Frontera de Temuco • Av. F.Salazar, #01145, Casilla 54-D. Temuco

CHILE (the Republic of) • Biblioteca, Facultad de Medicina, Universidad Austral de Chile • Casilla 39-A. Valdivia

CHILE (the Republic of) • Servicio de Bibliotecas, Facultat de Medicina, Universidad de Valparaiso • Hontaneda 2653, Casilla 92-V. Valparaiso

CHINA (the People's Republic of) • The Library, Capital Institute of Medicine, Beijing Capital College • You an Men. Beijing, 100054

CHINA (the People's Republic of) • Library, Institute of Epidemiol. and Microbiology Chinese, Academy of Preventive Medicine • Building 5, 9-301, Zhi Chun Dong Li, Haidian District. Beijing, 100086

CHINA (the People's Republic of) • Library, Binzhou Medical College • 522 Yellow River Third Road. Binzhou Shandong, 256603

CHINA (the People's Republic of) • The Library, Norman Bethune University of Medical Sciences • 30 Qinghua Rd. Changchun Jilin, 130021

CHINA (the People's Republic of) • Library, Chengde School of Medicine • Cui Qiao South Road, PO Box 6. Chengde Hebei, 067000

CHINA (the People's Republic of) • Library, Chengdu College of Traditional Chinese Medicine • 317 Twelve Bridge Street. Chengdu Sichuan, 610072

CHINA (the People's Republic of) • Library, West China Medical University • Chengdu. Sichuan Province, 610041

CHINA (the People's Republic of) • Library, Chongqing Medical College, Chongqing University of Medical Sciences • Xie Taizi, Yixieyuan Lu. Chongqing Sichuan, 630046

CHINA (the People's Republic of) • Library, Datong Medical College • 4 Yi Wei Street, South Xin Jian Rd. Datong Shanxi, 037008

CHINA (the People's Republic of) • Library, The Enshi College of Medicine • Enshi Hubei, 445000

CHINA (the People's Republic of) • Library, Fujian College of Traditional Chinese Medicine • No.53 Wu Si North Road. Fuzhou Fujian, 350003

CHINA (the People's Republic of) • Library, Guangzhou Medical College • 195 Dongfengxilu. Guangzhou Guangdong, 510182

CHINA (the People's Republic of) • Library, Sun Yat-Sen University of Medical Sciences • 74 Zhongshan Road, 2. Guangzhou, 510089

CHINA (the People's Republic of) • Library, Guangdong College of Medicine and Pharmacy • 40 Bao Gang Guang Han Zhi. Guangzhou Guangdong, 510224

CHINA (the People's Republic of) • Library, Medical College Jinan University • Shi Pai. Guangzhou Guangdong, 510632

CHINA (the People's Republic of) • Library, Guilin Medical College • Le Qun Road 56, Mailbox 63rd. Guilin Guangxi, 541001

CHINA (the People's Republic of) • The Library, Hainan School of Medicine • Haikou Hainan Island, 570005

CHINA (the People's Republic of) • Library, College of Traditional Chinese Medicine • Qing Chun Street. Hangzhou Zhejiang, 310009

CHINA (the People's Republic of) • Library, Zhejiang Medical University • 157 Yan An Road. Hangzhou City, Zhejiang, 310006

CHINA (the People's Republic of) • Library, Harbin Medical University • Xiefulu. Harbin Heilongjiang, 150086

CHINA (the People's Republic of) • Library, Department of Chinese Traditional Medicine, Anhui Chinese Medicine College • Hefei Anhui, 230038

CHINA (the People's Republic of) • Library, Hengyang Medical College, West College Village • Hengyang Hunan, 421001

CHINA (the People's Republic of) • Library, Heze Medical College • Kang Fu Road. Heze Shandong, 274030

CHINA (the People's Republic of) • Department of Foreign Languages, Jiamusi Medical College • Jiamusi Heilongjiang, 154002

CHINA (the People's Republic of) • Library, Jining Medical College • 38 Jian She Road. Jining Shandong, 272113

CHINA (the People's Republic of) • Library, Kaifeng School of Medicine • 65 Qian Ying Men Street. Kaifeng Henan, 475001

CHINA (the People's Republic of) • Library, Institute of Traditional Chinese Medicine and Materia Medica • Kunming Yunnan, 650223

CHINA (the People's Republic of) • Library, Kunming Medical College • Renmin Western Road. Kunming Yunnan, 650031

CHINA (the People's Republic of) • Library, Medical Department, Northwest Nationalities University • 1 Xibeixincun. Lanzhou Gansu, 730030

CHINA (the People's Republic of) • Library, Luoyang School of Medicine • 6 Anhui Road. Luoyang Jian Xi, Dist. Henan, 471003

CHINA (the People's Republic of) • Library, Luzhou School of Medicine • Zhong Shan. Luzhou Sichuan, 646000

CHINA (the People's Republic of) • Library, Jiangxi College of Traditional Chinese Medicine • 20 Yangmin Road. Nanchang Jiangxi, 330006

CHINA (the People's Republic of) • Library and Information Division, Guangxi Institute of Parasitic Diseases • Nanning Guangxi

CHINA (the People's Republic of) • Library, Guangxi Medical University • 6 Bin Hu Rd. Nanning Guangxi, 530021

CHINA (the People's Republic of) • Library, Qingdao Medical College • 10 Huangtailu. Qingdao Shandong, 266012

CHINA (the People's Republic of) • Library, Medical Center of Fudan University • 138 Yi Xue Yuan Road. Shanghai, 200032

CHINA (the People's Republic of) • Library, Shanghai College of Traditional Chinese Medicine • 530 Lingling Road. Shanghai, 200032

CHINA (the People's Republic of) • Library, Shanghai Medical Information Centre • 602 Juan Guo Road (west). Shanghai, 200031

CHINA (the People's Republic of) • Health Sciences Library and Information Center, Shanghai Second Medical University • 280 Chong Qing Southern Road. Shanghai, 200025

CHINA (the People's Republic of) • Library, Changzhi Medical College • 46 South Yanan Road. Shangzhi Shanxi, 046000

CHINA (the People's Republic of) • Library, College of Traditional Chinese Medicine • 79 Congshun Bei Ling Street. Shenyang Liaoning, 110032

CHINA (the People's Republic of) • Library, China Medical University • No. 92, Bei 2 Rd., Heping District. Shenyang Liaoning, 110001

CHINA (the People's Republic of) • Library, Shihezi Medical College • North Second Road. Shihezi Xinjiang, 832002

CHINA (the People's Republic of) • Library, Hebei College of Traditional Chinese Medicine • South Xin Shi Road. Shijiazhuang Hebei, 050091

CHINA (the People's Republic of) • Library, Tianjin Medical College • 22 Qixiangtai Rd. Tianjin, 300070

CHINA (the People's Republic of) • Library, Tianjin Second Medical College • 1 Guangdong Rd, Hexi District . Tianjin, 300203

CHINA (the People's Republic of) • Library, Tianjin College of Traditional Chinese Medicine • 20 Yu Quan Road, West Lake Village. Tianjin Nankai District, 300193

CHINA (the People's Republic of) • Library, The Inner Mongolia Traditional Mongolian Medical College • 16 Huo Lin He Street. Tongliao Inner Mongolia, 028041

CHINA (the People's Republic of) • Library, Weifang Medical College • 68 Shenghi Street. Weifang Shandong, 261042

CHINA (the People's Republic of) • Library, Wenzhou Medical College • Wenzhou Zhejiang, 325003

CHINA (the People's Republic of) • Library, Tongji Medical University • Wuhan Hubei, 430030

CHINA (the People's Republic of) • Library, Wannan Medical College • 2 Nang-Wu Road. Wuhu Anhui, 241001

CHINA (the People's Republic of) • Library, Shaanxi College of Traditional Chinese Medicine • Weiyang Road. Xianyang Shaanxi, 712083

CHINA (the People's Republic of) • Library, Xuzhou Medical College • 84 West Huai Hai Road. Xuzhou Jiangsu, 221002

CHINA (the People's Republic of) • Library, Yanan Medical College • Du Pu Chuan. Yanan Shaanxi, 716000

CHINA (the People's Republic of) • Library, Yangzhou Medical College • 6 Huaihai Lu. Yangzhou Jiangsu

CHINA (the People's Republic of) • Library, Zhangjiakou School of Medicine • Zhangjiakou Hebei, 075000

CHINA (the People's Republic of) • Library, Guangdong Medical College • Wenming Road, Xiashan District. Zhanjiang Guangdong, 524023

CHINA (the People's Republic of) • Library, Henan Medical University • 40 Daxue Road. Zhengzhou Henan, 450052

CHINA (the People's Republic of) • Library, Henan College of Traditional Chinese Medicine • East Jin Shui Road. Zhengzhou Henan, 450003

CHINA (the People's Republic of) • Library, Zunyi Medical College • Wai Huan Road. Zunyi Guizhou, 563003

COLOMBIA (the Republic of) • Biblioteca, Facultad de Medicina, Universidad del Quindio • Avda Bolivar Calle 12-N, APDO 460. Armenia Quindio

COLOMBIA (the Republic of) • Biblioteca, Facultad de Medicina, Universidad Seccional Barranquilla • Km. 7 Antigua Via Puerto Colon, Apartado Aereo 1752. Barranquilla Atlantico

COLOMBIA (the Republic of) • Biblioteca Central, Universidad del Norte • Km 5 Carretera a Puerto Colombia, Apartado Aereo 1569. Barranquilla Atlantico

COLOMBIA (the Republic of) • Biblioteca, Facultad de Ciencias de la Salud, Universidad Industrial de Santander • Apartado Aereo 678. Bucaramanga

COLOMBIA (the Republic of) • Departamento de Bibliotecas, Universidad del Valle, Ciudad Universitaria Melendez • Apartado Aereo 25360. Cali Valle Del Cauca

COLOMBIA (the Republic of) • Biblioteca, Facultad de Medicina • Universidad Libre • Diagonal 37a No. 3-29, Apdo 1040. Cali

COLOMBIA (the Republic of) • Biblioteca, Facultad de Medicina, Universidad de Cartagena • Cra.6 No.36-100, APDO 3210. Cartagena, 195

COLOMBIA (the Republic of) • Biblioteca Medica • Facultad de Medicina • Universidad de Antioquia • Apartado Aereo 1226. Medellin Antioquia

COLOMBIA (the Republic of) • Biblioteca Medica • Universidad Pontificia Bolivariana • Apartado Aereo 56006. Medellin Antioquia

COLOMBIA (the Republic of) • Biblioteca • Facultad de Medicina • Instituto de Ciencias de la Salud • Calle 10A No. 2204, Apdo aereo 054591. Medellin

COLOMBIA (the Republic of) • Biblioteca • Facultad de Medicina y Ciencias de la Salud • Universidad Sur Colombiana • Av. P. Borrero, Cra 1a, AA 385. Neiva Huila

COLOMBIA (the Republic of) • Biblioteca Ciencias de la Salud • Universidad Del Cauca • Carrera 6a Calle 13 Norte. Popayan Cauca

COLOMBIA (the Republic of) • Grupo de Documentacion Cientifica • Direccion de Planeacion Corporativa • Instituto de Seguro Social • Barrio Chapinero, Carrera 10a. 64-60, Piso 2, Apartado 5053. Santafé de Bogota DC

COLOMBIA (the Republic of) • Biblioteca • Jorge Bejarano • Ministerio de Salud • Carrera 13 No. 32-76. Santafé de Bogota

COLOMBIA (the Republic of) • Biblioteca • Facultad de Medicina • Pontificia Universidad Javeriana • Carrera 7a, No 41-00. Santafé de Bogota DE

COLOMBIA (the Republic of) • Biblioteca • Escuela de Medicina Juan N. Corpas • Avenida Corpas Km.3- Suba. Santafé de Bogota DC

COLOMBIA (the Republic of) • Biblioteca • Escuela Colombiana de Medicina • Universidad El Bosque • Transversal 9A bis No. 133-25, APDO 100998. Santafé de Bogota DE

COLOMBIA (the Republic of) • Biblioteca • Facultad de Medicina • Colegio Mayor de Nuestra Senora del Rosario • Calle 10 No.18-75, 1 Piso, AP 24743. Santafé de Bogota

COLOMBIA (the Republic of) • Biblioteca • Escuela Militar de Medicina y Ciencias de la Salud • Universidad Militar Nueva Granada • Transv. 5a. No. 49-00. Santafé de Bogota DE

COSTA RICA (the Republic of) • Biblioteca • Escuela Autonoma de Ciencias Medicas de Centro • America • Centro Colon, APDO 638-1007. San José

CUBA (the Republic of) • Biblioteca • Instituto Superior de Ciencias Medicas • Cra. Central Oeste, Apartado 144. C amaguey, 70700

CUBA (the Republic of) • Centro Nacional de Informacion en Ciencias Medicas • Viceministerio de Ciencia y Tecnica • Ministerio de Salud Publica MIN-SAP • Calle E No.454 c/ 19 y 21 Vedado. Habana Ciudad de la Habana, 10400

CUBA (the Republic of) • Facultad de Ciencias Medicas • Centro Provincial de Informacion de Ciencias Medicas • Av. Lenin 4, Esq. Aguilera. Holguin, 80700

CUBA (the Republic of) • Biblioteca, Instituto Superior Ciencias Medicas • Ave. de las Americas y Calle E. Santiago de Cuba

CZECH REPUBLIC • Library, Department of Social Medicine, Medical Faculty, Masaryk University • Jostova 10. Brno, 662 43

CZECH REPUBLIC • Library, Lekarska Fakulta, Universita Karlova • Simkova 870. Hradec Kralove, 500 38

CZECH REPUBLIC • Information Centre, Medical Faculty • Palacky University, Hnevotinska 3. Olomouc, 775 03

CZECH REPUBLIC • Narodni Lekarska Knihovna, National Medical Library • Sokolska 54. Praha 2, 121 32

CZECH REPUBLIC • United Nations Information Centre • Nam. Kinskych 6. Praha 5, 150 00

CZECH REPUBLIC • Library, Univerzita Karlova v Praze, 3. lékarská fakulta (3rd Medical Faculty) • Srobarova 48. Praha 10, 100 42

CZECH REPUBLIC • Library, 2. Lekarska Fakulta, Universita Karlova • V. Uvalu 84. Praha 5 Motol, 150 18

DEMOCRATIC REPUBLIC OF THE CONGO (the Republic of) • Bibliothèque, Faculté de Médecine, Université Kongo • Campus de Kisantu, BP 166. Inkisi (Bas Congo)

DEMOCRATIC REPUBLIC OF THE CONGO (the Republic of) • Bibliothèque, Faculté de Médecine, Université de Kinshasa • BP 834. Kinshasa XI

DEMOCRATIC REPUBLIC OF THE CONGO (the Republic of) • Bibliothèque, Faculté de Médecine, Université de Kisangani • BP 2012. Kisangani Haut-Zaire

DEMOCRATIC REPUBLIC OF THE CONGO (the Republic of) • Bibliothèque, Faculté de Médecine, Université de Lubumbashi • BP 1825. Lubumbashi Shaba

DENMARK (the Kingdom of) • United Nations Information Centre • Midtermolen 3. Kobenhavn, DK-2100

DOMINICA • Health Resource Library, Primary Health Care Center • Upper Lane, Roseau Commonwealth

DOMINICA (the Commonwealth of) • Library, School of Medicine, Ross University • PO Box 266. Roseau

DOMINICAN REPUBLIC • Biblioteca, Universidad Tecnologica del Cibao • Calle Autopista Duarte Km.1, Avenida Universitaria, AP 401. La Vega

DOMINICAN REPUBLIC • Biblioteca, Escuela de Medicina, Facultad de Ciencias Medicas, Universidad Central del Este (UCE) • Avenida de Circunvalacion. San Pedro de Macoris

DOMINICAN REPUBLIC • Biblioteca Central, Pontificia Universidad Catolica Madre y Maestra • Autopista Duarte Km 1 1/2, Apartado Postal 822. Santiago de los Caballeros

DOMINICAN REPUBLIC • Biblioteca, Escuela de Medicina, Universidad Nacional Pedro Henriquez Urena • Av. J.F. Kennedy, Km 5 1/2, AA 1423. Santo Domingo

DOMINICAN REPUBLIC • Centro de Documentacion en Salud "Rogelio Lamarche Soto", Facultad de Ciencias de la Salud, Universidad Autonoma de Santo Domingo • Zona Universitaria, Apdo 4355. Santo Domingo

DOMINICAN REPUBLIC • Biblioteca, Escuela de Medicina Universidad Henriquez y Carvajal • Isabel Aguiar 100, Herrera. Santo Domingo

DOMINICAN REPUBLIC • Biblioteca, Escuela de Medicina, Universidad Tecnologica de Santiago (UTESA) • M. Gomez Esq. Jose Contreras, AA 21423. Santo Domingo

ECUADOR (the Republic of) • Biblioteca, Facultad de Ciencias Medicas, Universidad de Cuenca • Av. 12 de Abril s/n, Casilla 01-01-1891. Cuenca

ECUADOR (the Republic of) • Biblioteca, Facultad de Medicina y Ciencias de la Salud, Universidad Catolica de Cuenca • Pio Bravo 2-56, Apartado 19 A. Cuenca Azuay

ECUADOR (the Republic of) • Biblioteca Dr Alfredo J. Valenzuela, Facultad de Ciencias Medicas, Universidad de Guayaquil • Ciudadela Salvador Allende. Av. J.F. Kennedy, Apartado 471. Guayaquil

ECUADOR (the Republic of) • Biblioteca, Facultad de Ciencias Medicas, Universidad Nacional de Loja • Miguel Angel y Av. Iberamericana, Casilla 349.Loja

Senor Jefe • Instituto Nacional de Higiene Leopoldo Izquieta • Perez , quique 2045 y Yaguachi . Quito

ECUADOR (the Republic of) • Biblioteca, Facultad de Ciencias Medicas, Universidad Central del Ecuador (the Republic of) • Iquique y Sodiro s/n, APDO 6120. Quito

EGYPT (the Arab Republic of) • The Library, Faculty of Medicine • Alexandria El-Messalah, 21521

EGYPT (the Arab Republic of) • The Library, Faculty of Medicine, Assiut University • Assiut

EGYPT (the Arab Republic of) • Library, Behna Faculty of Medicine • Benha El-Kalubia

EGYPT (the Arab Republic of) • Exchange and Gifts Division, National Information and Documentation Centre (NIDOC) • Al-Tahrir St., Dokki. Cairo

EGYPT (the Arab Republic of) • The Library, Faculty of Medicine • Al-Azhar University • Madinet Nasr. Cairo

EGYPT (the Arab Republic of) • Medical Documentation Administration (Library of the Ministry of Health and Population), Medical Education Technology Centre • 21 Abdelazizi Alsioud St. Roda. Cairo

EGYPT (the Arab Republic of) • Bibliotheca Alexandrina • El-Shatby. Alexandria, 21526

EGYPT (the Arab Republic of) • Library, Faculty of Medicine, Mansura University • Mansura

EL SALVADOR (the Republic of) • Biblioteca, Facultad de Medicina, Universidad Evangelica • 63 Av. Sur Pasaje 1 No.138, Apartado 1789. San Salvador, 01186

EL SALVADOR (the Republic of) • Biblioteca, Facultad de Medicina, Universidad Autonoma de Santa Ana • 5a Calle Pte entre 6a y 8a Av.Sur #28. Santa Ana

ERITREA • Library, College of Health Sciences, University of Asmara • PO Box 1220. Asmara

ETHIOPIA (the Federal Democratic Republic of) • Library, Ministry of Health • PO Box 1234. Addis Ababa

ETHIOPIA (the Federal Democratic Republic of) • Library, Gondar College of Medical Sciences • PO Box 196. Gondar

ETHIOPIA (the Federal Democratic Republic of) • Library, Department of Community Health • Jimma Health Sciences Institute. PO Box 378. Jimma Keffa Region

FINLAND (the Republic of) • National Library of Health Sciences • Haartmaninkatu 4. Helsinki, FIN-00290

FRANCE (the Republic of) • Bibliothèque Centrale, Institut Pasteur • 25-28 Rue du Dr Roux. Paris Cedex 15, F-75724

GERMANY (the Federal Republic of) • Senatsbibliothek Berlin • Strasse des 17 Juni 112. Berlin, D-10623

GHANA (the Republic of) • Medical and Dental Council • PO Box 10586. Accra North

GHANA (the Republic of) • Library, Ghana Institute of Management and Public Administration • PO Box 50. Achimota

GHANA (the Republic of) • The Library, University of Science and Technology • PMB 3201. Kumasi

GHANA (the Republic of) • Library, School of Public Health, University of Ghana • PO Box LG 13. Legon Accra

GRENADA • The Library, School of Medicine, St. George's University • St George's

GUATEMALA (the Republic of) • Biblioteca, Facultad de Ciencias Medicas, Universidade de San Carlos de Guatemala • Ciudad Universitaria, Edificio M-4. Guatemala 12

GUATEMALA (the Republic of) • Biblioteca, Facultad de Medicina, Universidad Francisco Marroquin • 6a Avenida 7-55. Guatemala 10

GUYANA • Library, Faculty of Health Sciences, University of Guyana • Turkey Campus. PO Box 10-1110. Georgetown

HAITI (the Republic of) • Bibliothèque, Ecole de Médecine et de Pharmacie, Université d'Etat d'Haiti • Rue Oswald Durand. Port-Au-Prince

HONDURAS (the Republic of) • Biblioteca Medica Nacional, Facultad de Ciencias Medicas atras del Hospital, Escuela Universidad Nacional Autonoma de Honduras • Tegucigalpa DC

HUNGARY (the Republic of) • Orszagos Orvostudomanyi Informacios Intezet • PO Box 278. Budapest , H-1444

HUNGARY (the Republic of) • Library, Debreceni Orvostudomanyi Egyetem • Nagyerdei Krt. 98. Debrecen 12, H-4012

HUNGARY (the Republic of) • Library, Pecs University Medical School • Szigeti ut. 12. Pecs, H-7643

HUNGARY (the Republic of) • Central Library, Albert Szent-Gyorgyi Medical University • PO Box 109. Szeged, H-6701

INDIA (the Republic of) • Library, Department of Preventive and Social Medicine, S.N. Medical College • Agra-282001. Uttar Pradesh

INDIA (the Republic of) • Departmental Library, Department of Preventive and Social Medicine, SMT. N.H.L. Municipal Medical College • Ellis Bridge, Ahmedabad-380006. Gujarat

INDIA (the Republic of) • Library, Department of Preventive and Social Medicine, J.L.N. Medical College • Ajmer-305001. Rajasthan

INDIA (the Republic of) • Library, Department of Community Medicine, Jawaharlal Nehru Medical College, Aligarh Muslim University • Aligarh-202002. Uttar Pradesh

INDIA (the Republic of) • Central Library, Motilal Nehru Medical College • Allahabad-211001. Uttar Pradesh

INDIA (the Republic of) • The Library, Swami Ramanand Teerth Rural Medical College • Dist. Beed, Ambajogai-431517. Maharashtra

INDIA (the Republic of) • Library Section, Department of Preventive and Social Medicine, Medical College • Amritsar-143001. Punjab

INDIA (the Republic of) • Library, Medical College • Aurangabad-431001. Maharashtra

INDIA (the Republic of) • Central Library, Goa University • Taleigaum Plateau. Bambolim-403202. Goa, Daman and Diu

INDIA (the Republic of) • Library, Department of Preventive and Social Medicine, B.S. Medical College • Calcutta University • Bankura-722101. West Bengal

INDIA (the Republic of) • Library, Department of Community Medicine, Medical College • Baroda-390001. Gujarat

INDIA (the Republic of) • Department of Community Medicine, Jawaharlal Nehru Medical College • Poona-Bangalore Road. Belgaum-590010. Karnataka

INDIA (the Republic of) • Library, Department of Preventive and Social Medicine, Government Medical College • South Central Railway, Bellary-583104. Karnataka

INDIA (the Republic of) • Library, Department of Preventive and Social Medicine, Sardar Patel Medical College • Shiv Bari Road, Bikaner-334001. Rajasthan

INDIA (the Republic of) • Library, Department of Community Medicine, Burdwan Medical College • Burdwan-713104. West Bengal

INDIA (the Republic of) • Library, Department of Preventive and Social Medicine, Medical College • Calicut-673008. Kerala

INDIA (the Republic of) • The Library, University of Madras, University Building • Chennai-600005. Tamil Nadu

INDIA (the Republic of) • Community Medicine Department Library, PSG Institute of Medical Sciences and Research • Peelamedu, Coimbatore-641004. Tamil Nadu

INDIA (the Republic of) • The Library, Patliputra Medical College • PO BCCL Township, Dhanbad-826005. Bihar

INDIA (the Republic of) • Departmental Library, Department of Social and Preventive Medicine, Assam Medical College • Dibrugarh-786002. Assam

INDIA (the Republic of) • Library, Department of Social and Preventive Medicine • B.R.D. Medical College • Medical College Campus • Gorakhpur-273013. Uttar Pradesh

INDIA (the Republic of) • Department of Preventive and Social Medicine, Guntur Medical College • Guntur-522004. Andhra Pradesh

INDIA (the Republic of) • Library, Department of Preventive and Social Medicine, Guwahati Medical College • Guwahati-781032. Assam

INDIA (the Republic of) • Library, Department of Preventive and Social Medicine, Gajra Raja Medical College • Gwalior-474009. Madhya Pradesh

INDIA (the Republic of) • Library, Department of Preventive and Social Medicine, Karnatak Medical College (Karnatak University) • K.M.C. Campus, Hubli-580022. Karnataka

INDIA (the Republic of) • Library, N.E. Regional Medical College • Lamphel, Imphal-795004. Manipur

INDIA (the Republic of) • Library, Department of Preventive and Social Medicine, M.G.M. Medical College • Bombay Agra Road, Indore-452001. Madhya Pradesh

INDIA (the Republic of) • Dr Robert Heilig Library, S.M.S. Medical College • Jaipur-302004. Rajasthan

INDIA (the Republic of) • Library, Department of Community Medicine, Government Medical College • Jammu-180001. Jammu and Kashmir

INDIA (the Republic of) • Central Library, M.L.B. Medical College Jhansi • Jhansi-284128. Uttar Pradesh

INDIA (the Republic of) • Library, Department of Preventive and Social Medicine, Dr S.N. Medical College, Rajasthan University • Jodhpur-342001. Rajasthan

INDIA (the Republic of) • Department of Preventive and Social Medicine, Rangaraya Medical College, Andhra University • East Godavari St. Kakinada-533001. Andhra Pradesh

INDIA (the Republic of) • Library, Department of Social and Preventive Medicine, G.S.V.M. Medical College • Kanpur-208002. Uttar Pradesh

INDIA (the Republic of) • Library, Department of Community Medicine, Medical College • 88 College Street, Kolkata-700012. West Bengal

INDIA (the Republic of) • Library, Department of Preventive and Social Medicine, R.G. Kar Medical College, Calcutta University • Kolkata-700004. West Bengal

INDIA (the Republic of) • Nilratan Sircar Medical College, Calcutta University • Academic Bldg (Central Library). 138 Acharya Jagidish Chandra Bose Rd, Kolkata-700014. West Bengal

INDIA (the Republic of) • Library, Department of Community Medicine, Kottayam Medical College • Gandhinagar, Kottayam-686008. Kerala

INDIA (the Republic of) • Library, Department of Preventive and Social Medicine, Kurnool Medical College • Budhavar Pet., Kurnool-518002. Andhra Pradesh

INDIA (the Republic of) • Library, Department of Preventive and Social Medicine, Christian Medical College, Punjab University • Ludhiana-141008. Punjab

INDIA (the Republic of) • Department of Preventive and Social Medicine, Dayanand Medical College and Hospital, Punjab University • Civil Lines, PO Box 265, Ludhiana-141001. Punjab

INDIA (the Republic of) • Library Committee, Madurai Medical College • Madurai-625020. Tamil Nadu

INDIA (the Republic of) • Library, Kasturba Medical College, Mangalore University • PO Box No. 8, Manipal-576119. Karnataka

INDIA (the Republic of) • Library, Department of Preventive and Social Medicine, Government Medical College, Shivahi University • Miraj-416410. Maharashtra

INDIA (the Republic of) • Library, Topiwala National Medical College, Municipal Corporation of Greater Bombay • Dr A.L. Nair Road, Mumbai-400008. Maharashtra

INDIA (the Republic of) • The Library, Department of Preventive and Social Medicine, Grant Medical College, Bombay University • Byculla, Mumbai-400008. Maharashtra

INDIA (the Republic of) • Library, Department of Preventive and Social Medicine, Govt. Medical College, Mysore University • Mysore-570001. Karnataka

INDIA (the Republic of) • Library, Centre for Community Medicine, All-India Institute of Medical Sciences • Ansari Nagar, New Delhi-110029

INDIA (the Republic of) • National Medical Library, Directorate General of Health Services • Ansari Nagar, Ring Road. New Delhi, 110029

INDIA (the Republic of) • Central Library, Lady Hardinge Medical College and associated KSC and SK Hospitals • Bhagat Singh Marg. New Delhi,110001

INDIA (the Republic of) • Central Library, Maulana Azad Medical College, Delhi University • Bahadur Shah Zafar Marg. New Delhi,110002

INDIA (the Republic of) • Library, Department of Preventive and Social Medicine, B.J. Medical College Poona University • Pune-411001. Maharashtra

INDIA (the Republic of) • Library, PT. J.N.M. Medical College, Ganj., Jail Road • Raipur-492001. Madhya Pradesh

INDIA (the Republic of) • Library Department of Preventive and Social Medicine, Medical College • Rohtak-124001. Haryana

INDIA (the Republic of) • The Library, Department of Preventive and Social Medicine, Indira Gandhi Medical College • Simla-171001. Himachal Pradesh

INDIA (the Republic of) • The Library Department of Social and Preventive Medicine, Government Medical College • PO Box 673. Srinagar 190001. Jammu and Kashmir

INDIA (the Republic of) • The Library, Department of Preventive and Social Medicine, Government Medical College • Majura Gate, Surat-395001. Gujarat

INDIA (the Republic of) • Library, Department of Preventive and Social Medicine, S.V. Medical College • Tirupati-517502. Andhra Pradesh

INDIA (the Republic of) • Central Library, Trichur Medical College • Velappaya, Trichur-680581. Kerala

INDIA (the Republic of) • Dodd Memorial Library, Christian Medical College and Hospital, Madras University • Vellore-632004. Tamil Nadu

INDIA (the Republic of) • Library, Department of Preventive and Social Medicine, Andhra Medical College • Maharanipata, Visakhapatnam-530002. Andhra Pradesh

INDIA (the Republic of) • Library, Department of Preventive and Social Medicine, Kakatiya Medical College, Osmania University • Warangal-506007. Andhra Pradesh

INDIA (the Republic of) • Library, Department of Community Medicine, Mahatma Gandhi Institute of Medical Sciences, Sevagram • Wardha-442102. Maharashtra

INDONESIA (the Republic of) • Library, Department of Public Health, Medical Faculty, Universitas Udayana • Jl. Pb. Sudirman-Sanglah. Denpasar Bali

INDONESIA (the Republic of) • Perpustakaan Kanwil Depkes, Kantwil Depkes Propinsi Timor Timur • Jl. Kaikoli, PO Box 117. Dili Propinsi Timor Timur

INDONESIA (the Republic of) • Library, Faculty of Medicine, Tarumanagara University • Jl. Jend. S. Parman I . Jakarta Barat, 11440

INDONESIA (the Republic of) • Division of Scientific Documentation and Data Processing, National Institute of Health Research and Development • Jl Percetakan Negara 29, POB 226. Jakarta

INDONESIA (the Republic of) • Ministry of Health Provincial Office • Abepura, PO Box 288. Jayapura, 99225

INDONESIA (the Republic of) • Library, Fakultas Kedokteran, Universitas Brawijaya • Jalan Mayor Jenderal Haryono 171. Malang East Java

INDONESIA (the Republic of) • Department of Public Health (Laborat. Ilmu Kesehatan Masyarakat), Fakultas Kedokteran, Universitas Sam Ratulangi • Kampus Unsrat, PO Box 1333. Manado 9115

INDONESIA (the Republic of) • Library, Department of Public Health, University of North Sumatra School of Medicine USU • Jl. Dr Mansur No. 5 . Medan North Sumatra

INDONESIA (the Republic of) • The Library, Perpustakaan Fakultas Kedokteran, Sriwijaya University Faculty of Medicine. Komplek RSU/FK.UNSRI • Jl. Mayor Mahidin Km 3 1/2. Sumatra Selatan, 30126

INDONESIA (the Republic of) • Library, Health Services and Technology Research and Development Centre, Ministry of Health • 17 Jalan Indrapura. Surabaya, 60176

INDONESIA (the Republic of) • Library, Faculty of Medicine, Hasanuddin University • Kampus Tamalanrea Km.10, Jl. Perintis Kemerdekaan. Ujungpandang, 90245

INDONESIA (the Republic of) • Library and Health Informatics Unit, Fakultas Kedokteran, Universitas Gadjah Mada • Jl. Farmako,k Sekip. Yogyakarta Java, 55281

IRAN (the Islamic Republic of) (ISLAMIC REPUBLIC) • Morteza Motahari Central Library, Razi University (Bakhtaran University) • Azadi Sq. Bakhtaran

IRAN (the Islamic Republic of) • Library, Shiraz Medical Sciences University • Fassa, 74615-168

IRAN (the Islamic Republic of) • Library, The University of Medical Sciences of Ghazvin • PO Box 34185-745. Ghazvine

IRAN (the Islamic Republic of) • Central Library and Medical Documentation, Hamadan University of Medical Sciences • Ayetollah Kashani Blvd., PO Box 518. Hamadan

IRAN (the Islamic Republic of) • Library, Medical School, Kerman University of Medical Sciences • BP 444. Kerman

IRAN (the Islamic Republic of) • Library, Meshed Medical Sciences University • Daneshgah Ave. Meshed

IRAN (the Islamic Republic of) • Library, School of Medicine Rafsanjan, University of Medical Sciences • Rafsanjan

IRAN (the Islamic Republic of) • Central Library, Tabriz Medical Sciences University • 29 Bahman Blvd. Tabriz

IRAN (the Islamic Republic of) • Library, Shahid Beheshti Medical Sciences University • Even. Teheran, 19395-4139

IRAN (the Islamic Republic of) • Library, School of Public Health and Institute of Public Health Research • PO Box 6446. Teheran, 14155

IRAQ (the Republic of) • Medical Library, College of Medicine-Basrah University-BASRAH • c/o The WHO Representative, Alwiyah Post Office. PO Box 2048. Baghdad

IRAQ (the Republic of) • Library-Department of Community Medicine, College of Medicine-Mosul University-MOSUL • c/o The WHO Representative, Alwiyah Post Office. PO Box 2048. Baghdad

IRAQ (the Republic of) • Library • Salahadin Medical School • University of Salahadin (ERBIL) • c/o The WHO Representative, Alwiyah Post Office. PO Box 2048. Baghdad

IRAQ (the Republic of) • Library, College of Medicine, Kufa University (PO Box 18), NAJEF KUFA • c/o The WHO Representative, Alwiyah Post Office. PO Box 2048. Baghdad

IRELAND • Official Publications Librarian, Trinity College Library • College Street. Dublin 2

ISRAEL (the State of) • Library, College of Medical Professions, Al-Quds University • PO Box 3523. Al-Bireh West Bank Via

ISRAEL (the State of) • Resource Center, Institute of Community and Public Health, Birzeit University • PO Box 14. Birzeit Via

ISRAEL (the State of) • Central Library, Islamic University of Gaza • PO Box 108. Gaza El-Rimal via

ISRAEL (the State of) • Central Administration, Hadassah Medical Organization • Ein-Kerem. PO BOX 12-000. Jerusalem, 91 120

ISRAEL (the State of) • Library of Life Sciences and Medicine, Tel-Aviv University • Ramat-Aviv, PO Box 39345. Tel Aviv-Yafo, 61392

ITALY (the italian Republic of) • Library (Serials), Food and Agriculture Organization of the United Nations • Via delle Terme di Caracalla. Roma, I-00100

ITALY (the italian Republic of) • Societa Italiana per l'Organizzazione Internazionale • Palazzetto di Venezia, Piazza di San Marco 51. Roma, I-00186

JAMAICA • Library, Cornwall County Health Administration • PO Box 472. Montego Bay

JORDAN (the Hashemite Kingdom of) • Library, Faculty of Medicine, Jordan (the Hashemite Kingdom of) University of Science and Technology • PO Box 3030. Irbid

KENYA (the Republic of) • Mahler Library, African Medical and Research Foundation International • Wilson Airport. PO Box 30125. Nairobi

KENYA (the Republic of) • Library, Department of Community Health, University of Nairobi • PO Box 19676. Nairobi

KENYA (the Republic of) • Library and Documentation Centre, United Nations Environment Programme, Headquarters Gigiri • PO Box 30552. Nairobi

KENYA (the Republic of) National Scientific and Technology Information and Documentation Centre, National Council for Science and Technology • PO Box 30623. Nairobi

KUWAIT (the State of) • Health Science Centre Library, Faculty of Medicine, Kuwait University • PO Box 24923. Safat 13110

LAO PEOPLE'S DEMOCRATIC REPUBLIC • Library, Ministry for Science and Technology Environmental Service • Ban Sisavat. Vientiane Lao PDR

LEBANON (the Lebanese Republic of) • Saab Medical Library, Faculty of Medicine, American University of Beirut • PO Box 11-0236/36. Beyrouth

LEBANON (the Lebanese Republic of) • Bibliothèque, Faculté de Médecine, Université Saint-Joseph • Campus des Sciences médicales. Rue de Damas, BP 11-5076. Beyrouth

LEBANON (the Lebanese Republic of) • Library, Faculty of Health Sciences University of Balamand • Youssef Sorsok St. Facing St. Georges Hospital • Ashrafieh, PO Box 166378-6417. Beyrouth

LEBANON (the Lebanese Republic of) • La Bibliothèque, Université Antonine • BP 40016. Hadath-Baabda

LITHUANIA (the Republic of) • Vilnius University Library • Universiteto 3. Vilnius, 232633

MACAO • Medical and Health Department of Macau, Servicos de Saude de Macau, Biblioteca-Nucleo Centro Hospitalar • CP 3002. Macau

MADAGASCAR (the Republic of) • Bibliothèque, Faculté de Medecine, Etablissement d'Enseignement Supérieur des Sciences de la Santé, Université de Madagascar (the Republic of) • BP 652. Mahajanga, 401

MADAGASCAR (the Republic of) • Bibliothèque, Direction interrégionale du Développement sanitaire de Toliara • BP 239. Toliara, 601

MALAWI (the Republic of) • Library, College of Medicine, University of Malawi • Chichiri, Private Bag 360. Blantyre 3

MALAWI (the Republic of) • Library and Documentation Centre, Ministry of Health and Population • Capital City, PO Box 30377. Lilongwe 3

MALAYSIA • Medical Library, Universiti Sains Malaysia • Kubang Kerian, 16150 Kota Bharu. Kelantan

MALAYSIA • Division of Library Information and Publications, Institute for Medical Research • Jalan Pahang. Kuala Lumpur, 50588

MALAYSIA • The Medical Library, Universiti Kebangsaan Malaysia • Jalan Raja Muda Abd. Aziz. Kuala Lumpur, 50778

MALI (the Republic of) • Bibliothèque, Ecole nationale de Médecine et de Pharmacie du Mali • BP 1805. Bamako

MAURITIUS (the Republic of) • Library, The University of Mauritius • Reduit

MEXICO (The United Mexican States) • Biblioteca, Centro de Investigacion de Enfermedades Tropicales, Facultad de Medicina, Universidad Autonoma de Guerrero • APDO 25-A. Acapulco

MEXICO (The United Mexican States) • Biblioteca, Centro Biomedico, Universidad Autonoma de Aguascalientes • Avenida Universidad Km.2. Aguascalientes AGS, 20100

MEXICO (The United Mexican States) • Biblioteca, Escuela Superior de Medicina, Universidad Autonoma de Campeche • Ciudad Universitaria. Campeche Camp., 24030

MEXICO (The United Mexican States) • Biblioteca, Escuela de Medicina, Universidad de Colima, Direccion de Desarrollo • Av.Universidad #333 • APDO COR. 134. Colima Col., 28040

MEXICO (The United Mexican States) • Depto de Documentacion y Biblioteca, Instituto Nacional de Salud Publica • Av. Universidad 655, Col. Sta. Maria Ahuacatitlán. Cuernavaca Morelos, 62508

MEXICO (The United Mexican States) • Biblioteca, Facultad de Medicina, Universidad Autonoma de Estado de Morelos • Avenida Chamilpa #1001. Cuernavaca Mor., 62410

MEXICO (The United Mexican States) • Biblioteca, Escuela de Medicina, Universidad Autonoma de Sinaloa • Corregon/Ort.de Dominguez, APDO 1667. Culiacan Sinaloa

MEXICO (The United Mexican States) • Biblioteca, Centro de Estudios Universitarios Xochicalco • Ave. Lopez Mateos, APDO 1377. Ensenada Bc

MEXICO (The United Mexican States) • Biblioteca, Facultad de Medecina de Gomez Palacio, Universidad Juarez del Estado de Durango • Sixto Ugalde y Calzada la Salle I . Gomez Palacio Durango, 35050

MEXICO (The United Mexican States) • Biblioteca Dr Enrique Avalos Perez, Instituto de Ciencias Biologicas, Universidad Autonoma de Guadalajara • Calle Priv. Dr Banda #26, APDO 1-440. Guadalajara Jalisco, 44100

MEXICO (The United Mexican States) • Biblioteca, Facultad de Medicina de Leon, Universidad de Guanajuato • 20 de Enero 929, Apartado Postal 772. Leon de Guanajuato Gto., 37000

MEXICO (The United Mexican States) • Biblioteca, Facultad de Medicina, Universidad Veracruzana • Av.Hidalgo Esq.F.Carrillo Puerto, Apartado Aereo 6. Mendoza Veracruz, 94730

MEXICO (The United Mexican States) • Biblioteca Dr Ignacio Vado Lugo, Facultad de Medicina, Universidad Autonoma de Yucatan • Av. Itzaes No. 498, APDO 1225-A. Merida Yucatan, 97000

MEXICO (The United Mexican States) • Instituto Nacional de Higiene, Ministerio de Salud y Asistencia • Calz. Mariano Escobedo No 20. Mexico 17 DF, 11400

MEXICO (The United Mexican States) • Biblioteca Dr Miguel E. Bustamante, Depto de Medicina Social, Preventiva y Salud Publica, Facultad de Medicina, Universidad Nacional Autonoma de Mexico • Piso 6, Delegacion Coyoacan. Mexico DF, 04510

MEXICO (The United Mexican States) • Biblioteca, Escuela Mexicana de Medicina, Universidad la Salle • Fuentes 31, Tialpan, APDO 22271. Mexico, 14000

MEXICO (The United Mexican States) • Biblioteca, Escuela Nacional de Medicina y Homeopatia • Calle Guil. Massieu Helguera No.239, Fracc. La Escalera Col. Ticoman. Mexico DF, 07320

MEXICO (The United Mexican States) • Biblioteca, Centro Interdisciplinario de Ciencias de la Salud, Instituto Politecnico Nacional • Apartado Postal 5. Mexico 23 DF, 02060

MEXICO (The United Mexican States) • Biblioteca, Escuela Medico Militar • Bd Avila Camacho/Batalla de Celaya. Mexico DF, 11649

MEXICO (The United Mexican States) • Library, Facultad de Medicina, Unidad de Ciencias de la Salud, Universidad Veracruzana • Atenas y Managua. Minatitlan Ver. , 96760

MEXICO (The United Mexican States) • Biblioteca, Escuela de Medicina, Universidad de Montemorelos • APARTADO 16-37. Montemorelos Nuevo Leon, 67500

MEXICO (The United Mexican States) • Biblioteca del Area Ciencias Salud, Escuela de Medicina Dr Ign. Chavez, Universidad Michoacana de San Nicolas de Hidalgo • Ventura Puente Y R. Carrillo. Morelia Mich.

MEXICO (The United Mexican States) • Biblioteca, Escuela de Medicina, Universidad Autonoma de Hidalgo • Dr Eliseo Ramirez Ulloa 400. Pachuca Hidalgo

MEXICO (The United Mexican States) • Biblioteca, Facultad de Medicina, Universidad Autonoma de Queretaro • Clavel No. 200, Fracc. La Capilla. Queretaro Qto., 76170

MEXICO (The United Mexican States) • Biblioteca, Escuela de Medicina, Universidad Valle del Bravo • Apartado Postal 331. Reynosa Tamaulipas

MEXICO (The United Mexican States) • Biblioteca, Escuela de Medicina, Universidad Mexico-Americana del Norte • Col. del Prado, Apdo Postal 1118. Reynosa Tamaulipas, 88500

MEXICO (The United Mexican States) • Biblioteca, Facultad de Medicina, Unidad Saltillo • Francisco Murguia Sur No. 205. Saltillo Coah. 25000

MEXICO (The United Mexican States) • Biblioteca, Division de Ciencias de la Salud, Universidad de Monterrey • Avenida I. Morones Prieto 4500 Poniente, Apdo 321, San Pedro Garza Garcia. Nuevo Leon, 66238

MEXICO (The United Mexican States) • Biblioteca, Escuela de Medicina, Universidad del Noreste • Prolong. Av. Hidalgo S/n, A.P. 469. Tampico Tam, 89339

MEXICO (The United Mexican States) • Biblioteca, Facultad de Medicina, Universidad Autonoma de Baja California • Mesa de Otay, Apartado Postal 113-A. Tijuana BC

MEXICO (The United Mexican States) • Biblioteca, Escuela Nacional de Estudios Profesionales Iztacala, Universidad Nacional Autonoma de Mexico • Ave. de los Barrios S/n, Apdo 314. Tlalnepantla, 54090

MEXICO (The United Mexican States) • Biblioteca, Facultad de Medicina, Universidad de Coahuila • Morelos 900 Oriente. Torreon Coahuila, 2700

MEXICO (The United Mexican States) • Biblioteca, Facultad de Medicina Humana, Universidad Autonoma de Chiapas • Calle Central y 10 sur s/n. Tuxtla Gutierrez Chiapas, 29000

MEXICO (The United Mexican States) • Hemeroteca Ciencias Biologicas, Universidad Veracruzana • Carmen Serdan e Iturbide S/n. Veracruz Ver., 97700

MEXICO (The United Mexican States) • Biblioteca, Division Acad. Ciencias de la Salud, Universidad Juarez Autonoma de Tabasco • Av. Gregorio Mendez #2838-a Col. Tamulte. Villahermosa Tabasco, 86150

MEXICO (The United Mexican States) • Biblioteca, Facultad de Medicina y Ciencias de la Salud, Universidad Autonoma de Zacatecas • Carretera a La Bufa S/n. Zacatecas Zac., 98000

MONGOLIA • National Public Library • Ulaanbaatar

MOROCCO (the Kingdom of) • Province Médicale d'Agadir • Rue du 29 Février Talborjt . Agadir

MOROCCO (the Kingdom of) • Bibliothèque, Faculté de Médecine et de Pharmacie, Université Hassan II • 19, rue Tarik Bnou Ziad. Casablanca

MOROCCO (the Kingdom of) • Bibliothèque Centrale, Ministère de la Santé • 335, avenue Mohammed V. Rabat

MOZAMBIQUE (the Republic of) • Biblioteca, Direccion Provincial de Saude de Sofala • Caixa Postal 583. Beira

MOZAMBIQUE (the Republic of) • Biblioteca, Faculdade de Medicina, Universidade Catolica de Mozambique (UCM) • Rua Marques de Soveral 960, Caixa Postal 821. Beira

MOZAMBIQUE (the Republic of) • Biblioteca Faculdade de Medicina, Universidade Eduardo Mondlane • CAIXA POSTAL 257. Maputo

MYANMAR • Institute of Medicine (II) • Mingaladon, 13th Mile Prome Road. Yangon

MYANMAR • The Library, Institute of Medicine (I) • 245 Myoma Kyaung Road, PO 11131. Yangon

NAMIBIA • Documentation Resource Centre, Directorate Policy, Planning and HRD • Private Bag 13198. Windhoek

NEPAL (the Kingdom of) • Library, Nepal Medical College • Jorpati, PO Box 13344. Kathmandu

NICARAGUA (the Republic of) • Biblioteca del Complejo Docente de la Salud, Facultad de Medicina • Universidad Nacional Autonoma de Nicaragua • Apdo 68. Leon

NIGERIA (the Federal Republic of) • The Library, College of Medical Sciences, University of Calabar • Calabar Cross River State

NIGERIA (the Federal Republic of) • Medical Library, College of Medicine, University of Nigeria • Enugu Campus. Enugu, Enugu State

NIGERIA (the Federal Republic of) • Library, National Postgraduate Medical College of Nigeria • Km 26, Badagry Expressway, PMB 2003. Ijanikin Lagos State

NIGERIA (the Federal Republic of) • The Library, Faculty of Health Sciences, Obafemi Awolowo University • Ile Ife Osun State

NIGERIA (the Federal Republic of) • The Medical Library, University of Ilorin • PMB 1515. Ilorin Kwara State

NIGERIA (the Federal Republic of) • Branch Medical Library, University of Jos • PMB 2084. Jos Plateau State

NIGERIA (the Federal Republic of) • The Library, College of Medicine, University of Lagos • PMB 12003. Lagos, Lagos State

NIGERIA (the Federal Republic of) • The Library, National Institute for Medical Research • Edmond Crescent (off City Way) Yaba. PMB 2013. Lagos, Lagos State

NIGERIA (the Federal Republic of) • Harold Scarborough Medical Library, College of Medical Sciences, University of Maiduguri • PMB 1069. Maiduguri Borno State

NIGERIA (the Federal Republic of) • The Medical Library, University of Port Harcourt • PMB 5323. Port Harcourt Rivers State

NIGERIA (the Federal Republic of) • Medical/Veterinary Sciences Library, Usmanu Danfodiyo University • Sultan Abubakar Road, PMB 2346. Sokoto, Sokoto State

NIGERIA (the Federal Republic of) • Medical Library, Ahmadu Bello University Hospital • Zaria Kaduna State

PAKISTAN (the Islamic Republic of) • Library, Ayub Medical College • Abbottabad

PAKISTAN (the Islamic Republic of) • Quaid-e-Azam Medical College, Islamia University • Bahawalpur

PAKISTAN (the Islamic Republic of) • The Library, Sind Medical College • Rafiqui H.J. Shaheed Road. Karachi, 75510

PAKISTAN (the Islamic Republic of) • Health Sciences Library, The Aga Khan University Medical College, Faculty of Health Sciences • Stadium Road PO Box 3500. Karachi, 74800

PAKISTAN (the Islamic Republic of) • Library, Dow Medical College • Baba-e-Urdu Road. Karachi, 74200

PAKISTAN (the Islamic Republic of) • The Library, Fatima Jinnah Medical College for Women, University of Punjab • Queen's Road. Lahore

PAKISTAN (the Islamic Republic of) • Library, College of Community Medicine • 6 Abdul Rehman Road (Birdwood Road). Lahore 54000

PAKISTAN (the Islamic Republic of) • Library, Chandka Medical College • Larkana Sindh, PO Box 8. Larkana, 77170

PAKISTAN (the Islamic Republic of) • Library, Nishtar Medical College, Bahuddin Zakaria University • Multan

PAKISTAN (the Islamic Republic of) • Directorate of Health Services, Azad Government of the State of Jammu and Kashmir • Muzaffarabad Azad Jammu and Kashmir

PAKISTAN (the Islamic Republic of) • Library, University of Balochistan • Sariab Road. Quetta

PAKISTAN (the Islamic Republic of) • The Library, Rawalpindi Medical College • Tipu Road. Rawalpindi

PAKISTAN (the Islamic Republic of) • Library, Armed Forces Medical College • Rawalpindi, 46000

PANAMA (the Republic of) • Biblioteca, Facultad de Medicina, Universidad de Panama • APDO 3368. Panama 9

PERU (the Republic of) • Biblioteca de Biomedicas, Universidad Nacional de San Agustin • Apartado 2726. Arequipa

PERU (the Republic of) • Biblioteca Central, Universidad Nacional de Cajamarca • Jr. Amazonas No.304, Apartado 16. Cajamarca

PERU (the Republic of) • Biblioteca, Programa Academico de Medicina Humana, Universidad Nacional San Antonio Abad • Ave. de la Cultura S/n, Apartado 367. Cuzco

PERU (the Republic of) • Biblioteca, Facultad de Medicina Humana D.A.C., Univ. Nacional san Luis Gonzaga • Av. D. Alcides Carrion S/n, APDO 106. Ica

PERU (the Republic of) • Biblioteca, Facultad de Medicina, Universidad Nacional Mayor de San Marcos • Av. Grau 755, APARTADO 529. Lima 100

PERU (the Republic of) • Biblioteca Central, Universidad Peru (the Republic of)ana Cayetano Heredia • Av. Honorio Delgado 430, Apartado 2563. Lima 100

PERU (the Republic of) • Biblioteca, Facultad de Medicina Humana, Universidad de San Martin de Porres • Av. Alameda del Corregidor Cdra.15, Las Vinas de la Molina. Lima

PERU (the Republic of) • Biblioteca, Facultad de Medicina Humana, Universidad Nacional de Piura • Campus Universitario, Urb.Miraflores, APDO 295. Piura

PHILIPPINES (the Republic of) • Health Sciences Library, Our Lady of Lourdes Hall, Angeles University Foundation • Angeles City, 2009

PHILIPPINES (the Republic of) • Medical and Health Science Library, Perpetual Help College of Laguna • Sto.Nino. Binan Laguna, 4024

PHILIPPINES (the Republic of) • Library, Dr Jose P. Rizal College of Medicine, Xavier University • Corrales Avenue. Cagayan de Oro City, 9000

PHILIPPINES (the Republic of) • Library, College of Medicine, Manila Central University (FDT), Medical Foundation • Samson Road. Caloocan City Metro Manila, 3108

PHILIPPINES (the Republic of) • Medical Library, Cebu Doctors' College of Medicine • Osmena Blvd. Cebu City, 6000

PHILIPPINES (the Republic of) • Library, Lyceum Northwestern, Dr Francisco Q. Duque Medical Foundation, College of Medicine • Dagupan City Pangasinan, 0701

PHILIPPINES (the Republic of) • Library, De la Salle University, College of Medicine • Dasmarinas Cavite, 4114

PHILIPPINES (the Republic of) • Library, Davao Medical School Foundation • Circumferential Road, PO BOX 251. Davao City Bajada, 8000

PHILIPPINES (the Republic of) • Library, Iloilo Doctors' College of Medicine • Molo, West Avenue. 5901 Iloilo City

PHILIPPINES (the Republic of) • Library, College of Medicine, University of the City of Manila • Muralla and General Luna Streets. Intramuros Manila, 2801

PHILIPPINES (the Republic of) • Library, Ago Medical and Educational Center, Bicol Christian College of Medicine • J. Rizal Street. Legaspi City, 4901

PHILIPPINES (the Republic of) • Library and Information Services Division, Nutrition Center of the Philippines (the Republic of) • MC P.O.BOX 1858. Makati Metro Manila, 1299

PHILIPPINES (the Republic of) • Medical Library, Faculty of Medicine and Surgery, University of Santo Tomas • Metro Manila Espana, 2801

PHILIPPINES (the Republic of) • Library, School of Health Sciences, University of the Philippines • Manila, Palo Leyte, 6501

PHILIPPINES (the Republic of) • Library, Ramon Magsaysay Memorial Medical Center, College of Medicine, University of the East • Quezon City Quezon City, 3008

PHILIPPINES (the Republic of) • Library, Virgen Milagrosa University Foundation, Institute of Medicine Foundation • San Carlos City Pangasinan, 2420

PHILIPPINES (the Republic of) • Library, College of Medicine, Fatima College • 120 Macarthur Highway. Valenzuela City of Manila, 2627

POLAND (the Republic of) • Biblioteka, Akademii Medycznej • Ul. Kilinskiego 1. Bialystok, PL-15-230

POLAND (the Republic of) • Library, The L. Rydygier University, School of Medical Science in Bydgoszcz • Ul. M. Skeodowskiey-Curie 9. Bydgoszcz, PL-85-094

POLAND (the Republic of) • Biblioteka Glowna, Akademia Medyczna W Gdansku • Ul. Debinki 1, SKR.POCZT.645. Gdansk, PL-80-952

POLAND (the Republic of) • Biblioteka Glowna, Akademii Medycznej • Ul. Medyczna 7. Krakow , PL-30-688

POLAND (the Republic of) • Biblioteka Glowna, Akademia Medyczna (Medical Library of Lodz, Main Library) • Ul. Muszynskiego 2. Lodz, PL-90-151

POLAND (the Republic of) • Dept of Health Care Organization, Faculty of Medicine, The Lodz Medical Academy • Piotrkowska 5. Lodz, PL-90-955

POLAND (the Republic of) • Biblioteka Glowna, Akademii Medycznej • ul. Szkolna 18, skr. poczt. 184. Lublin, PL-20-950

POLAND (the Republic of) • Biblioteka Glowna, Pomorska Akademia Medyczna • Ul. Rybacka 1. Szczecin, PL-70-204

POLAND (the Republic of) • Library, Medical Centre for Postgraduate Education (Centrum Medyczne Ksztalcenia Podyplomowego) • Ul. Schroegera 82. Warszawa, PL-01-828

POLAND (the Republic of) • Biblioteka Glowna, Akademia Medyczna • Ul. Oczki 1. Warszawa, PL-02-007

POLAND (the Republic of) • Biblioteka, Akademii Medycznej (Library of the Medical Academy) • Ul. Rosenbergow 1/3. Wroclaw 12, PL-51-616

PORTUGAL (The Portuguese Republic) • Centre de Documentation, Escola Nacional de Saude Publica • Avenida Padre Cruz . Lisboa, P-1699

PORTUGAL (The Portuguese Republic) • Biblioteca, Instituto Bacteriologico Camara Pestana • Rua do Instituto Bacteriologico. Lisboa, P-1169-1100

PORTUGAL (The Portuguese Republic) • Biblioteca, Faculdade de Medicina • Avenida Prof. Egas Moniz. Lisboa, P-1600

PORTUGAL (The Portuguese Republic) • Biblioteca, Instituto de Higiene e Medicina Tropical • Rua da Junqueira 96. Lisboa, P-1300-344

PORTUGAL (The Portuguese Republic) • Biblioteca, Faculdade de Medicina • Rue Alameda Prof. Hernani Monteiro. Porto, P-4200

REPUBLIC OF KOREA • Medical Library, Soonchunhyang University College of Medicine • 366-1 Ssangyong-Dong. Chunan, Choong-Nam, 330-090

REPUBLIC OF KOREA • Library, Faculty of Medicine, Hallym University • 1 Okchon-Dong, Chunchon 200. Kangwon-Do

REPUBLIC OF KOREA • Library, College of Medicine, Inha University • 253 Yong-Hyun Dong, Nam-Gu. Inchon, 402-751

REPUBLIC OF KOREA • Medical School Library, College of Medicine, Chonnam National University • 5 Hak 1, Dong. Kwangju, 501-190

REPUBLIC OF KOREA • Library, Institute of Population and Community Medicine, Soon Chun Hyang University • PO Box 97, Onyang 337-880. Chung Chung Nam Do

REPUBLIC OF KOREA • Library, College of Medicine, Pusan National University • 1-10 Amidong Suh-Ku. Pusan, 602-739

REPUBLIC OF KOREA • Library, Kosin Medical College • 34 Amnam-Dong, Suh-Ku. Pusan, 600

REPUBLIC OF KOREA • Medical Library, Korea University • 126-1, 5-Ka, Anam-Dong, Sungbuk-Ku. Seoul, 136-701

REPUBLIC OF KOREA • Library, College of Medicine, Ewha Women's University • 11-1 Daehyon, Sodaemun-Ku. Seoul

REPUBLIC OF KOREA • Library, College of Medicine, Hanyang University • 17 Haengdang-Dong, Sungdong-Ku. Seoul, 133-791

REPUBLIC OF KOREA • Medical Library, College of Medicine, Yonsei University • 134 Sinchon-Dong, Sodaemun-Ku, CPO Box 8044. Seoul, 120

REPUBLIC OF KOREA • Library, Yeungnam University Medical Center • Daemyungdong. Taegu, 705-035

ROMANIA • The Academy of Medical Sciences • 11 Boul. 1er Mai. Bucuresti 1, R-79173

ROMANIA • Library, Institute of Hygiene, Public Health, Health Services and Management • Str. Dr Leonte 1-3. Bucuresti, R-76256

ROMANIA • Bibliothèque, Institutul Cantacuzino • Spalaiul Independentei 103, CP 1-525. Bucuresti, R-76201

ROMANIA • United Nations Information Centre • 16 Aurel Vlaicu Street, PO Box 1-701. Bucuresti, R-79362

ROMANIA • Biblioteca Centrala, U.M.F. • Str. Avram Iancu 21. Cluj-Napoca, R-3400

ROMANIA • Biblioteca, Facultatea de Medicina Generala Din Craiova • Rua Petru Rares 4. Craiova Dolj , R-1100

ROMANIA • Library, Institutul de Sanatate Publica • Bv. Dr V. Babes 16-18, PO Box 5. Timisoara, R-1900

ROMANIA • Biblioteca, Universitatea de Medicina si Farmacie • Piata Eftimie Murgu nr. 2. Timisoara, R-1900

ROMANIA • Biblioteca Centrala, Institutul de Medicina si Farmacie • Str. Gheorghe Marinescu Nr.38 Tirgu Mures, R-4300

RUSSIAN FEDERATION • Russian Academy of Medical Sciences • Kamennoostrovsky Avenue 69/71. St Petersbourg, 197376

RWANDA (the Rwandese Republic) • Centre de Documentation, Ecole de Santé publique et Nutrition, Université nationale du Rwanda • Campus universitaire de Butare, B.P. 56. Butare

SAINT LUCIA • Library, Spartan Health Sciences University, School of Medicine • PO BOX 324. Vieux-Fort

SAMOA (The Independent State of) • The Director-General of Health, Health Department • Apia

Sao Tome and Principe (the Democratic Republic of) • Centre de Documentation, Ministère de la Santé • CP 23. Sao Tomé

SAUDI ARABIA (the Kingdom of) • Central Library, King Faisal University • PO Box 1982. Dammam, 31441

SAUDI ARABIA (the Kingdom of) • Library, College of Medicine and Allied Sciences, King Abdulaziz University • PO Box 9029. Jeddah, 21413

SAUDI ARABIA (the Kingdom of) • Medical Library, College of Medicine and King Khalid University, Hospital (44) King Saud University • PO Box 2925. Riyad, 11461

SAUDI ARABIA (the Kingdom of) • Central Medical Library, Ministry of Health • Airport Road, Main Ministry. Riyad, 11176

SENEGAL (the Republic of) • Centre de Documentation, Direction de l'Hygiène et de la Protection Sanitaire, Ministère de la Santé et de la Prévention • Boîte postale 4024. Dakar

SERBIA and MONTENEGRO • Central Medical Library, Medical Fakulty Skopje (Medicinski Fakultet) • Vodnjanska 17. Skopje, 91000

SERBIA and MONTENEGRO • Dr Milan Jovanovic Batut Biblioteka, Zavod Za Zastitu Zdravilja Srbije • Dr Subotica 5. Beograd, YU-11000

SIERRA LEONE (the Republic of) • Health Library, Endemic Diseases Control Unit, Ministry of Health • Baima Road. Bo

SIERRA LEONE (the Republic of) • Medical Library, Connaught Hospital • Lightfoot-Boston Street. Freetown

SLOVAKIA (the Slovak Republic) • Library, Medical Faculty, Comenius University • Odborarske Nam. C.14. Bratislava, 813 72

SLOVAKIA (the Slovak Republic) • Kniznica, UK Jeseniova Lekárska Fakulta • Novomeskeho 7. Martin, 036 45

SOMALIA (the Republic of) • The Documentation Center, Ministry of National Planning • PO Box 1742. Mogadiscio

SOUTH AFRICA • Medical Library Faculty of Medicine, University of Natal • P. Bag 7. Congella KZN, 4013

SOUTH AFRICA • Library, Faculty of Health Sciences, University of Durban Westville • Private Bag X54001. Durban N, 4000

SOUTH AFRICA • Department of Community Health, Medical University of Southern Africa • PO Box 13. Medunsa, 0204

SOUTH AFRICA • Health Sciences Library, University of the North • Private Bag X1112. Sovenga T, 0727

SOUTH AFRICA • Library, University of Transkei • Private Bag X2. Umtata K/C, 5100

SRI LANKA (The Democratic Socialist Republic of) • Library, Postgraduate Institute of Medicine, University of Colombo • 160 Norris Canal Road. Colombo 8

SRI LANKA (the Democratic Socialist Republic of) • Medical Library, University of Jaffna • Thirunelvely. Jaffna

SRI LANKA (the Democratic Socialist Republic of) • Medical Library, Faculty of Medicine, University of Peradeniya • Peradeniya

SRI LANKA (the Democratic Socialist Republic of) - Library • North Colombo Medical College, Faculty of Medicine, University of Kelaniya • Talagolla Road, PO Box 6. Ragama

SUDAN (the Republic of the) • Library, Faculty of Medicine, Shendi University • PO Box 10. Shendi

SURINAME (the Republic of the) • Medical Library, University of Suriname • Kernkampweg 5. Paramaribo

SWEDEN (the Kingdom of) • Library Parliament, Riksdagsbiblioteket • Stockholm, S-10012

SWITZERLAND (the Swiss Confederation) • Bibliothèque Publique et Universitaire, Service des Périodiques • Promenade des Bastions. Genève 4, 1211

SYRIAN ARAB REPUBLIC • The Library, Faculty of Medicine, University of Damascus. Damascus

THAILAND (the Kingdom of) • Library, Phramongkutklao College of Medicine • 315 Rajavithi Road. Bangkok, 10400

THAILAND (the Kingdom of) • UNICEF, East Asia and Pacific Regional Office • 19 Phra Atit Road, PO Box 2-154. Bangkok, 10200

THAILAND (the Kingdom of) • Library, Faculty of Medicine, Chulalongkorn University • Rama VI Road. Bangkok, 10330

THAILAND (the Kingdom of) • Department of Preventive and Social Medicine, Faculty of Medicine, Mahidol University • Ramathibodi Hospital. Rama VI Road. Bangkok, 10400

THAILAND (the Kingdom of) • Library, Faculty of Medicine, Chiang Mai University • 110 Intravaroros Road. Chiang Mai, 50002

THAILAND (the Kingdom of) • Library, Faculty of Medicine, Prince of Songkla University • PO Box 84, Hatyai. Songkla, 90110

THAILAND (the Kingdom of) • Library, Faculty of Medicine, Khon Kaen University • 123 Mitraparp Highway, Amphur Muang. Khon Kaen, 40002

THAILAND (the Kingdom of) • Library, Sirindhorn College of Public Health • 90/1 Anamai Road, A. Muang. Khon Kaen, 40000

THAILAND (the Kingdom of) • Director, Bureau of Health Policy and Planning Office of the Permanent Secretary, Ministry of Public Health, Royal Thai Government • Tiwanond Road. Nonthaburi, 11000

TOGO (the Togolese Republic) • Bibliothèque, Faculté de Médecine, Université de Benin • BP 1515. Lomé

Trinidad and Tobago (the Republic of) • Medical Sciences Library, The University of the West Indies, Eric Williams Medical Sciences Complex • Champs Fleurs. Trinidad

TUNISIA (the Republic of) • Bibliothèque, Faculté de Médicine de Sfax • Sfax, 3000

TUNISIA (the Republic of) • Bibliotheque, Deptartement de Médecine Communautaire, Faculté de Médecine de Sousse • Sousse, 4000

TUNISIA (the Republic of) • Bibliothèque, Faculté de Médecine Ibn el Jazzar, Université du Centre • Ave Mohamed Karoui. BP 126. Sousse, 4002

TUNISIA (the Republic of) • Bibliothèque, Faculté de Médecine de Tunis • 9 Rue Professeur Zouheir Essafi. Tunis, 1006

TURKEY (the Republic of) • Kitapligi, Tip Fakultesi, Ankara Universitesi • Ankara, TR-06100

TURKEY (the Republic of) • Kutuphanesi, Department of Public Health, Tip Fakultesi, Hacettepe Universitesi • Ankara, TR-06100

TURKEY (the Republic of) • Kutuphanesi, Gulhane Askeri Tip Akademisi Askeri, Tip Fakultesi, Dr Tevfik Saglam Cad. • Ankara ETLIK, TR-06018

TURKEY (the Republic of) • Merkez Kutuphanesi, Gazi Universitesi • Ankara Besevler, TR-06500

TURKEY (the Republic of) • Kutuphanesi • Ege Universitesi, Tip Fakültesi • Bornova Izmir

TURKEY (the Republic of) • Kitapligi, Tip Fakultesi, Uludag University • Bursa, TR-16059

TURKEY (the Republic of) • Halk Sagligi Anabilim Dali Kitapligi, Dicle Universitesi, Tip Fakultesi • Diyarbakir, TR-21280

TURKEY (the Republic of) • Kitapligina, Trakya Universitesi, Tip Fakültesi • Edirne, TR-22030

TURKEY (the Republic of) • Kutuphanesi, Tip Fakultesi, Atatürk Üniversitesi • Erzurum, TR-25050

TURKEY (the Republic of) • Medical Library, Osmangazi University, Eskisehir Osmangazi Kampüsü Meselik • Eskisehir , TR-26480

TURKEY (the Republic of) • Kutuphanesi, Halk Sagligi Anabilim Dali, Cerrahpasa Tip Fakultesi, Istanbul Universitesi • Istanbul Cerrahpasa, TR-34303

TURKEY (the Republic of) • Kitapligi (Library), Tip Fakultesi (Faculty of Medicine), Marmara Üniversitesi • Istanbul Haydarpasa, TR-34413

TURKEY (the Republic of) • Kutuphanesi, Tip Fakultesi, Dokuz Eylul Universitesi • Izmir , TR-35210

TURKEY (the Republic of) • Kütüphane ve Dokümantasyon Dairesi, Erciyes Üniversitesi • Kayseri, 38039

TURKEY (the Republic of) • Kutuphanesi, Tip Fakultesi, Selcuk Universitesi • Konya, TR-42151

TURKEY (the Republic of) • Kutuphanesi, Tip Fakültesi, Celal Bayar Üniversitesi • Manisa, TR-45020

TURKEY (the Republic of) • Kutuphanesi, Cumhuriyet University • Kampus/sivas. Sivas, TR-58140

TURKEY (the Republic of) • Kutuphanesi, Karadeniz Teknik Universitesi, Tip Fakultesi • Trabzon, TR-61080

UGANDA (the Republic of) • Library, National Research Council • Plot 12 Johnstone Street, PO Box 6884. Kampala

UGANDA (the Republic of) • Library, Faculty of Medicine, Mbarara University • PO Box 1410. Mbarara

UNITED ARAB EMIRATES • Library • Dubai Medical College for Girls • PO Box 19964. Dubai

UNITED KINGDOM • University Library, Cambridge University • West Road. Cambridge, UK CB3 9DR

UNITED KINGDOM • Library, Welsh Office • Cathays Park. Cardiff Wales, UK CF1 3NQ

UNITED KINGDOM • Official Publication Unit, National Library of Scotland • George IV Bridge. Edinburgh, UK EH1 1EW

UNITED KINGDOM • Radcliffe Science Library • Parks Road. Oxford, UK OX1 3QP

UNITED REPUBLIC TANZANIA (the United Republic of) • The Library, Centre on Integrated Rural Development for Africa (CIRDAFRICA) • PO Box 6115. Arusha

UNITED REPUBLIC TANZANIA (the United Republic of) • Director General, Tanzania Library Service • PO Box 9283. Dar Es Salaam

UNITED STATES OF AMERICA • Library, National Institutes of Health • Building 10, Room 1-l 13, 10 Center Drive, Msc1150. Bethesda, MD 20892-1150

UNITED STATES OF AMERICA • Serials Department, University of Hawaii Library • 2550 The Mall. Honolulu, HI 96822-2233

URUGUAY (the Eastern Republic of) • Biblioteca, Facultad de Medicina, Universidad de la Republica • Avenida Gral Flores 2125, Casilla de Correo 24049. Montevideo

VENEZUELA (the Bolivarian Republic of) • Biblioteca, Escuela de Medicina, Universidad Centro Occidental Lisandro Alvarado • Apdo 516. Barquisimeto Lara

VENEZUELA (the Bolivarian Republic of) • Biblioteca Francisco Urdaneta, Escuela de Salud Publica, El Algodonal • Antimano, UCV APDO 62231 A. Caracas, 1060 DF

VENEZUELA (the Bolivarian Republic of) • Sistema Nacional de Documentacion et Informacion, Biomedica (SINADIB), Instituto de Medicina Experimental (IME), Facultad de Medicina, Universidad Central de Venezuela • APDO 50587. Caracas Sabana Grande, 1051

VENEZUELA (the Bolivarian Republic of) • Biblioteca, Escuela de Medicina, Universidad de Oriente • Avenida Jose Mendez, Apdo Postal 94. Ciudad Bolivar, 80001A

VENEZUELA (the Bolivarian Republic of) • Biblioteca Dr Joaquin Esteva Parra, Facultad de Medicina, Universidad del Zulia • Av. 20 con calle 65, Apartado Postal 526. Maracaibo, 4003-A

VENEZUELA (the Bolivarian Republic of) • Biblioteca Antonio Perez Romero, Facultad de Ciencias de la Salud, Universidad de Carabobo (Nucleo Aragua) • La Morita II, Apdo 4944. Maracay, Aragua

VIET NAM (the Socialist republic of) • Library, Technical School of Medicine • No.2 , 97 Hung Vuong. Danang City

VIET NAM (the Socialist republic of) • Ecole de la Sante Publique (thu Vien Truong Can Bo-Quan Ly Nganh y Te) • 138 Rue Gianj Vo. Ha Noi, 10000

VIET NAM (the Socialist republic of) • Library, Faculty of Medicine Haiphong • 213 Bd. Tran Quoc Toan (Iach Tray). Hai Phong, 35000

VIET NAM (the Socialist republic of) • Bibliotheque, Faculte de Medicine • 217 An Duong Vuong. Ho Chi Minh-Ville, 15000

VIET NAM (the Socialist republic of) • Bibliothèque, Faculté de Médecine, Université de Hue • 1 Ngo Quyen. Hue, 43100

VIET NAM (the Socialist republic of) • Library, Bac Thai Medical University • Dong Anang. Thai Nguyen, 23000

YEMEN (the Republic of) • Dhamar Hospital and Primary Health Care Project • PO Box 87189. Dhamar

YEMEN (the Republic of) • The Library, Sana'a University, Faculty of Medicine and Health Sciences • Wadi Dhahar Rd., PO Box 13078. Sana'a

ZAMBIA (the Republic of) • Medical Library, School of Medicine, University of Zambia • PO Box 50110. Lusaka, 10101

ZAMBIA (the Republic of) • Library, Tropical Disease Research Centre • PO Box 71769. Ndola

SALES AGENTS

WHO official sales agents world wide

Global Sales

SWITZERLAND (THE SWISS CONFEDERATION) • World Health Organization, Marketing and Dissemination, • Avenue Appia, 20. CH-1211 Geneva 27 • Telephone: (+41-22) 7912476 • Fax: (+41-22) 7914857 • To place orders, please write to: bookorders@who.int; For any questions about publications, please write to: publications@who.int

Local Sales Agents

For countries not listed, please refer to global sales. For an updated list of local sales agents where this title, as well as all WHO publications, can be purchased, please consult the Internet Catalogue of WHO publications at the following address: http://bookorders.who.int

ARGENTINA • World Publications S.A. • Av. Córdoba, 1877. Buenos Aires, C1120AAA • Tel: (+54-11) 4815 8156 • Fax: (+54-11) 4815 8156 • Email: ventaswp@wpbooks.com.ar • Web site: http://www.worldpublications.com.ar

AUSTRALIA • Hunter Publications - Tek Imaging, P.O. Box 404. Abbotsford, VIC 3067 • Tel: (+61-3) 94175361 • Fax: (+61-3) 94197154 • Email: admin@tekimaging.com.au

BANGLADESH • Refer to WHO Regional Office (India (the Republic of)) or Global Sales.

BELGIUM (the Kingdom of) • Patrimoine sprl • Rue du Noyer 168. Bruxelles, 1030. • Tel: (+32-2) 7366847 • Fax: (+32-2) 7366847 • Email: Patrimoine@chello.be

BUTHAN (the Kingdom of) • Refer to WHO Regional Office (India (the Republic of)) or Global Sales.

BOTSWANA (the Republic of) • Botsalo Books (Pty) Ltd • P.O. Box 1532, Gaborone • Tel: (+267) 312576 • Fax: (+267) 372608

CAMEROON (the Republic of) • FAS Foundation International • Fon's Street, (Former SOPECAM Building), P.O. Box 443. Bamenda, NWP • Tel: (237) 361023 • Fax: (237) 361023 • Email: allied.engineers@lom.camnet.cm

CANADA • Canadian Public Health Association • 1565 Carling Avenue, Suite 400. Ottawa, Ont. K1Z 8R1 • Tel: (+1-613) 7253769 • Fax: (+1-613) 7259826 • Email: hrc/cds@cpha.ca

CHILE (the Republic of) • Libros Médicos en Chile (the Republic of) • Miguel Concha Caldera, Casilla 7 Correo 22. Providencia, Santiago • Tel: (+56-2) 6551545 • Fax: (+56-2) 2746655 • Email: internac.ional001@chilnet.cl • Web site: http://www.internacional.cl

CHILE (the Republic of) • Internacional Libros Miguel Concha S.A. • Alférez Real 14614. Providencia

DENMARK (the Kingdom of) • GAD Import Booksellers • c/o Gad Direct 31-33 Fiolstraede. Kobenhavn K ,DK-1171 • Tel: (+45-33) 137233 • Fax: (+45-32) 542368 • Email: info@gaddirect.dk

EGYPT (the Arab Republic of) • 2 Bahgataly street , EL-Masri Towers Building D, Apt. 24. Cairo, Zamalek • Tel: (+202) 7363824 • _ Fax: (+202) 7369355 • Web site: http://www.meric-co.com

EL SALVADOR (the Republic of) • Libreria Estudiantil • Edificio Comercial B, No 3, Avenida Libertad, Centro Urbano. Libertad, San Salvador

FINLAND (the Republic of) • Stockmann/Akateeminen Kirjakauppa • PL 128, Keskuskatu. Helsinki, 100101 • Tel: (+358-9) 1214403 • Fax: (+358-9) 12144 50 • Email: sps@akateeminen.com • Web site: http://www.akateeminen.com

FRANCE (the Republic of) • Librairie Privat Arnette • 2, rue Casimir Delavigne. PARIS, F-75006 • Tel: (+33-1) 55428787 • Fax: (33-1) 55428788 • Email: arnette@privat.fr

FRANCE (the Republic of) • Librairie Lavoisier • 14 rue de Provigny. Cachan Cedex, 94236 • Tel: (+33-1) 47406700 • Fax: (+33-1) 47406702 • Email: edition@Lavoisier.fr

FRANCE (the Republic of) • Sauramps Médical • 11, Boulevard Henri IV. Montpellier, 34000 • Tel: (+33-4) 67636880 • Fax: (+33-4) 67525905 • Email: sauramps.medical@livres-medicaux.com

GERMANY (the Federal Republic of) • Buchhandlung Alexander Horn • Friedrichstrasse 34. Wiesbaden, 65185 • Tel: (+49-611) 9923540/41 • Fax: (+49-611) 9923543 • Email: alexhorn1@aol.com

GERMANY (the Federal Republic of) • Govi-Verlag GmbH • Ginnheimerstrasse 26, POSTFACH 5360. Eschborn, 65728 • Tel: (+49-619) 6928250 • Fax: (+49-619) 6928259

GERMANY (the Federal Republic of) • UNO-Verlag GmbH • Am Hofgarten 10. Bonn, 53113 • Tel: (+49-2) 2894902-0 • Fax: (+ 49-2) 2894902-22 • Email: bestellung@uno-verlag.de • Web site: http://www.uno-verlag.de

GREECE (THE HELLENIC REPUBLIC OF) • G.C. Eleftheroudakis S.A - Librairie internationale • 17, Panepistimiou. Athens, 105-634, • Tel: (+30-1) 3314180 • Fax: (+30-1) 3239821

GUINEA (the Republic of) • Librairie de Guinée • BP 542 Conakry. Guinea (the Republic of) • Tel: (224) 463507 • Fax: (224) 412012

HUNGARY (the Republic of) • Librotrade KFT • Periodicall Import/K Pesti Ut 237. Budapest, H-1173 • Tel: (+36-11) 574417 • Fax: (+36-11) 574318

ICELAND (the Republic of) • Bókabúd Máls and Menningar • Laugavegi 18, Box 392. Reykjavik, 101 • Tel: (+354-1) 5152500 • Fax: (+354-1) 5152505 • Email: erlent@mm.is • Web site: http://www.mm.is

INDIA (the Republic of) • World Health Organization, Regional Office for South-East Asia • World Health House, Indraprastha Estate, Mahatma Gandhi Road. New Delhi, 110002 • Tel: (+91-11) 3370804 • Fax: (+91-11) 3370639 • Email: publications@whosea.org • Web site: http://w3.whosea.org/rdoc/

ISRAEL (the State of) • Yozmot Ltd • P.O. Box 56055. Tel Aviv, 61560 • Tel: (+972-3) 5284851 • Fax: (+972-3) 5285397 • Email: books@yozmot.com

ISRAEL (the State of) • Educational Bookshop • 22 Salah Eddin Street, PO Box 54008. Jerusalem, 91513 • Tel: (+972) 26283704 • Fax: (+972) 26280814

ITALY (THE ITALIAN REPUBLIC OF) • Edizioni Minerva Medica Corso • Bramante 83-85. Turin, 10126 • Tel: (+39-011) 678282 • Fax: (+39-011) 674502 • Email: minmed@tin.it

JAPAN • Maruzen Co., Ltd. • Information Resources Navigation Division • 2-3-10, Nihombashi, Chuo-ku. Tokyo 103-8245. • Tel: (+81-3) 32758595 • Fax: (+81-3) 32750655 • Email: irneisui3@maruzen.co.jp

JORDAN (THE HASHEMITE KINGDOM OF) • Jordan (the Hashemite Kingdom of) Book Center Co., Ltd. (Al-Jubeiha) • P.O. Box 301. Amman • Tel: (+962) 6676882 • Fax: (+962) 6602016

JORDAN (THE HASHEMITE KINGDOM OF) • Global Development Forum • PO Box 941488. Amman, 11194 • Tel: (+962) 64656124 • Fax: (+962) 64656123 • Email: gdf@index.com.jo • Web site: http\\www.ngoglobalforum.org

KENYA (the Republic of) • Text Book Center Ltd • P.O. Box 47540. Nairobi • Tel: (+254) 2330340 • Fax: (+254) 2338110

KUWAIT (the State of) • The Kuwait (the State of) Bookshop Co. Ltd. • P.O. Box 2942. Safat, 13030 • Tel: (+965) 2424266 • Fax: (+965) 2420558

MEXICO (The United Mexican States) • Librería Internacional de C.V. • Av. Sonora 206. Mexico (the United Mexican States), 06100 D.F. • Tel: (+52-5) 2651165 • Fax: (+52-5) 2651164 • Email: libinter@compuserve.com.mx

NETHERLANDS (the Kingdom of) • Swets Blackwell B.V. • P.O. Box 830. SZ. Lisse, 2160 • Tel: (+31) 252435111 • Fax: (+31) 252415 888 • Email: infoho@nl.swetsblackwell.com • Web site: http://www.swetsblackwell.com

NEW-ZEALAND • Medical Books, Ltd • P.O. Box 7389. Wellington South • Tel: (+64-9) 3733772 • Fax: (+64-9) 3733282

NIGERIA (the Federal Republic of) • Mr Godfrey O. Obiaga • 28 Onitsha Road, P.O. Box 370. Nnewi, Anambra State • Tel: (+234) 46460273 • Fax: (+234) 46460273 • Email: obiaga@infoweb.abs.net

NORWAY (the Kingdom of) • Academic Book Center • P.O. Box 2728, St. Hanshaugen 0131. Oslo • Tel: (+47) 22994840 • Fax: (+47) 22208971 • Email: abc@fribokhandel.no

PERU (the Republic of) • Euroamerican Bussines S.A. • Ca. Las Begonias No. 183 Dpto.202, Urb. J.C. Mariategui. Lima, 35 • Tel: (+51-1) 7259152 • Fax: (+51-1) 2830129 • Email: euroamerican@terra.com.pe

PHILIPPINES (the Republic of) • World Health Organization • Regional Office for the Western Pacific Publications Office • P.O. Box 2932. Manila, 1099 • Tel: (+63-2) 5288001 • Fax: (+63-2) 5211036

POLAND (the Republic of) • Foreign Trade Enterprise - ARS Polona Joint Stock Company • Ul. Krakowskie Przedmiescie 7. Warszawa, PL-00 068, • Tel: (+48-22) 8261201 • Fax: (+48-22) 8264763 • Email: Books119@arspolona.com.pl

PORTUGAL (THE PORTUGUESE REPUBLIC) • Lusodoc Documentacao - Tecnico-Cientifica Lda • Rua Cruzado Osberno Lote 3, 5 Dto. Lisboa, 1900 • Tel: (+351-21) 8153312 • Fax: (+351-21) 8130641 • Email: postmaster@lusodoc.pt

PORTUGAL (THE PORTUGUESE REPUBLIC) • Prata e Rodrigues Publicacoes Lda • Estraca da Luz, nº 90-11ºH. Lisboa, 1600 –160 • Tel: (+351-21) 7223528 • Fax: (+351 21) 722 3531 • Email: prpublicacoes@clix.pt

RWANDA (THE RWANDESE REPULIC) • Bufmar ASBL • B.P. 716. Kigali • Tel: (+250) 86176 • Fax: (+250) 83008

SPAIN (the Kingdom of) • Librería Díaz de Santos Lagasca, 95. Madrid, 28006 • Tel: (+34-91) 7819480 • Fax: (+34-91) 5755563 • Email: librerias@diazdesantos.es

SPAIN (the Kingdom of) • Librería Díaz de Santos • Balmes 417 y 419. Barcelona, 08022 • Tel: (+34-3) 2128647 • Fax: (+34-3) 2114991 • Email: librerias@diazdesantos.es

SENEGAL (the Republic of) • Librarie Clairafrique • 2 rue El Hadj Mbaye Gueye, BP 2005. Dakar • Tel: (+221) 82221 69 • Fax: (+221) 8218409

SINGAPORE (the Republic of) • Select Books • 19 Tanglin Road, 03-15, Tanglin Shopping Center. Singapore (the Republic of), 247909 • Tel: (+65) 7321515 • Fax: (+65) 7360855 • Email: info@selectbooks.com.sg • Web site: http://www.selectbooks.com.sg

SLOVENIA (the Republic of) • Cankarjeva Zalozba Kopitarjeva 2. Ljubljana, 1512 • Tel: (+386-1) 2310791 • Fax: (+386-1) 2301435

• Email: nada.sever@cankarjeva-z.si • Web site: http://www.cankarjeva-z.si

SOUTH AFRICA • Democratic Nursing Organization of South Africa • P.O. Box 1280. Pretoria, (T) 001 • Tel: (+27-12) 3432315 • Fax: (+27-12) 3440750 • Email: info@denosa.org.za

SOUTH AFRICA • South African Medical Association • Private Bag X1. Pinelands, 7430 • Tel: (+27-21) 5306527 • Fax: (+27-21) 531 4126 • Email: jstrydom@samedical.org

SWEDEN (the Kingdom of) • PrioInfocenter AB Traktorvagen 11-13. Lund, S-22182 • Tel: +(46-46) 180420 • Fax: (+46-46) 180441 • Email: gunnar.sjolin@prioinfo.se • Web site: http://www.prioinfo.se

SWEDEN (the Kingdom of) • Akademibokhandeln • Mäster Samuelsgatan 32, Box 7634. Stockholm, 103 94 • Tel: (+46-8) 6136130 • Fax: (+46-8) 242543 • Email: marikka.lindahl@city.akademibokhandeln.se

SWITZERLAND (THE SWISS CONFEDERATION) • Huber and Lang - Hans Huber AG • Länggass Strasse 76. Bern 9, CH 3000 • Tel: (+41-31) 3004500 • Fax: (+41-31) 3004590 • Email: who@hanshuber.com

TRINIDAD AND TOBAGO (the Republic of) • Systematic Studies Limited • St. Augustine Shopping Centre Eastern Main Road. St. Augustine • Tel: (+868) 6458466 • Fax: (+868) 6458467 • Email: tobe@trinidad.net

UNITED KINGDOM • The Stationery Office Ltd (Customer Services) • 51 Nine Elms Lane London, SW8 5DR • Tel: (+44-870) 6005522 • Fax: (+44-870) 6005533 • E-mail (for orders) customer.services@theso.co.uk

UNITED STATES OF AMERICA • WHO Publications Center UNITED STATES OF AMERICA • 49 Sheridan Ave. Albany. NY, 12210 • Tel: (+1-518) 4369686 • Fax: (+1-518) 43674 33 • Email: QCORP@compuserve.com

URUGUAY (THE EASTERN REPUBLIC OF) • Libreria Tecnica Uruguaya Ltu • Casilla De Correo 1518. Montevideo, 11000 • Tel: (+598-2) 490072 • Fax: (+598-2) 413448

VENEZUELA (THE BOLIVARIAN REPUBLIC OF) • Librería Médica Paris • Apartado 60.681. Caracas, 1060-A • Tel: (+58-212) 7819045 • Fax: (+58-212) 7931753 • Email: libreriamp@cantv.net

OTHER BOOKS

Selected WHO publications of related interest

Active Ageing – a policy framework. Geneva, World Health Organization, 2002. WHO/NMH/NPH/02.8

Epilepsy. A manual for medical and clinical officers in Africa. Geneva, World Health Organization, 2002. 124 pages. WHO/MSD/MBD/02.02

Innovative Care for Chronic Conditions: Building Blocks for Action. Geneva, World Health Organization, 2002. ISBN 92 4 159017 3, 112 pages, Order no. 1150500

Integrated management of cardiovascular risk. Report of a WHO meeting, Geneva, 9-12 July, World Health Organization, 2002. ISBN 92 4 156224 2, 35 pages, Order no. 1151523

National cancer control programmes: policies and managerial guidelines. 2nd ed. Geneva, World Health Organization, 2002. 92 4 154557 7, 180 pages, Order no. 1152422

Secondary prevention of noncommunicable diseases in low and middle income countries through community based and health service interventions WHO – Wellcome Trust Meeting report. Geneva, 1-3 August 2001, World Health Organization, 2002. ISBN 92 4 159026 2, 25 pages, Electronic access: http://whqlibdoc.who.int/hq/2002/WHO_MPN_CVD_2002.01.pdf

Treatment of tuberculosis: guidelines for national programmes. 3rd edition. WHO/CDS/TB/2003.313

WHO CVD-risk management package for low and medium resource settings. Geneva, World Health Organization, 2003. ISBN 92 4 154585 2, 40 pages, Order no. 1152523

World Health Report 2001- Mental Health: new understanding, new hope. Geneva, World Health Organization, 2001. ISBN 92 4 156201 3, 178 pages, Order no. 1242001

JUST PUBLISHED!

World Health Organization

Adherence to Long-term Therapies
Evidence for action

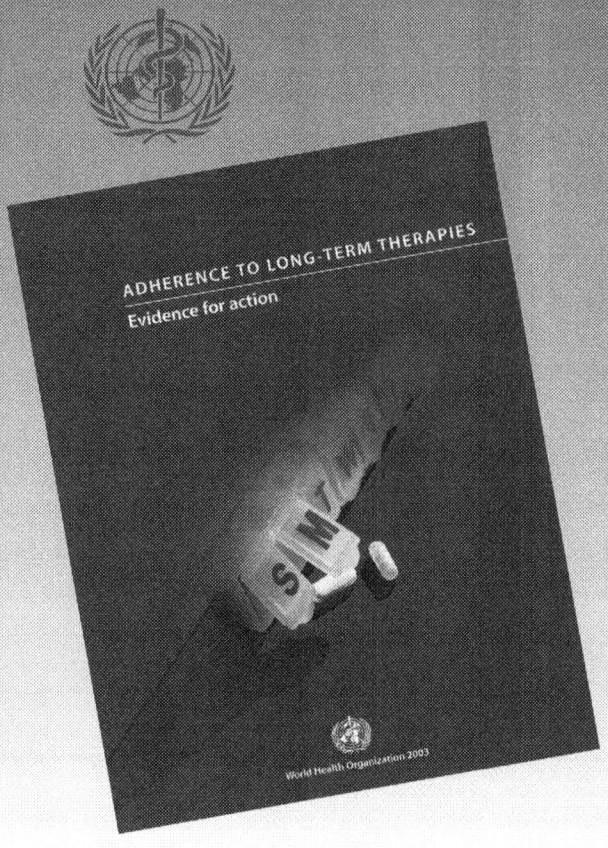

Adherence to therapies is a primary determinant of treatment success. Poor adherence attenuates optimum clinical benefits and therefore reduces the overall effectiveness of health systems.

"Medicines will not work if you do not take them" – Medicines will not be effective if patients do not follow prescribed treatment, yet in developed countries only 50% of patients who suffer from chronic diseases adhere to treatment recommendations. In developing countries, when taken together with poor access to health care, lack of appropriate diagnosis and limited access to medicines, poor adherence is threatening to render futile any effort to tackle chronic conditions, such as diabetes, depression and HIV/AIDS.

This report is based on an exhaustive review of the published literature on the definitions, measurements, epidemiology, economics and interventions applied to nine chronic conditions and risk factors. These are asthma, cancer (palliative care), depression, diabetes, epilepsy, HIV/AIDS, hypertension, tobacco smoking and tuberculosis.

Intended for health managers, policy-makers and clinical practitioners this report provides a concise summary of the consequences of poor adherence for health and economics. It also discusses the options available for improving adherence, and demonstrates the potential impact on desired health outcomes and health care budgets. It is hoped that this report will lead to new thinking on policy development and action on adherence to long-term therapies.

World Health Organization
2003, 216 pages [E]
ISBN 92 4 154599 2
Swiss francs: 30.-/US$ 27.00
In developing countries: Sw. 15.-/US$ 13.50
Order no. 1150526

ORDER FORM

MDI.DIV.526

Contact Information

Name: _____

Job Title: _____

Institution: _____

Address: _____

_____

_____

Tel/Fax: _____

E-mail: _____

Payement Information

☐ Please send a free reference copy to the library of my public institution (developing countries only, full contact information is required)

☐ Please send me ___ copies of Adherence to Long-Term Therapies (order no. 1150526) at the price of US$27; In developing countries US$13.50.

☐ Payment enclosed

☐ Visa ☐ Mastercard ☐ Diners Club ☐ American Express

Card N°: _____

Expiry date: _____

Date of order: _____

Signature: _____

WHO, Marketing and Dissemination, 1211 Geneva 27, Switzerland.
Tel: +41 (22) 791-2476; Fax: +41 (22) 791-4857; Email: publications@who.int
You may also order online at: http://bookorders.who.int

Please send this form by fax or mail to your collegues